Critical Perspectives on **Schooling** and **Fertility** in the Developing World

Caroline H. Bledsoe, John B. Casterline,
Jennifer A. Johnson-Kuhn, and John G. Haaga, editors

Committee on Population

Commission on Behavioral and Social Sciences and Education

National Research Council

NATIONAL ACADEMY PRESS
Washington, D.C 1999

NATIONAL ACADEMY PRESS • 2101 Constitution Ave., N.W. • Washington, D.C. 20418

NOTICE: The project that is the subject of this report was approved by the Governing Board of the National Research Council, whose members are drawn from the councils of the National Academy of Sciences, the National Academy of Engineering, and the Institute of Medicine. The members of the committee responsible for the report were chosen for their special competences and with regard for appropriate balance.

This project was supported by the United States Agency for International Development's Office of Population, under award no. CCP-A-0095-00024-02, the Andrew W. Mellon Foundation, and the William and Flora Hewlett Foundation. The opinions expressed herein are those of the authors and do not necessarily reflect the views of the U.S. Agency for International Development.

Library of Congress Cataloging-in-Publication Data

Critical perspectives on schooling and fertility in the developing world / Caroline H. Bledsoe ... [et al.] editors.
p. cm.
"Committee on Population, Commission on Behavioral and Social Sciences and Education, National Research Council."
ISBN 0-309-06191-1 (pbk.)
1. Birth control—Study and teaching—Developing countries. 2. Fertility, Human—Study and teaching—Developing countries. 3. Teenage girls—Education—Developing countries. I. Bledsoe, Caroline H. II. National Research Council (U.S.). Committee on Population.
HQ766.5.D44 C75 1999
363.9′6′07101724—dc21 98-40216

Additional copies of this report are available from: National Academy Press, 2101 Constitution Avenue, N.W., Washington, D.C. 20418.
Call 800-624-6242 or 202-334-3313 (in the Washington Metropolitan Area).

This report is also available online at **http://www.nap.edu**.

Printed in the United States of America.

COMMITTEE ON POPULATION
1998

The National Academy of Sciences is a private, nonprofit, self-perpetuating society of distinguished scholars engaged in scientific and engineering research, dedicated to the furtherance of science and technology and to their use for the general welfare. Upon the authority of the charter granted to it by the Congress in 1863, the Academy has a mandate that requires it to advise the federal government on scientific and technical matters. Dr. Bruce M. Alberts is president of the National Academy of Sciences.

The National Academy of Engineering was established in 1964, under the charter of the National Academy of Sciences, as a parallel organization of outstanding engineers. It is autonomous in its administration and in the selection of its members, sharing with the National Academy of Sciences the responsibility for advising the federal government. The National Academy of Engineering also sponsors engineering programs aimed at meeting national needs, encourages education and research, and recognizes the superior achievements of engineers. Dr. William A. Wulf is president of the National Academy of Engineering.

The Institute of Medicine was established in 1970 by the National Academy of Sciences to secure the services of eminent members of appropriate professions in the examination of policy matters pertaining to the health of the public. The Institute acts under the responsibility given to the National Academy of Sciences by its congressional charter to be an adviser to the federal government and, upon its own initiative, to identify issues of medical care, research, and education. Dr. Kenneth I. Shine is president of the Institute of Medicine.

The National Research Council was organized by the National Academy of Sciences in 1916 to associate the broad community of science and technology with the Academy's purposes of furthering knowledge and advising the federal government. Functioning in accordance with general policies determined by the Academy, the Council has become the principal operating agency of both the National Academy of Sciences and the National Academy of Engineering in providing services to the government, the public, and the scientific and engineering communities. The Council is administered jointly by both Academies and the Institute of Medicine. Dr. Bruce M. Alberts and Dr. William A. Wulf are chairman and vice chairman, respectively, of the National Research Council.

CONTRIBUTORS

ALAKA M. BASU, Division of Nutritional Sciences, Cornell University
CAROLINE H. BLEDSOE, Department of Anthropology, Northwestern University
ANTHONY T. CARTER, Department of Anthropology, University of Rochester
JOHN B. CASTERLINE, The Population Council, New York
IAN DIAMOND, Department of Social Statistics, University of Southampton
PARFAIT M. ELOUNDOU-ENYEGUE, RAND, Santa Monica, California
BRUCE FULLER, School of Education, University of California, Berkeley
PAUL GLEWWE, The World Bank
JOHN G. HAAGA, Population Reference Bureau, Washington, D.C.
JENNIFER A. JOHNSON-KUHN, Department of Anthropology, Northwestern University
XIAOYAN LIANG, The World Bank
CYNTHIA B. LLOYD, The Population Council, New York
BARBARA MENSCH, The Population Council, New York
MARK R. MONTGOMERY, Department of Economics, State University of New York, Stony Brook, and The Population Council, New York
MARGARET NEWBY, Department of Social Statistics, University of Southampton
DUNCAN THOMAS, RAND, Santa Monica, California
SARAH VARLE, Department of Social Statistics, University of Southampton

Acknowledgments

The committee is grateful to the many individuals who made substantive and productive contributions to the project. Most important, we are indebted to the authors of the papers for their willingness to participate and to contribute with their special knowledge. Primary organization and planning for the workshop and this report was overseen by committee member Caroline Bledsoe, former committee member John Casterline, and former staff director John Haaga. The committee would also like to thank Barney Cohen, project director; LaTanya Johnson, project assistant; and Rona Briere, contract editor.

These papers have been reviewed by individuals chosen for their diverse perspectives and technical expertise, in accordance with procedures approved by the Report Review Committee of the National Research Council (NRC). The purpose of this independent review is to provide candid and critical comments to assist the authors and the NRC in making the published report as sound as possible and to ensure that the report meets institutional standards for objectivity, evidence, and responsiveness to the purpose of the activity. The committee thanks the following individuals for their participation in the review of the papers in this report: William Axinn, Pennsylvania State University; Jere Behrman, University of Pennsylvania; Caroline Bledsoe, Northwestern University; John Casterline, Population Council; Teresa Castro-Martín, United Nations; Orieji Chimere-Dan, University of Witwatersrand; Elizabeth Colson, University of California, Berkeley; Barbara Entwisle, University of North Carolina; Bruce Fuller, University of California, Berkeley; Eugene A. Hammel, University of California, Berkeley; Jennifer Johnson-Kuhn, Northwestern University; Elizabeth King, World Bank; Anjini Kochar, Stanford University; David Lam, University of

Michigan; Thomas Pullum, University of Texas at Austin; Brian Street, University of Sussex; Stephen Tollman, London School of Hygiene and Tropical Medicine; and Nicholas Townsend, Brown University. While these individuals provided constructive comments and suggestions, responsibility for the final content of this volume rests solely with the authoring committee and the NRC.

Finally, the committee gratefully acknowledges the United States Agency for International Development, the Andrew W. Mellon Foundation, and the William and Flora Hewlett Foundation for their generous financial support.

Contents

Critical Perspectives on
Schooling and Fertility
in the Developing World

1

Introduction

Caroline H. Bledsoe, Jennifer A. Johnson-Kuhn, and John G. Haaga

Over the last century and a half, organized mass education in the Western style has spread across the world. The second half of the twentieth century in particular has seen immense transformations in both the educational and reproductive expectations of young people in the developing world. As of the end of World War II, women in Asia, Latin America, and Africa had few opportunities to attend school and little access to what are commonly referred to as modern methods of fertility control. Today, after two decades of dramatic rises in literacy and gross enrollment ratios (Craig, 1981; Hill and King, 1993; United Nations, 1995:15), formal Western education enjoys a position of global prestige. Throughout virtually every country in the world, Western-style schooling has become the most coveted type of preparation for adult female life. Whether she aspires to life as a secretary, a doctor, or the wife of an urban man with rising prospects, almost any young woman in the world, if she had the choice, would probably go to school.

During the same decades in which this revolution in mass education was creating a new social climate of career possibilities for young women, a reproductive revolution was occurring in many parts of the world: early and rapid childbearing were no longer assumed to be the inevitable or enviable patterns of life. Almost half the married couples in developing nations now use some form of modern contraception. The desired family sizes reported by both women and men in survey responses are notably smaller almost everywhere outside Africa than was the case two decades ago. It is unlikely that these two virtually simultaneous changes in educational opportunities and fertility have no causal links. Yet under what circumstances can a causal relationship in the conventionally expected direction—education influencing fertility—actually be identified? Through what mechanisms does it operate?

In cross-country analyses, a generally consistent inverse relationship appears: women with more schooling have lower fertility than those with less (Adamchack and Ntseane, 1992; Ainsworth et al., 1996; Castro Martín, 1995; United Nations, 1995; Jejeebhoy, 1995).[1] The assumption of a causal flow from education to fertility has led many governments to support women's education not only to foster human rights and national development, but also to reduce fertility rates, promote the use of modern contraception, and improve child health. Indeed, a pressing need to educate girls for precisely these reasons was one of the strongest messages emerging from the 1994 International Conference on Population and Development in Cairo:

> The increase in the education of women and girls contributes to greater empowerment of women, to a postponement of the age of marriage, and to a reduction in the size of families (United Nations, 1994:Ch. XI, Para. 11.3).

This statement is appropriately concise. A Programme of Action agreed upon by more than 180 nations and other signatories is not the right place for nuance, qualification, or counterexample. However, the empirical record does not support the idea that such a simple causal process operates everywhere. Understanding the nature and strength of the relationship between education and fertility remains a central challenge both for scholars seeking to explain demographic and social change and for policy makers who must decide on the allocation of scarce public resources.[2] This volume takes up that challenge by bringing together analyses from several research perspectives to reexamine the education-fertility relationship and to rethink conventional lines of logic in the education-fertility paradigm. Although the geographical focus of most of the case studies is Africa, the papers, as well as this introduction, draw from a wider world literature.

EMPIRICAL ASSOCIATION BETWEEN EDUCATION AND FERTILITY

The effects of education on fertility have held enduring interest in demography. Aside from a woman's age and marital status, educational attainment is

[1]The distinction between schooling (number of years spent in school) and education (amount or content of learning actually acquired) is a critical one; see Jeffery and Basu (1996) for a cogent discussion. Because the thrust of this volume does not rest on this distinction (with the exception of the chapter by Glewwe), we have not tried to disentangle the vocabulary in all cases.

[2]For some important recent discussions, see, e.g., Adamchack and Ntseane, 1992; Schultz, 1993a; Ainsworth et al., 1996; Castro Martín, 1995; United Nations, 1995; and Jejeebhoy, 1995.

probably the variable most frequently included in fertility analyses in developing countries. If the relationship between an individual's education and fertility were consistent across time and place, and if its temporal trajectory at the societal level proceeded in the generally assumed direction—changes in schooling precede changes in fertility (or perhaps, the expectations of reproductive behavior—the matter would appear to be straightforward: because an individual's education is almost always finished by the time childbearing begins, education must lower fertility (or perhaps the expectations of reproductive behaviors) and not vice versa. Of course, the question of who receives schooling would remain pressing, as would the question of why education seems to have this effect on fertility. As noted above, however, the assumption of a simple causal relationship between higher levels of female schooling and lower fertility is not universally supported by the empirical record.

Those who see girls' education as a route to lower fertility can point to countries on both ends of the education-fertility continuum as evidence. Sri Lanka has unusually low fertility rates for a low-income country (total fertility rate [TFR] of 2.3 children per woman) and an unusually high female literacy rate (87 percent of women over age 15). Pakistan, with a much lower literacy rate (24 percent of adult women) has a much higher fertility rate (5.6 children per woman). But there are also anomalous populations in which high female literacy rates coexist with high fertility rates. Jordan, with 86 percent of women literate, has a TFR of 5.6, while in Bangladesh, a relatively low TFR of 3.3 coexists with a low female literacy rate of 26 percent.

In Jejeebhoy's (1995) analyses, the inverse association was found to be monotonic and significant in fewer than half (26) of the countries examined, including only 1 of 21 countries in sub-Saharan Africa. In those countries where the expected negative association did prevail, fertility differences were often small; the negative relationship appeared in regions such as Latin America that have more-developed economies and well-established schooling systems (see also Cochrane, 1979; Cochrane and Farid, 1989; Castro Martín, 1995). The expected pattern held least often where levels of per capita income and literacy were low and where there was gender imbalance in literacy levels (see also Diamond et al., this volume). Cross-sectional analyses of 6 of 26 countries in which Demographic and Health Surveys (DHS) were conducted (Burundi, Kenya, Liberia, Indonesia, Sri Lanka, and Bolivia) even show a reversal of the overall negative association between educational levels and fertility at lower levels of education: TFRs were higher among women with 1 to 3 years of schooling than among those with no schooling (United Nations, 1995:29). In 9 countries, almost all of them in sub-Saharan Africa, women with some education had higher completed fertility than did those with no schooling. Comparing the relationships between education and both fertility and child mortality, Cleland and Kaufmann (1998) report a highly consistent, almost straight dose-response relationship with child mortality.[3] With respect to female fertility, however, they report considerably more variation, and they argue that the fertility-education relationship appears far more context-dependent than is the case for child mortality.

Various explanations for such results have been advanced. In high-fertility contexts, for example, small amounts of education have been hypothesized to undermine lengthy postpartum breastfeeding and sexual abstinence that in previous times would have delayed a new pregnancy (see, e.g., Lesthaeghe et al., 1981:16-21). Alternatively, these unexpected findings may reflect the ability of educated women to achieve their numerical reproductive goals, whether these are goals of high or low fertility (Cleland and Kaufmann, 1998).[4]

As Diamond et al. (this volume) point out, the most recent DHS surveys show that the inverse relationship between education and fertility is emerging more strongly than ever; most of the contrary cases have begun to fall away. However, the pattern that has emerged has not always followed the temporal order that a straightforward thesis of education causing fertility decline would imply. Rodriguez and Aravena (1991) show, for example, that fertility differentials by education were low in Latin American countries early in the transition, then opened up, then narrowed again during the 1960s and 1970s. In Indonesia, education increased and fertility declined simultaneously (Oey-Gardiner and Sejahtera, 1996), and most of the Asian fertility decline has occurred among populations that are not literate or, for that matter, wealthy or urban (Caldwell, 1993; see also Freedman 1995, on the case of Bangladesh). These findings suggest either that education may be only one of many possible precipitates of fertility decline or that it may co-occur with fertility decline and other societal changes.

As with the effects of formal education, or training, on cognition or fertility,

---

[3]The children of educated women appear to have significantly lower morbidity and mortality risks (for recent analyses, see some of the contributions to National Research Council, 1998). Because the associations among maternal education, fertility, and infant mortality are not independent (Cleland and Kaufmann, 1998; Pitt, 1995), educated women, who are less likely to lose their children, may feel they need bear fewer children to replace those who die. Schultz (1993b) found that in a cross-national time-series analysis, a significant part of the effect of education on fertility could be explained by the effect of education on infant mortality, with lower mortality rates in turn leading to lower fertility. (See, however, Desai and Alva [1998] for reservations about the relationship between maternal education and child health.)

[4]One of the more interesting puzzles among these findings is why per capita income per se might condition the relationship. Most scholars agree that educated women usually have markedly different options in the labor market than do uneducated women. Able to command higher salaries, they forgo greater earnings when they cannot work. Insofar as childbearing reduces time spent in the labor market and domestic labor cannot be substituted, educated women are hypothesized to be more inclined to limit their childbearing (Willis, 1973; Blanc and Lloyd, 1990; cf. Delancy, 1980). Recently, the inverse association between work outside the home and childbearing has broken down in wealthier countries (Rindfuss and Brewster, 1996).

assertions about the effect of education in conveying accurate information about the biology of fertility must be made cautiously.[5] It has been shown (United Nations, 1995:71) that larger proportions of women correctly identify the most fertile period in the ovulatory cycle in countries where average levels of schooling are higher. Yet across countries, the correspondence between knowledge of the fertile period and fertility rates is quite low. In Thailand, with a TFR of 2.2, 13 percent of women identified the middle of the cycle as the most fertile, compared with 44 percent in Sri Lanka, with a TFR of 2.7. In sub-Saharan Africa, where fewer than 10 percent of women in 5 of 10 DHS countries analyzed by the United Nations (1995) identified the middle of the cycle as the most fertile, two of those countries with very low knowledge, Botswana and Zimbabwe, were two of the first three countries in all of Africa to undergo a fertility transition. In Botswana, with the lowest TFR of all the United Nations' 10 African countries, knowledge of the ovulatory cycle was the lowest among all 26 countries analyzed: 3.3 percent.

A number of researchers are careful to point out that education need not necessarily cause a fertility decline (e.g., Cochrane, 1979:7,31-32; Mason, 1993; United Nations, 1995:103; Castro Martín, 1995:194; Ahlburg et al., 1996) or produce behaviors considered conducive to lowering fertility. Roudi (1995:16) observes that in Jordan, which was found in the 1990 DHS to have the most closely spaced births in the Middle Eastern region, women with at least a secondary education, despite their later age at first marriage and higher levels of modern contraception, were more likely to have closely spaced births than those with less education. Analogous patterns have been in observed as well in Taiwan. Freedman (1995:22), pointing to a marked increase in births among educated Taiwanese women who delay marriage and childbearing, argues that "period measures such as the TFR are likely to exaggerate the fertility decline, which is made up when postponed births occur at a later age." Clearly, Western education, whether or not it played a key role in lowering fertility initially, may now be exerting pressures or offering inducements to keep fertility low. Yet given such variation in observed empirical results, education cannot be a necessary cause for fertility decline at either the individual or the societal level. The question is under what conditions education or some aspect of it might be a sufficient cause.

The following discussion is organized under two rubrics: cognition and social influence. As for the first, there is a long tradition of work behind the demographic view that schooling transforms the way individuals think or gives them access to new information; as educated people, they will more likely want fewer

---

[5]Family-life education programs, which have grown in number and scope over the past two decades, are designed to help girls make choices that will help them to avoid pregnancy so they can continue their schooling and to pursue a low-fertility adult life. However, there have been no systematic studies on the effects of these programs on fertility or on life chances.

children and have the personal knowledge or skills needed to be able to implement their desires. Accordingly, education is often hypothesized to have its greatest influence over young women's future reproductive lives by making them significantly different from uneducated women. What evidence is there of such cognitive effects that might bear on fertility?

With regard to social influence, behind many discussions of education as a key variable in fertility research is the Parsonian view of the individual as a socialized actor (Parsons, 1964:207-226). In this view, individuals' actions stem from the values they are imbued with by institutions in the external world. As individuals internalize the values of new social institutions and cultural patterns, they gain skills and behavioral norms that allow them to adopt new practices differing from those of previous generations who were not imbued with these values. This view of the socialized actor pervades descriptions of modernization and its impacts on individuals (see especially Inkeles, 1969). Quoting from Inkeles, Easterlin (1983:563) describes the personality changes that modernization appears to entail as "an increased openness to new experience, increased independence from parental authority, belief in the efficacy of science, and greater ambition for oneself and one's children." Applied to fertility, education is said to break down traditional beliefs and customs, inducing couples to make conscious efforts to limit family size. It may also alter cultural norms that oppose the use of birth control, shift consumer tastes to goods rather than children, present new lifestyle possibilities that compete with children, raise healthcare standards for those children one does bear, and (in general) encourage a problem-solving approach to life (Easterlin, 1983:63).

These speculations about the conventionally expected impact of modernization on individuals make intuitive sense. The problem is that the literature provides little direct evidence for these speculations or, indeed, for the socialized-actor explanation of innovations in fertility behavior. More serious is a logical conundrum concerning the perceptions of those who send children to school: Why would parents enroll their children in school if they know it is a forum where children will be encouraged to reject parental values? The issue is particularly acute in the case of girls: Why would parents enroll their daughters in school knowing that doing so may very well result in rejection of the society's high-fertility values? A number of answers might be advanced. For example: (1) parents are aware of the likely transformation to come and are willing to accept it; (2) whatever changes in behavior schooling entails are not as drastic as outsiders perceive; and (3) parents are willing for some of their daughters, though not necessarily all, to become transformed in the ways they expect schooling to effect.

While individual women are usually the exclusive focus of studies of the education-fertility relationship, the issue of the perceptions not only of the educated individual, but also the wider body of consumers of education raises a set of questions that have received far less attention in fertility studies. These questions relate to how the groups in which a woman lives and acts affect the relationship between her education and childbearing. Of particular interest are relationships involving generational and conjugal links. To address these questions, we pay particular attention in what follows to the notion of "selection," a term generally used to describe sources of error in demographic statistical calculations. Here we put the notion to a highly sociological purpose in order to understand how young women may be recruited into or withdrawn from groups whose members are more likely to have lower or higher fertility.

COGNITION AND SOCIAL INFLUENCE AND THE EDUCATION-FERTILITY RELATIONSHIP

Fertility and the Cognitive Effects of Schooling

While education may indeed impart knowledge and skills that bear directly on fertility, research on this specific point is surprisingly sparse. As a result, LeVine et al. (1994:304) point out, the processes by which learning experiences may produce demographic behaviors remain mysterious:

> Among the least understood processes are those that mediate the effects of school experience during childhood on the behavior of adult women as mothers and reproductive decision makers in Third World countries. This is the "black box" in survey data linking years spent in school with demographic and health outcomes; it is often covered by speculative assumptions and interpretations, but rarely investigated.

The question of how Western-type schooling may transform thinking is a subject that sparks great controversy among those who study the sociology of education and literacy. Yet it seems quite paradoxical that almost no one in the field of education has displayed any interest in the demographic implications of a phenomenon of such historic importance as the global spread of mass education (cf. LeVine et al., 1991). Indeed, the presumed capability of education to transform individuals in ways that seem so intuitively compelling in the domain of population research are seen in more problematic terms by most of those in the field of international education and literacy (see, e.g., Graff, 1979, 1981, 1987; Heath, 1982; Street, 1984, 1993; Willis, 1977; Wagner, 1983; Meyer et al., 1992; and Daniels and Bright, 1996).

In the domain of studies that see literacy as transformative of society, comparative and historical psychological studies have explored what is regarded as a cognitive divide between literate and nonliterate people whereby the schemata people use to evaluate the world are transformed by the process of education (Goody and Watt, 1963; Ong, 1967, 1982; Clammer, 1976; see Collins, 1995:77-78, for a review of such work). In this framework, writing, because of its clarity, endurance, and precision—attributes that advocates of the position see as a logical consequence of the medium itself—is described as superior to traditional oral modes of communication for transmitting ideas across space and time (e.g., Goody and Watt, 1963; Goody, 1968, 1977; Goody et al., 1977; Olson et al., 1985). Text and the written word can therefore replace reliance on memory and oral communication because their meaning can be understood independently of context.

In this view, education and its effects on social institutions and cognitive processes are taken as central objects of study: literacy is seen as increasing individualism, writing is seen as creating detachment because it is not context dependent, and literacy is seen as enhancing communication in extending it beyond face-to-face interaction and reducing dependence on memory for storing and retrieving information. Variants of this theory of cognitive modernization regard education, especially in its function of teaching literacy, as fundamentally altering basic forms of thought. These changes are said to allow people to calculate along longer time frames; to distinguish between opinion and truth on the basis of critical, externally informed evaluation; and to pursue autonomous courses of action instead of accepting received tradition or adhering to authority. LeVine and White (1986), for example, suggest that schools provide new decontextualized modes of communication that can be useful in confronting complex bureaucracies, as well as didactic models for childrearing practices. This formulation of language use is not meant to imply that nonliterate cultures are deficient or that people living in them give up traditional aspirations upon adopting Western institutions. Rather, local institutions of socialization create new combinations of indigenous and imported meanings, and schooling allows new modes of communication, new concepts of self-perception, and new kinds of thought.

In recent years, however, numerous critiques of the thesis of the primacy of literacy have emerged. One of the most visible critics, Street (1984:2-3), ". . . treats skeptically claims by western liberal educators for the 'openness,' 'rationality' and critical awareness of what they teach . . . [concentrating] on the overlap and interaction of oral and literate modes rather than stressing a 'great divide.'" According to such critics, to believe literacy has qualities that surpass those of oral communication is to neglect the equally logical potential of writing to provide "cultural capital" in the creation of elite status (Bourdieu, 1984) or to obfuscate (Bledsoe and Robey, 1986).

Against the idea that literacy both marks and creates an intellectual or evolutionary divide between those with and without the ability to read (Levy-Bruhl, 1926), most recent studies argue that Western education has no particular monopoly on efficacy or application (e.g., Halverson, 1992; Street, 1993). As Collins (1995:80) notes, Goody (1968) has modified his original stance to distinguish between full and restricted literacy. Goody has also ". . . steadily weakened his claims about literacy and logic, turning instead to arguments about literacy and social organization; Olson's [1994] latest treatment of the subject concedes that alphabetic literacy is not inherently superior to other scripts, and literacy does not by itself cause cognitive or cultural development. . . ."

In the framework in which the meaning and impact of education are seen as deriving more from context than from inherent qualities, education is seen as imparting special skills, such as reading, that a child may be unable to acquire elsewhere. Yet neither the forms of logical thinking nor the kinds of knowledge that are imparted have an intrinsic advantage over those children might acquire through other modes of training. As McDermott and Peiu (n.d.) observe, most scholarship based on work conducted in the field instead of in the laboratory has by now concluded that it is difficult, if not impossible, to separate the effects of literacy from the social contexts in which literacy arises (see, for example, Lave and Wenger, 1991; Scribner and Cole 1981; Street, 1984; and McDermott and Peiu, n.d; cf. Havelock, 1986). It is instead the political and economic setting, including its existing societal hierarchies, that determines how skills will be evaluated and how they will be put to use. With respect to issues of fertility, these observations imply that students who learn their national language may well become better equipped to acquire family planning/economic resources by employing their language skills or gaining bureaucratic connections. Yet information on issues such as fertility regulation can travel independently of education and even of the national language, if the context demands.[6]

An example of how the local context shapes the meaning and fertility impact of education (or, more broadly, training) is that of trade apprenticeships in West Africa. Through the work of Guyer (n.d.), the National Research Council (1993) found that although secondary education is generally associated with later first birth for young women in African countries, very different levels of secondary education can be associated with similar patterns of entry into childbearing if other forms of training have delaying effects. Young women in Ghana, a country with vast trade industries and high levels of informal-sector female employment, including an established tradition of female apprenticeship, showed almost the same age distribution at first birth as did young women in Botswana, a country with a strong industrial base, despite very large differences in levels of secondary education (7 percent in Ghana versus 38 percent in Botswana). Such findings on the varied pathways into the reproductive years suggest that the structure of training or its content per se may be less important in delaying the initiation of a sexual and reproductive career than a more general extension of supervised training into young adulthood, combined with certain relationships with a mindful mentor, in ways that discourage early fertility.

Situational factors may even effectively reverse the usual assumptions of

[6]This may help explain why older African women tend to know more about Western contraceptives than do younger women. Although few are educated, they encounter mounting problems of reproductive morbidity that motivate them to manage their births carefully (Bledsoe et al., 1994).

causality implied in the education-fertility relationship. Research on the effect of education on fertility frequently takes as the object of study one person's life course, with a first period characterized by preparation for adulthood and a second by roles that are seen as adult in nature, particularly childbearing. While this ordered division allows formal modeling of schooling as an investment in human capital, it can be misleading. Schoolgirls who get pregnant may be forced by social pressures to leave school, an effect that some might call reverse causation (for the case of Africa, see National Research Council, 1993). In such instances, strong social opinions about the proper timing of childbearing may cause childbearing to influence education, rather than the reverse.

The possibility that context fundamentally determines the meaning and impact of schooling is also seen in power dynamics. One of the most prominent aspects of theory that seeks to explain the inverse relationship between education and fertility is the possibility that education may bestow power on women, who generally express a desire to stop childbearing earlier than do their husbands (e.g., Mason and Taj, 1987). While individuals may acquire special knowledge or skills in school, the mere fact of having attended school may evoke deference from others, a phenomenon analogous to the employment theory notion of credentialism (e.g., Knight and Sabot, 1990). (For discussion of more substantial questions of whether schooling inevitably confers power on women, see Jeffery and Basu [1996] and Shah and Bulatao [1981].) In fact, education may even have negative consequences in the education-fertility relationship: in a society with highly unequal access to literacy, those who lack literacy may experience discrimination. As McDermott and Varenne (1995:341) have noted in a sobering description of the effects of adult literacy programs in the United States, "the more people believe that literacy is cognitively and culturally transformative, the more they can find reasons to degrade those without such powers. . . ."

Finally, a fundamental problem with assuming that education produces modern behavior is the question of what, precisely, constitutes modern behavior. It has been noted repeatedly, for example, that education is strongly related to the use of modern contraceptives, itself one of the strongest correlates of reduced fertility rates (for some recent figures, see United Nations, 1995:69). What has gone virtually unnoticed in such analyses is a clear increase as well with education in the use of "traditional" forms of contraception. Although traditional methods are typically considered less effective than "modern" ones and are thus seldom included in contraceptive analyses, virtually all 26 countries included in the U.N. analysis showed a monotonic increase with education in the use of traditional contraception. With the exception of Zimbabwe, there is more use of traditional contraception among the most educated women (10 or more years) than among women as a whole (United Nations, 1995:74). Education may indeed allow women to adopt rational behaviors that break the bonds of custom and superstition. Yet if modern contraceptive use is a key indicator of rational action, it is not clear why educated women across the developing world should be using traditional contraceptives more often than women with less education unless "traditional" methods are more "rational" than we believed.

The mystery can be solved in part simply by acknowledging the enduring semantic problems involved in coding and interpreting survey responses. The U.N. figures combine the DHS category of "traditional" methods (abstinence and withdrawal) with that of "folkloric" methods, which includes everything from imbibing herbs to wearing Islamic scriptures around the waist in an amulet pouch. Hence, use of the word "traditional" to describe what is probably largely abstinence and, to a lesser extent, withdrawal with respect to the behaviors of educated women is hiding more than it reveals (see Curtis and Neitzel, 1996, for a similar observation; see especially Tables D.9 through D.11, pp. 86-88). This stark example implies that traditional methods should be taken seriously in analyses of fertility control (see also Santow, 1995, on the importance of withdrawal as a contraceptive method in the European fertility decline). Furthermore, while it is tempting to see as rational the kinds of behaviors that Western schooling is said to induce, few analysts would argue that educated women, though more frequent users of traditional contraception than uneducated women, are more "irrational" in their reproductive decision making than are their uneducated counterparts. The bottom line, to which everyone would likely ascribe, is that women from all walks of life take steps to stop childbearing or control its timing when they need to do so. How they can do so is determined less by custom than by circumstance and resources.

Social Influences on the Education-Fertility Relationship: Who Is Sent to School and by Whom?

Seen as an instrument of modernity, education is most commonly assumed to bring about lower fertility by inculcating those who acquire it with new ways of thinking and perceiving. Yet social forces intrude upon this relationship at every point. Among the most powerful are those operating across generations. Young children seldom make choices about their own education. The implication is that if educational experiences are important in shaping fertility careers, the educational choices adults make for their daughters are as important as the choices the children eventually make for themselves.[7]

Among the most subtle yet pervasive domains of social influence is mass

---

[7]Some analysts see parents with limited resources as confronting what economists have termed a "quality-quantity" trade-off, in which parents with a limited and nonelastic supply of resources must choose between investing more in each of a few or less in each of many children. The choice to invest more heavily in fewer children is strongly associated with income (Blake, 1981), particularly given severe economic inequalities (Mueller and Short, 1983). This finding led Eloundou-Enyegue (1994) to argue that parents' aspirations for their children, rather than current income per se, spurs investment choices.

education, whereby all members of the population, including those who have not attended school, may be affected by the changes that a new cultural climate of an educated populace entails (e.g., Caldwell, 1980). Mass schooling clearly changes parents' expectations about the circumstances their children and future grandchildren will confront. Prior to this societal change, having little or no education might suffice to establish one's progeny in a respectable economic situation and secure them advantageous marriages. In the new situation created by mass schooling, this is no longer the case. The paradoxical result is often that young couples in rapidly developing economies perceive a need to educate all their children. Though clearly better off in material terms than their parents, these couples decide they cannot "afford" as many children as their parents somehow afforded a generation earlier (see the discussions of Thai villagers reported by Knodel et al., 1987: Ch. 7). In such situations, education may affect fertility, but hardly by imparting new cognitive skills. The implication is that the education-fertility association may sometimes arise less from a process by which modernity is imprinted on individuals whose student years precede their reproductive careers than from pressures on the preceding generation, for whom the anticipated costs of educating any future children may act to discourage high fertility (see, e.g., Caldwell, 1980, and Axinn, 1993).

For most wealthy countries in the 1990s, parents who do not provide formal schooling (or make equivalent arrangements) for all their children well into the teenage years are considered negligent and are liable for legal prosecution. In less fortunate countries, parents who manage to educate some of their children into the teenage years are either rich or unusually determined. In some circumstances, the children themselves, by showing exceptional talent, may go further in school than their parents had planned. This means the characteristics of the situation that result in certain children attaining more schooling and others less may well lead to lower fertility, independently of what actually happens in school.

Situations such as this, in which levels of two variables are affected by unobserved characteristics of individuals or groups that are known to those involved but not to the researcher, are termed "selection" effects. Invisible selection effects can render groups noncomparable and lead to spurious correlations. Prominent examples come from the realms of employment and marriage (Heckman, 1976; Smith, 1980; Axinn and Thornton, 1992). Yet beyond its application to the question of sampling errors, the notion of selection offers a sociological handle for addressing the question of education and fertility in the developing world, insofar as it may reflect the outcome of intentional social actions to recruit certain people into, or filter others out of, one pool or another. Such processes lie at the heart of Guyer's (1996) work on life pathways in the development of "singularity" in Equatorial Africa, in which youthful abilities are constantly being cultivated for different career path potentials in a volatile economy (see also Guyer, 1993, and Guyer and Eno Belinga, 1995). Parents may choose formal schooling for children with certain attributes, such as intellectual aptitude or a willingness to follow instructions. Other children may be seen as suited for local alternatives to schooling, such as trade apprenticeships.

Across the world, unequal access to higher levels of education, whether by gender, by perceived ability, or by class (e.g., Knodel and Jones, 1996), is the rule rather than the exception. In national education systems that offer limited numbers of places on a competitive basis, decisions must be made to invest in the education of certain children and not others. Such pressures strongly shape the outcomes of competition for places in secondary schools, a process Bourdieu and Passeron (1971) vividly document for the selection and cultivation of members of the French elite. Individuals may or may not be transformed by processes of pedagogy and communication in education, but they clearly are measured at a point in time after their different unobservable characteristics affected their selection into or out of the pool of continuing students.

Whether this broadened view of selection refers to a passive process of being filtered out of a particular group by forces beyond one's control or to a process of entering another group by individual choice (or by some combination of the two), it captures the situation in many contemporary developing countries in which the number of women who can complete a certain level of education is sharply reduced at each successive level. Pressures exerted by social class, notions of propriety, or academic ability that influence which individual women will continue in school and which will be withdrawn for early marriage and motherhood may mean that reproduction effectively influences education. Such forces of selection are particularly important in light of the vast variation in the quality and cost of schooling both within and across countries. A family may send an academically gifted daughter to an expensive school with high academic standards: she is thus selected to attend a school whose students are likely to delay fertility because they are firmly established in a professional career track. A girl whose character or talents are not judged worthy, however, may not be enrolled in school at all or may be withdrawn as soon as marriage becomes possible. Her parents may even seek to avoid the very outcomes that schools are said to promote—female autonomy, shifts of loyalty from the family toward the outside world, late marriage, and low fertility.

The possibility that observed sortings may represent outcomes of intentional social actions implies that the removal by families of certain women from the elite pool of continuing students may even occur with the intent that their future life will be channeled toward high fertility. Similar forces of selection arise with respect to admission standards for students seeking transfer to a new school or reentry after a hiatus, issues of singular importance to women who seek to resume their schooling after childbirth. They may also apply to situations involving girls from low-status families, children from large families, or children whose births were unwanted.

Besides the complications posed for the education-fertility relationship by selection and associated generational forces are those involving the dynamics of marriage. Women's choices about schooling and childbearing are inevitably shaped by the kinds of support available to them from men who may provide them with economic assistance, father their children, or protect them from other men. A variety of studies have shown that educated African women marry later; marry more educated men; and, at high levels of education, are less likely to marry (Gage-Brandon, 1993; Stambach, 1996). Yet powerful selection factors may affect fertility. The husbands of educated women, as Basu (this volume) points out for India, differ from those of uneducated women; as such they represent a distinct selected subset of men. This means that a certain fertility dynamic has been set up well before the women themselves take any reproductive decisions.

The forces by which young women are drawn into groups characterized by certain patterns of reproduction have been thinly documented and conceptualized. All deserve greater attention in both empirical research and theory building.

OVERVIEW OF THIS VOLUME

The chapters that follow contribute to our understanding of the above associations between education and fertility. Chapter 2, by Ian Diamond, Margaret Newby, and Sarah Varle, summarizes some recent empirical evidence, primarily from the DHS on the education-fertility relationship. The authors review a broad array of studies, positing that while primary education may affect fertility indirectly, by mediating the effect of various factors, secondary and higher education may influence fertility more directly by making people "more able to make independent decisions based on an assessment of the likely costs and benefits of different actions." They also ask, however, how the same measure of schooling can lead to very different fertility outcomes depending on the social, economic, and political circumstances. They identify multiple possible pathways to explain the influence of education on fertility: employment/opportunity costs, the nature of marriage, familiarity with bureaucratic institutions, and reference communities.

Most studies of education and fertility see schooling as imbuing students not with unthinking adherence to what they are taught, but with the ability to evaluate information and problems for themselves, and in particular to break loose from traditional beliefs. In Chapter 3, however, Anthony Carter shows that such models see students as passive recipients of educational messages, with education imprinting itself upon them in some way that will induce them to bear fewer children. If this is so, he shows, the students themselves need no discussion; they are the bearers of family planning messages and followers of new reproductive expectations. Drawing on theory from linguistic anthropology, Carter describes a model of schooling as social practice in which education and childbearing represent transformative moments in a life course shaped by the communities of practice in which the individual, by virtue of his or her educational experience, becomes a participant. In this model, schools do not simply transmit ideas or cause women to bear fewer children through some series of prior or external forces. Rather, students actively select from among disparate pieces of knowledge from many different sources, including but not exclusive to the classroom, for use in different contexts.

Although education may in some way affect fertility, direct evidence on this question remains thin. Four of the chapters, those by Cynthia Lloyd and Barbara Mensch, Paul Glewwe, Duncan Thomas, and Bruce Fuller and Xiaoyan Liang, make significant contributions to the question of what specific forces may bring about such results and through what channels their effects may be felt. In Chapter 4, Lloyd and Mensch, asking what young women learn or experience in school that may bear on their entry into parenthood, review a wide range of literature on schooling and adolescence from the developing world, including their own recent study in Kenya. They examine the transition to adulthood for young women in terms of the possible links between schooling and low fertility, and shed light on the potentially fertility-relevant content of schooling. Their chapter brings together work on a variety of factors that may facilitate or constrain continued schooling for girls. Among these factors are school policies regarding marriage and pregnancy, school quality and academic achievement, gender-biased differences in study time, punishments, material investments, curriculum, and teacher attitudes.

In Chapter 5, Glewwe addresses the issue of comparability among schools. He suggests that if schools have a significant impact on demographic change, the specific cause of that impact is far less identifiably one of cognitive development among students than a simple measure of years of school attended or highest grade completed would imply. The use of such measures assumes that schools provide universally some comparable "dose" of learning in a year; school quality is treated as a constant and as having no bearing on parental choices regarding the length of their children's schooling. Using a neoclassical economic model, Glewwe demonstrates that a simplistic model of investment fails to explain parents' educational choices. He finds that parents are likely to invest in more schooling for their children if they perceive the available school to be of high quality. Because students will probably attend longer the kinds of schools likely to provide them with more cognitive skills, this observation confounds a presumed relationship between years of schooling and the amount of knowledge students acquire. Glewwe's work makes clear the need to ask why parents educate their children for certain numbers of years. His work also suggests that school quality cannot be taken as given; rather, empirical research is needed on what occurs in schools.

In Chapter 6, Thomas examines important empirical evidence concerning a possible mechanism through which the negative association between education and fertility might develop. He finds that among women in South Africa, reading comprehension skills are strongly associated with lower fertility, quite independently of earnings (see also Oliver, in press). Thomas is thus able to argue that what makes a difference for fertility is not schooling in general, or even its duration, but specific comprehension skills learned in school. He argues that these results lend support to the thesis that women with stronger comprehension skills may be able to acquire and incorporate family planning information, although the specific mechanisms may vary across contexts. At the same time, Thomas' data reveal that cognitive skills alone cannot explain the variations in fertility. Women who leave school at natural breaks, such as those between primary and secondary school, have lower fertility than would be predicted if the schooling-fertility relationship followed a linear dose-response pattern. Thomas suggests that the women who leave school at natural breaks differ in systematic ways from women who leave at other times, meaning that processes of selection out of school may constitute a significant factor in the education-fertility relationship.

In Chapter 7, another study of South Africa, Fuller and Liang address the key question of who receives schooling. Using data from three South African provinces, they find that personal, family, and community characteristics all influence the likelihood that girls will stay in school. They also find support for a family model of household economics in which short-term economic resources and social obligations, rather than long-term investment strategies, predict the school attainment of eldest daughters. Their findings suggest that the community of educated women is both shaped and differentiated from that of uneducated women in ways that predate their schooling.

As for the possible effects of generational ties on the education and fertility relationship, Chapter 8, by Mark Montgomery and Cynthia Lloyd, offers an intriguing analysis of what might be labeled reverse causation through the notion of the "wantedness" of a child or a birth. Using DHS data, they find instances in which educational outcomes may be shaped by "exogenous" fertility at least as heavily as fertility is affected by education. They argue that in some instances, unintended or excess fertility may lead parents to withdraw children from school or to enroll them late. Their analysis also underscores the value of a situational view of childbearing and education choices, in which parents constantly revise their choices on the basis of changing circumstances. By focusing on births that women report they did not want, Montgomery and Lloyd transcend the simplistic assumption that any quantity-quality trade-off made by parents in childbearing decisions is a decision "made once-and-for-all, generally at the beginning of the reproductive lifespan" (Greenhalgh, 1995:22). Their findings suggest that the immediate constellation of the family is critical in this process.

Much research on education and fertility focuses on how schooling affects women's participation in labor markets. Yet marriage markets also figure critically in a couple's fertility. Schooling transforms or bolsters social positions in ways that affect profoundly who ends up marrying whom; thus the most important fertility decisions may be settled for all intents and purposes before the couple actually meets. Certainly in the case of South Asia, where so many marriages continue to be arranged, the logic of assuming that schooling gives women power that might allow them to counter men's high-fertility demands must be weighed against the realization that most women in developing countries have partners who are more educated than they are. Thus, even if a woman has power conferred on her by education, her husband is likely to have more education than she does, meaning that the most powerful partner in a union is very likely to remain the man. The power of marriage markets in affecting subsequent fertility outcomes is central to Alaka Basu's analysis in Chapter 9. Countering the idea that educated women choose to reduce their fertility independently of their husbands, she argues that in India, men's education is nearly universally desired, so it cannot serve as a marker of particular values or preferences. However, men who choose to marry educated women differ systematically from other men. Coming from families that value women's education, these men were raised to seek the same in a spouse. Men who marry educated women, therefore, are largely in agreement with the low fertility aspirations of their educated wives well before the marriage.

In a concluding review in Chapter 10, Parfait Eloundou-Enyegue notes the parallels and contrasts in some of the themes of this volume with regard to questions raised 20 years ago in Cochrane's (1979) seminal book, *Fertility and Education: What Do We Really Know?*. In contrast to Cochrane's work, he attributes the cautions expressed here about how education may affect fertility to several factors. These factors include changes in demography as a discipline, its broadened geographical coverage from which generalizations must be drawn, its increasing sophistication as a social science, and the expansion of theoretical and statistical demographic models to grapple with the challenges posed by increasingly rich and complex data sources. As his observations reveal, the seemingly simple question of Cochrane's subtitle has grown into a set of deeper challenges to the field.

REFERENCES

Adamchak, D., and P. Gabo Ntseane

1992 Gender, education and fertility: A cross-national analysis of Sub-Saharan nations. *Sociological Spectrum* 12:167-182.

Ahlburg, D.A., A.C. Kelley, and K.O. Mason, eds.

1996 *The Impact of Population Growth on Well-being in Developing Countries.* New York/ Berlin, Germany: Springer-Verlag.

Ainsworth, M., K. Beegle, and A. Nyamete

1996 The impact of women's schooling on fertility and contraceptive use: A study of 14 Sub-Saharan African countries. *World Bank Economic Review* 10(1):85-122.

Axinn, W.G.

1993 The effects of children's schooling on fertility limitation. *Population Studies* 47(3):481-493.

Axinn, W.G., and A. Thorton

1992 The relationship between cohabitation and divorce: Selectivity or causal influence? *Demography* 29(3):357-374.

Blake, J.

1981 Family size and the quality of children. *Demography* 18(4):421-442.

Blanc, A., and C. Lloyd

1990 *Women's Childrearing Strategies in Relation to Fertility and Employment in Ghana.* Policy Research Division Working Paper No. 16. New York: The Population Council.

Bledsoe, C., and K. Robey

1986 Arabic literacy and secrecy among the Mende of Sierra Leone. *Man* 21:202-226.

Bledsoe, C., A.G. Hill, U. d'Alessandro, and P. Langerock

1994 Constructing natural fertility: The use of Western contraceptive technologies in rural Gambia. *Population and Development Review* 20(1):81-113.

Bourdieu, P.

1984 *Distinction: A Social Critique of the Judgment of Taste.* Cambridge, Mass.: Harvard University Press.

Bourdieu, P., and J-C. Passeron

1971 *Reproduction in Education, Society and Culture.* London: Sage Publications.

Caldwell, J.C.

1980 Mass education as a determinant of the timing of fertility decline. *Population and Development Review* 6(2):225-255.

1993 The Asian fertility revolution: its implications for transition theories. Pp. 299-316 in R. Leete and I. Alam, eds., *The Revolution in Asian Fertility: Dimensions, Causes, and Implications.* Oxford: Clarendon Press.

Castro Martín, T.

1995 Women's education and fertility: Results from 26 Demographic and Health Surveys. *Studies in Family Planning* 26(4):187-202.

Clammer, J.R.

1976 *Literacy and Social Change: A Case Study of Fiji.* Leiden: Brill.

Cleland, J., and G. Kaufmann

1998 Education, fertility and child survival: Unraveling the links. In A. Basu and P. Aaby, eds., *The Methods and Uses of Anthropological Demography.* Oxford: Clarendon.

Cochrane, S.H.

1979 *Fertility and Education: What Do We Really Know*? Baltimore, Md.: Johns Hopkins University Press.

Cochrane, S.H., and S.M. Farid

1989 *Fertility in Sub-Saharan Africa: Analysis and Explanation.* World Bank Discussion Paper, No. 43. Washington, D.C.: The World Bank.

Collins, J.

1995 Literacy and literacies. *Annual Review of Anthropology* 24:75-93.

Craig, J.

1981 The expansion of education. *Review of Research in Education* 8:151-210.

Curtis, S.L., and K. Neitzel

1996 *Contraceptive Knowledge, Use, and Sources.* Demographic and Health Surveys Comparative Studies No. 19. Calverton, Md.: Macro International, Inc.

Daniels, P., and W. Bright, eds.

1996 *The World's Writing Systems.* Oxford: Oxford University Press.

Delancy, V.H.

1980 *The Relationship Between Female Wage Employment and Fertility in Africa: An Example from Cameroon.* Unpublished Doctoral Dissertation. Department of Economics, University of South Carolina.

Desai, S., and S. Alva

1998 Maternal education and child health: Is there a strong causal relationship? *Demography* 35(1):71-81.

Easterlin, R.A.

1983 Modernization and fertility: A critical essay. Pp. 562-586 in R.A. Bulatao and R.D. Lee, eds., *Determinants of Fertility in Developing Countries.* Volume 2. New York: Academic Press.

Eloundou-Enyegue, P.

1994 Why Trade Quantity for Child Quality? A "Family Mobility" Thesis. Working Paper 94-15. University Park, Pa.: Pennsylvania State University Population Research Institute.

Freedman, R.

1995 Asia's recent fertility decline and prospects for future demographic change. *Asia-Pacific Population Research Reports*, No. 1.

Gage-Brandon, A.J.

1993 The formation and stability of informal unions in Côte d'Ivoire. *Journal of Comparative Family Studies* 24(2):219-233.

Goody, J.

1968 Introduction. Pp. 1-26 in J. Goody, ed., *Literacy in Traditional Societies.* Cambridge: Cambridge University Press.

1977 *The Domestication of the Savage Mind.* Cambridge: Cambridge University Press.

Goody, J., and I. Watt

1963 The consequences of literacy. *Comparative Studies in Society and History* 5:304-345.

Goody, J., M. Cole, and S. Scribner

1977 Writing and formal operations: A case study among the Vai. *Africa* 47:289-304.

Graff, H.J.

1979 Literacy, education and fertility, past and present: A critical review. *Population and Development Review* 5(1):105-140.

1981 *Literacy and Social Development in the West.* Cambridge: Cambridge University Press.

1987 *The Legacies of Literacy.* Bloomington, Ind.: Indiana University Press.

Greenhalgh, S.

1995 Anthropology theorizes reproduction: Integrating practice, political economic, and feminist perspectives. Pp. 3-28 in *Situating Fertility: Anthropology and Demographic Inquiry.* Cambridge: Cambridge University Press.

Guyer, J.I.

n.d. The economics of adolescent fertility in Africa. Background paper for the National Research Council Report on the Social Dynamics of African Population. Working Group on the Social Dynamics of Adolescent Fertility in Sub-Saharan Africa, Panel on the Population Dynamics of Africa, National Academy of Sciences. Washington, D.C.

1993 Wealth in people and self-realization in Equatorial Africa. *Man* 28:243-265.

1996 Traditions of invention in Equatorial Africa. *African Studies Review* 39(3):1-28.

Guyer, J., and S.M. Eno Belinga

1995 Wealth in people as wealth in knowledge: Accumulation and composition in Equatorial Africa. *Journal of African History* 36:91-120.

Halverson, J.

1992 Goody and the implosion of the literacy thesis. *Man (NS)* 27:301-317.

Havelock, E.A.

1986 *The Muse Learns To Write: Reflections on Orality and Literacy from Antiquity to the Present.* New Haven, Conn.: Yale University Press.

Heath, S.
1982 *Ways with Words: Language, Life, and Work in Communities and Classrooms.* New York: Cambridge University Press.
Heckman, J.
1976 The common structure of statistical models of truncation, sample selection and limited dependent variables and a simple estimator for such models. *Annals of Economic and Social Measurement* 5(4):475-492.
Hill, M.A., and E.M. King
1993 Women's education in developing countries: An overview. Pp. 1-50 in E.M. King and M.A. Hill, eds., *Women's Education in Developing Countries: Barriers, Benefits, and Policies.* Baltimore, Md.: The Johns Hopkins University Press.
Inkeles, A.
1969 Making men modern: On the causes and consequences of individual change in six developing countries. *American Journal of Sociology* 75:208-225.
Jeffery, R., and A.M. Basu
1996 Schooling as contraception? Pp. 15-47 in R. Jeffery and A.M. Basu, eds., *Girls' Schooling, Women's Autonomy and Fertility Change in South Asia.* New Delhi: Sage Publications.
Jejeebhoy, S.J.
1995 *Women's Education, Autonomy, and Reproductive Behavior: Experience from Developing Countries.* Oxford: Clarendon Press.
Knight, J.B., and R.H. Sabot
1990 *Education, Productivity, and Inequality: The East African Natural Experiment.* Oxford: Oxford University Press.
Knodel, J., and G.W. Jones
1996 Post-Cairo population policy: Does promoting girls' schooling miss the mark? *Population and Development Review* 22(4):683-702.
Knodel, J., A. Chamratrithirong, and N. Debavalya
1987 *Thailand's Reproductive Revolution: Rapid Fertility Decline in a Third-World Setting.* Madison, Wisc.: University of Wisconsin Press.
Lave, J., and E. Wenger
1991 *Situated Learning: Legitimate Peripheral Participation.* Cambridge: Cambridge University Press.
Lesthaeghe, R., P.O. Ohadike, J. Kocher, and H.J. Page
1981 Child-spacing and fertility in sub-Saharan Africa: An overview of the issues. Pp. 3-23 in H.J. Page and R. Lesthaeghe, eds., *Child-Spacing in Tropical Africa: Traditions and Change.* London: Academic Press.
Levy-Bruhl, L.
1926 *How Natives Think.* Princeton, N.J.: Princeton University Press.
LeVine, R.A., S.E. LeVine, A. Richman, F.M. Tapia Uribe, C.S. Correa, and P.M. Miller
1991 Women's schooling and child care in the demographic transition: A Mexican case study. *Population and Development Review* 17(3):459-496.
LeVine, R.A., S.E. LeVine, A. Richman, F.M. Tapia Uribe, and C.S. Correa
1994 Schooling and survival: The impact of maternal education on health and reproduction in the Third World. Pp. 303-338 in L. Chen, A. Kleinman, and N.C. Ware, eds., *Health and Social Change in International Perspective.* Boston, Mass.: Harvard University Press.
LeVine, R., and M. White
1986 *Human Conditions: The Cultural Basis of Educational Developments.* New York: Kegan Paul.

Mason, K.O.
1993 How female education affects reproductive behavior in urban Pakistan. *Asian and Pacific Population Forum* 6(4):93-103.
Mason, K.O., and A.M. Taj
1987 Differences between women's and men's reproductive goals in developing countries. *Population and Development Review* 13(4):611-638.
McDermott, R. and H. Varenne
1995 Culture as disability. *Anthropology & Education Quarterly* 26(3):324-348.
McDermott, R., and A. Peiu
n.d. The cognitive consequences of Greek literacy. Unpublished manuscript.
Meyer, J.W., D.H. Kamens, and A. Benavot
1992 *School Knowledge for the Masses: World Models and National Primary Curricular Categories in the Twentieth Century.* Studies in Curriculum History Series: 19. Washington, D.C.: The Falmer Press.
Mueller, E., and K. Short
1983 Effects of income and wealth on demand for children. Pp. 590-642 in R.A. Butalao and R.D. Lee, eds., *Determinants of Fertility in Developing Countries.* New York: Academic Press.
National Research Council
1993 *The Social Dynamics of Adolescent Fertility in Sub-Saharan Africa.* Washington, D.C.: National Academy Press.
1998 *From Death to Birth: Mortality Decline and Reproductive Change.* Washington, D.C.: National Academy Press.
Oey-Gardiner, M., and I.H. Sejahtera
1996 Indonesian girls, too, get at least some education. Paper presented at National Research Council workshop on Education and Fertility in the Developing World. Washington D.C., February 29 - March 1, 1996.
Oliver, R.
In press Fertility and women's schooling in Ghana. In P. Glewwe, ed., *The Economics of School Quality Investments in Developing Countries: An Empirical Study of Ghana.* United Kingdom: Macmillan.
Olson, D.R.
1994 *The World on Paper: The Conceptual and Cognitive Implications of Writing and Reading.* Cambridge: Cambridge University Press.
Olson, D.R., N. Torrance, and A. Hildyard
1985 *Literacy, Language, and Learning: The Nature and Consequences of Reading and Writing.* Cambridge: Cambridge University Press.
Ong, W.
1967 *The Presence of the Word.* New Haven, Conn.: Yale University Press.
1982 *Orality and Literacy: The Technologization of the Word.* London: Methuen Press.
Parsons, T.
1964 *The Social System.* New York: The Free Press.
Pitt, M.
1995 *Women's Schooling, the Selectivity of Fertility, and Child Mortality in Sub-Saharan Africa.* Washington, D.C.: The World Bank.
Rindfuss, R.R., and K.L. Brewster
1996 Childrearing and fertility. *Population and Development Review* 22(Suppl.):297-324.
Rodriguez, G., and R. Aravena
1991 Socio-economic factors and the transition to low fertility in less developed countries: A comparative analysis. Pp. 39-72 in *Demographic and Health Surveys World Conference Proceedings, Volume 1.* Columbia, Md.: Institute for Resource Development/Macro International.

Roudi, F.
1995 *An Analysis of Birth Spacing in the Near East.* Prepared for the Asia/Near East Bureau of USAID by the OPTIONS Project. Washington, D.C.: Population Reference Bureau.

Santow, G.
1995 *Coitus interruptus* and the control of natural fertility. *Population Studies* 49(1):19-43.

Schultz, T.P.
1993a Investments in the schooling and health of women and men: Quantities and returns. *Journal of Human Resources* 28(4):694-725.
1993b Returns to women's education. Pp. 51-99 in E.M. King and M.A. Hill, eds., *Women's Education in Developing Countries: Barriers, Benefits, and Policies.* Baltimore, Md.: The Johns Hopkins University Press.

Scribner, S., and M. Cole
1981 *The Psychology of Literacy.* Cambridge, Mass.: Harvard University Press.

Shah, N., and R. Bulatao
1981 Purdah and family planning in Pakistan. *International Family Planning Perspectives* 7:32-36.

Smith, J.P., ed.
1980 *Female Labor Supply: Theory and Estimation.* Princeton, N.J.: Princeton University Press.

Stambach, A.
1996 'Seeded' in the market economy: Schooling and social transformations on Mount Kilimanjaro. *Anthropology and Education Quarterly* 28(4):545-567.

Street, B.
1984 *Literacy and Theory in Practice.* Cambridge: Cambridge University Press.
1993 *Cross-Cultural Perspectives on Literacy.* Cambridge: Cambridge University Press.

United Nations
1994 *International Conference on Population and Development (ICPD) (New York).* Report of the International Conference on Population and Development (Cairo, 5-13 September 1994). No. A/Conf.171/13, October 18, 1994. New York: United Nations.
1995 *Women's Education and Fertility Behaviour: Recent Evidence from the Demographic and Health Surveys.* New York: United Nations.

Wagner, D.A., ed.
1983 *Child Development and International Development: Research-Policy Interfaces.* San Francisco, Calif.: Jossey-Bass.

Willis, P.
1977 *Learning to Labour: How Working-Class Kids Get Working-Class Jobs.* London: Routledge & Kegan Paul.

Willis, R.J.
1973 A new approach to the economic theory of fertility behavior. *Journal of Political Economy* 81(2, pt. 2):S14-S64.

2

Female Education and Fertility: Examining the Links

Ian Diamond, Margaret Newby, and Sarah Varle

INTRODUCTION

In the past 20 years a large amount of both theoretical and empirical research has investigated the relationship between women's education and fertility. The results of this work suggest that, unlike the relationship between a woman's years of schooling and infant mortality, which tends to be linear (Cleland and van Ginneken, 1988), the relationship between education and fertility is much more complex. The underlying pattern most commonly shows a negative relationship, although positive relationships at very low and very high levels of schooling have been demonstrated.

In a comprehensive review of empirical research on the relationship between women's schooling and fertility, Jejeebhoy (1995) usefully categorizes education-fertility relationship into four types, based on the results of 59 studies (see Figure 2-1). The first pattern (a) is one in which fertility falls monotonically with increased years of schooling. This pattern occurs in 26 of the 59 studies. There is a similar pattern in (c), but rather than a constant decrease in fertility, the relationship is "seven-shaped," and the first few years of schooling have either no effect on or produce a slight rise in fertility (13/59). Pattern (b) shows an inverted U or J-shaped curve, indicating that a few years of schooling increases fertility initially, but eventually fertility declines (13/59). The final relationship (d) is one in which there is no relationship or fertility rises monotonically with education (7/59), although it should be noted that there are no examples of this latter relationship in recent studies.

Comparisons based on a large number of international studies are risky given

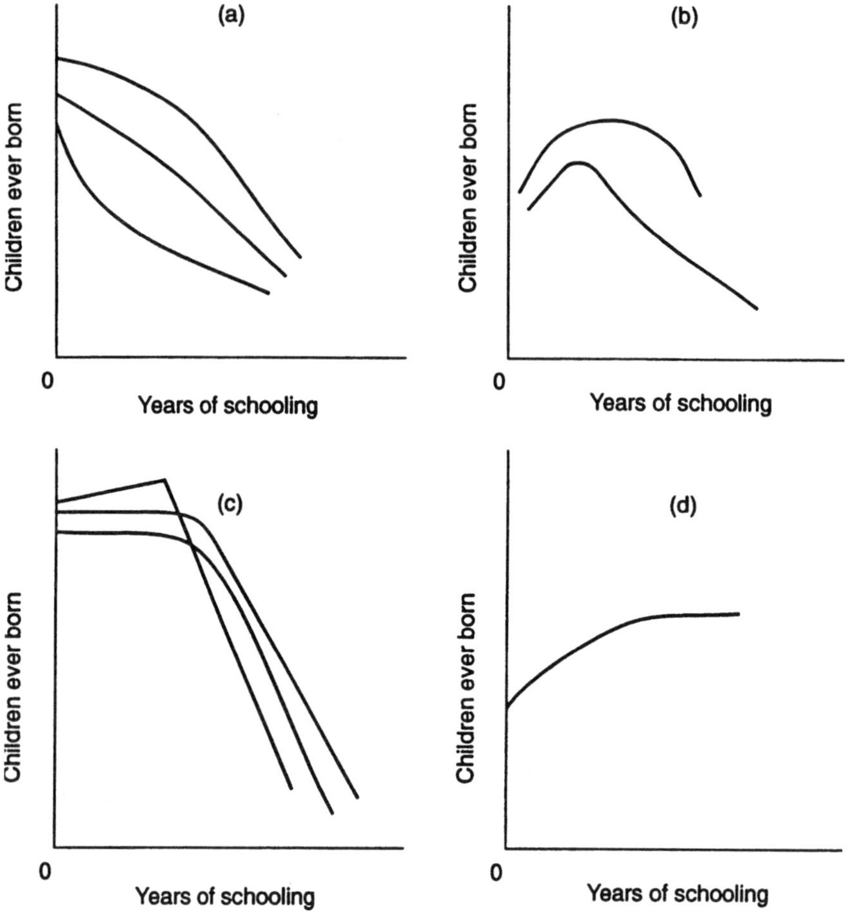

FIGURE 2-1 Illustrative patterns in the relationship between women's education and the number of children ever born: (a) Inverse relationships; (b) Curvilinear: Reversed-U and reversed-J relationships; (c) 7-shaped relationships; (d) Positive relationships. SOURCE: Reprinted from Jejeebhoy (1995:20) with permission of Oxford University Press.

compositional differences in the demographic and socioeconomic structure of the populations, as well as in the period to which the studies refer. Nevertheless, Jejeebhoy's review demonstrates clearly that for women with just a few years of education, there is little evidence of a systematic relationship between education and fertility, although a number of recent studies indicate a moderate negative effect. At the secondary level or above, however, the relationship is always negative. The countries in which there is either no or a positive relationship are almost exclusively in sub-Saharan Africa (6/7), as are the majority of inverted U or J-shaped relationships (8/13) and seven-shaped relationships (6/11). Therefore, with the exception of sub-Saharan Africa, the education-fertility relationship has a strong tendency to be negative. It should also be noted that a number of the sub-Saharan African studies included in Jejeebhoy's review are now relatively dated, and the incidence of a positive effect is now much rarer than was observed using World Fertility Survey data. For example, Muhuri et al. (1994) find a positive association between fertility and a small amount of education in only 4 of 14 sub-Saharan African countries in which Demographic and Health Surveys were conducted during 1985-1992.

An important question is the extent to which there is a simple macro-level relationship between Jejeebhoy's categorization of the education-fertility relationship and the country's level of economic and educational development (see Singh and Casterline, 1985; Entwisle and Mason, 1985). Jejeebhoy's data show that negative relationships characterize countries that have both higher per capita income and a higher level of female literacy. This finding supports the view that both economic development and mass education influence childbearing behavior. However, it would be extremely naive not to recognize the large amount of heterogeneity at the individual level.

Therefore, it is important to consider individual-level data when attempting to identify the ways in which women's education influences fertility. Throughout the 1980s and 1990s, a large number of studies, often based on data from the World Fertility Surveys and Demographic and Health Surveys, have addressed the issue. Many of these studies have tried to explain the impact of education on fertility through the proximate determinants of fertility, most notably by quantifying education's relationship with age at marriage and use of contraception. These studies typically show, not surprisingly, that educated women tend to marry later and are more likely to use modern methods of contraception.

Indeed, educated women generally also have a lower desired family size. Cleland and Kaufmann (1993) point out, however, that after controlling for age and existing family size, educational differentials in desired family size are relatively modest and much smaller than the actual fertility differentials. This finding leads them to conclude that the key question to be addressed is why more-educated women are more likely to act on their reproductive preferences, rather than why they want smaller numbers of children (see also Sathar, 1996). Cleland and Kaufmann (1993) go on to argue that attempts to explain the education-fertility relationship should focus more on identifying the determinants of reproductive decision making. The studies that look at proximate determinants are all extremely useful, then, but ultimately one needs to know what it is about education that leads to these behavioral changes. Answering the question of the pathways through which education influences fertility is the primary aim of this paper.

Many of the pathways identified relate to how educated women are, for example, better able to appreciate and interpret media messages, deal with bureaucracy, enter the labor market, and have better dialogues with their spouses than their less-educated counterparts. More-educated women also (tend to) belong to groups with different social norms than those of the less educated. Each of these factors has implications for effective reproductive decision making, and each is associated what can be described as ‘women’s autonomy’ (although see Jeffery and Basu [1996] for a critique of the education-autonomy viewpoint).

In her review, Jejeebhoy (1995) develops a framework in which education influences fertility first through five types of autonomy—knowledge, decision making, physical (in interacting with the outside world), emotional, and economic and social—and then through the proximate determinants. All five types of autonomy are influenced by education, and all have an important effect on fertility behavior, particularly through ensuring that women have an increased ability to make decisions, to move freely, and to have control over their actions. It should be noted that there are a number of complexities within this framework. For example, it is often assumed that there is a close positive relationship between autonomy and status. However, while the ability to move freely is often cited as a key indicator of autonomy (see, for example, Steele et al., 1996), freedom of movement may not always be associated with increased status. Caldwell (1986) argues that women who move around of their own volition may have lower status in their society, and Amin (1996) describes how in Bangladesh, family planning workers often wear an elaborate burqa or veil to compensate for any loss in status due to moving around.

The framework proposed by Jejeebhoy (1995) is essentially of the path analytic type. A comprehensive illustration of such a framework is provided by Jeffery and Basu (1996) and is adapted in Figure 2-2. This framework could be used as the base for a multivariate analysis aimed at identifying the factors that influence fertility directly as opposed to doing so only indirectly. For example, Mason (1984) suggests that women’s education may affect fertility only through other factors. However, those who have undertaken individual-level analyses of large data sets have typically found that there remains an effect of years of schooling even after controlling for many other socioeconomic and behavioral factors (Rodriguez and Cleland, 1980; United Nations, 1987; Cleland and Rodriguez, 1988; Rodriguez and Aravena, 1991; Castro Martín and Juárez, 1995; United Nations, 1995), although as Jejeebhoy (1995) points out, few of these analyses have addressed the pathways through women’s autonomy.

Another important concern is the impact of national and regional norms and culture. To take an example, a particularly strong state could alter childbearing norms across all social strata with little individual choice; one could argue that China provides such an example. Yet it is rare that a state can have such a strong and widespread impact on the norms and values of its people, nor is it likely that individuals will be completely unaffected by their normative and cultural context. Moreover, the impact of such contextual factors may vary with the individual’s level of educational attainment. For example, an educated woman may be more

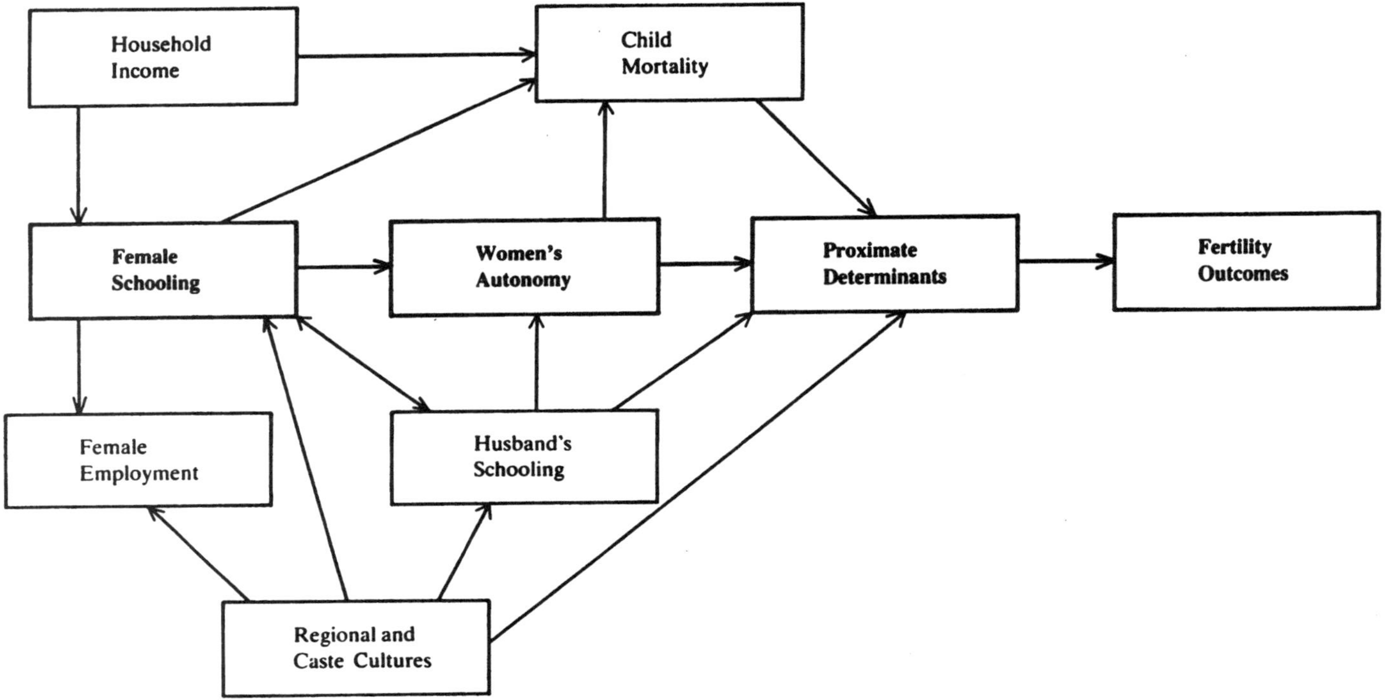

FIGURE 2-2 Possible relationships between girls' schooling and later fertility reduction. SOURCE: Reprinted from Jeffery and Basu (1996:29) with permission. Copyright Roger Jeffery and Alaka Basu, New Delhi, 1996.

inclined to act counter to local norms or more likely to marry at a social level at which lower childbearing norms prevail (see Basu, this volume).

In summary, there is no global relationship between education and fertility; rather, the linkages are both variable and complex. Yet given this essential caveat, it can be said that the relationship between the two is largely negative, and some common associations between different levels of education and reduced fertility can be identified. Before the discussion of these associations proceeds, however, four additional caveats must be noted. First, the education to which we refer is formal academic schooling received by children and young people. The suggested associations with fertility should not be generalized to special adult education programs or training within the workplace, although they clearly have implications for these other forms of education. Second, the discussion focuses on female education. Although we recognize that the influence of men is extremely important in reproductive decision making, this is a large topic that merits separate treatment and is not addressed in this chapter. Third, while years of schooling is used as the measure of education, it is essential to recognize that there is great variability in the quality and content of education that is acquired during a year of schooling in different parts of the world; hence the categorization should be seen in broad terms. Finally, this chapter focuses primarily on the linkages between education and fertility at the individual level, while bearing in mind that the education system also helps shape societal norms that may affect the fertility of women who do not themselves receive formal education.

The next section summarizes the ways which the education-fertility relationship varies with level of education (years of schooling). The chapter then examines specific factors that appear to influence the association between education and fertility. The final section presents a summary and conclusions.

THE EDUCATION-FERTILITY RELATIONSHIP AND YEARS OF SCHOOLING

In almost all countries, primary education is associated with lower numbers of children ever born than are found among those with no education, although, as noted earlier, a positive relationship has been observed in some countries, particularly for only 2 to 3 years of primary education (see Singh and Casterline, 1985). The relationship between primary education and desired family size, on the other hand, is almost universally negative, whether or not the primary education is completed (Jejeebhoy, 1995). Both incomplete and complete primary education also tend to be associated with later age at marriage and increased contraceptive use (see Westoff et al., 1994).

In contrast with primary education, almost every study reported by Jejeebhoy (1995) shows a marked decline in children ever born for women with secondary education. In many of the studies, the negative effect is substantial. The difference in total fertility rates (TFRs) between women with secondary education and those with no education is more than 50 percent in Latin America. In Asia the differential is smaller because the TFR among women with no education is relatively low (3.36 with no education versus 2.52 with secondary education in Indonesia; 4.90 and 3.64, respectively, in Pakistan). In many sub-Saharan African countries the differential is smaller still. Women in that region with secondary plus education have higher fertility than do women with no education in Asia.

It should be noted here that the association between secondary education and fertility may be attributable to the fact that in many developing countries, those girls who attend secondary school form a highly select group that might be expected to have lower fertility for other reasons, such as higher socioeconomic status. In the majority of developing countries, a woman who reaches and completes secondary education is rather a special case. Very few countries have achieved mass secondary education for women, and thus the influence on fertility will be largely at the level of the individual. For a girl to attend secondary school, her family must believe strongly in the value of education, which implies an investment in their daughter's future, and expectations and aspirations for her in terms of further education, employment, and marriage will be high. All this may act to delay marriage and reduce fertility. In addition, the woman may already be exposed to low family-size norms since, in general, the high cost of secondary schooling means that one would expect it to be biased toward small families in which there are fewer siblings competing for resources.

The relationship between higher education (beyond the secondary level) and fertility is undoubtedly negative. Jejeebhoy's (1995) data show that higher education is associated with large reductions in completed family size (percentage reductions over no schooling range from almost 20 to over 70 percent) and with substantially lower desired family size and higher age at marriage. In none of the studies is 10 or more years of education associated with higher fertility relative to women with no education.

At the same time, it is difficult to draw clear conclusions about the influence of higher education on fertility since the proportion of the female population involved is very small, and those women who have benefited from tertiary education in most developing countries are predominantly in the younger age groups. Thus it remains to be seen what influence higher education has on fertility over the full span of the childbearing career. As the work by Kiernan and Diamond (1983) in Great Britain suggests, it may be that in relatively low-fertility societies (as many societies will already be when they have widespread higher education), higher education influences the timing of childbearing as much as it affects completed family size. Further understanding will be possible only when the more highly educated cohorts complete their childbearing careers. It is possible to speculate that their completed fertility may be relatively high since they will have the economic resources to care for and educate a large number of children. It is equally possible to speculate that their completed fertility will be low because of the costs of rearing children, along with a shift toward social norms related to low fertility.

However, since educating these few women to the tertiary level will have small macro-demographic effects on fertility, the importance of higher education lies more in how these women will use their education in a position of influence than in the effects of that education on their personal fertility. This influence may be informal, with these women serving as role models for other family members, friends, and neighbors, or it may be institutionalized through their role as family planning workers, government ministers, and civil servants—careers to which their education gives them access. The informal role is more likely among upwardly mobile women from relatively disadvantaged backgrounds and the latter among the socioeconomic elite.

An important pathway through which higher education can influence declines in fertility is by delaying marriage. Choe (1996) has shown that highly educated women in Korea are much less likely to be married at any age. The reasons for this are that attendance at university usually delays marriage until the degree is completed, and higher education increases career aspirations and entry into employment. In addition, highly educated women may not be well positioned in the marriage market because some men may not wish to marry women who are more educated than themselves.

It is also important to note that those women from relatively lower socioeconomic groups who do receive tertiary education are likely to be extremely motivated and independently minded and to have high career aspirations, qualities that are inconsistent with the traditional norms and ways of life found in many developing countries. In addition, higher education usually can be obtained only in cities, so that those with higher education will be urban born or rural-urban migrants; in almost all countries, both these groups have lower fertility than rural dwellers. Thus women with higher education come from a very select socioeconomic group or tend to have exceptional personal characteristics and experience of urban living. As a result, it is difficult to be sure whether the lower fertility of highly educated women can be attributed to their education per se or to their other characteristics.

Finally, it must be noted that education does not work in isolation to affect fertility. There will probably be a certain degree of direct influence, but in many ways, education will also serve as a proxy for other factors. Increased education rarely occurs without concomitant changes to a society, such as increased health services, enhanced communication, and better infrastructure. The effects of these factors cannot easily be disentangled. The direct effects of education at the individual level, such as the increased employment prospects it affords, the transfer of knowledge about the costs of children, or an increase in social skills enabling better use of health services, are meaningless if other societal changes are not occurring in parallel. Thus, for example, health services cannot be used if they are not available, and one cannot aspire to different jobs or lifestyles if there is not some way, however remote, of being able to achieve them. Moreover, as discussed further below, "the notion that there is a linear relationship between length of schooling and degree of modernity or westernization is a gross oversimplification" (Cleland and Kaufmann, 1993:24).

FACTORS INFLUENCING THE EDUCATION-FERTILITY RELATIONSHIP

The available evidence suggests that the following factors help shape the relationship between education and fertility: key contextual factors, the skills and knowledge imparted by schooling, social and ideational influence, and enhanced employment opportunities for the educated.

Contextual Factors

Two contextual factors influence the relationship between education—particularly incomplete primary education—and fertility: the existence of mass education[1] and the presence of an active family planning program. It is likely, of course, that countries with a strong program of mass education will also have a strong family planning program, and thus it may be difficult to separate out the influence of each (Mauldin and Ross, 1991).

Presence of Mass Education

Countries in which a small amount of education (less than completed primary) is associated with a decline in fertility at the individual level tend to be those countries with mass education. This may be the case in part because in the latter countries, the influence of education extends beyond the individuals who attend school to the society at large. In general, a shift toward smaller families tends to occur in parallel with the introduction of mass education. Caldwell (1982) argues that this shift takes place as a result of not only the direct influence of education on individuals, but also the interaction among knowledge, ideas, and increased opportunities afforded by mass education through the restructuring of family and community relationships. Thus women with just a few years of schooling will tend to adopt norms of lower fertility and higher age at marriage that are characteristic of societies with mass education even if the influence of education on them as individuals is very small.

---

[1]As Caldwell (1982) argues, it is not possible to establish a dividing line between societies with mass education and those without. However, indicators of mass education are almost universal attendance by children of both sexes, compulsory education, and free education.

With a globally increasing emphasis on education, countries in which large proportions of the population have completed primary education are becoming more common. This is the case in many parts of Latin America, the Caribbean, and the Far East. By the 1980s, for example, gross primary enrollment rates for females exceeded 90 percent in all the countries of East Asia listed by King and Hill (1993). Among those who were of school age in the 1960s and 1970s, however, when completed primary education was rare in developing countries, individuals with completed primary education are likely to have been educational "pioneers" within their communities. In India in 1992-1993, for example, only 11.7 percent of women interviewed in the National Family Health Survey had completed primary schooling, and this percentage was even lower in some rural areas. At about the same time in Kenya, only 15.3 percent of women interviewed for the Demographic and Health Survey (National Council for Population and Development, 1993) had completed primary education. In such contexts, the influence of education on fertility is likely to be limited to those individuals who have completed primary schooling. As noted above, such contexts can be expected to become increasingly rare.

As the level of education increases within a community, norms concerning childbearing within that community will change. Thus, in situations where there is mass education, women who complete primary school may have lower than expected fertility because their reproductive decisions are influenced by lower community childbearing norms. Lower fertility will then result from changing societal norms, which will have occurred only partly as a result of mass education. Other changes that often occur in parallel with the development of education are that a nation moves toward a monetarized economy and becomes more industrial, less agricultural, and more urbanized. Thus the advent of mass education is just one aspect of a changing society that will influence the individual effects of education.

Presence of an Active Family Planning Program

Entwisle and Mason (1985) found that in poor countries, the relationship between education and fertility is negative when there is a family planning program, but positive when there is not. In most cases, countries in which women with incomplete primary education have a substantially lower total marital fertility rate than women with no education are those classified by Mauldin and Ross (1991) as having a strong or moderate family planning program effort in 1989 (see Table 2-1).[2] In Botswana, for example (Lesetedi et al., 1989), which was

---

[2]The relationship is not entirely consistent. Brazil, for example, had a family planning effort that was classified as weak, yet there was a 33.2 percent differential between women with incomplete primary education and those with no education. This finding reflects patterns of contraceptive use in Brazil, where the private sector has predominated in the absence of a strong government program.

TABLE 2-1 Mean difference between total marital fertility rate of women with no education and those with incomplete primary education by family planning program effort as a percentage of the total marital fertility rate with no education

Program effort[a]	% Difference in TMFR[b]
Strong	−8.79 (7)[c]
Moderate	−8.64 (12)
Weak	−1.97 (10)
Very weak or none	5.81 (2)

NOTES:
[a]Program effort data from Mauldin and Ross (1991).
[b]Total marital fertility rate (TMFR) of women married 0-19 years in the 0-4 years prior to the survey. Data are for 31 countries in which Demographic and Health Surveys were conducted during 1985-1992 (Muhuri et al., 1994).
[c]Numbers in parentheses are the number of countries in that category.

classified as having a strong family planning program effort, among women married for 0-19 years, those with incomplete primary education had a total marital fertility rate 8.8 percent below that of women with no education. In countries such as Nigeria, Burundi, and Liberia, where the marital fertility of women with incomplete primary education was found to be substantially higher than that of women with no education, family planning effort was classified as weak, very weak, or none. A strong family planning program will provide both the means to reduce fertility and the messages to encourage this reduction.

It is important to note, however, that family planning program effort may be related to a country's level of economic development. Thirty years ago, Carleton (1967, cited in Cochrane, 1979) argued that since none of the ways in which education affects fertility is completely independent of economic development, care must be taken in assigning causality to the family planning program. In addition, as family planning can influence all educational groups (Cleland and Kaufmann, 1993), it is possible that the influence of education on fertility may be weaker in the presence of a strong family planning program. An example here would be China, where a strong state family planning program influenced fertility across all socioeconomic and educational groups. At the same time, for reasons explained below, it is likely that the impact of a family planning program will be stronger in societies in which at least a small amount of education is usual, and that one effect of small amounts of education is to facilitate the effective use of family planning programs.

Skills and Knowledge Imparted

The quality of education provided at all levels (primary, secondary, and beyond) varies greatly among countries; moreover, the level of competence achieved varies greatly among countries, schools within countries, and pupils in the same school. Nevertheless, certain basic skills can be expected to be imparted by primary schooling. The most obvious skills transferred in the first few years of schooling are basic literacy and numeracy. The skills imparted are unlikely to meet high standards, and many of those who have received only 2 to 3 years of education may be functionally illiterate. Yet children who have had some education are better equipped than their noneducated counterparts to recognize written text and the fact that it is likely to contain some sort of message, and those who have completed primary education will probably have achieved a substantial level of literacy. These children are thereby brought into contact with health education, family planning, and other media information.

LeVine et al. (1994) examined the effects of literacy on the ability to read and listen to health announcements. A study in Nepal among a sample of women with a mean level of schooling of 1.4 years found comprehension of a health interview to be positively correlated with maternal schooling. This increased comprehension also appeared to have an effect on practice since there was a positive correlation between maternal schooling and a number of health outcomes, including contraceptive use. LeVine and colleagues also found that in Mexico and Zambia, where their samples had a higher mean number of years of schooling, literacy increased the ability to understand radio broadcasts through better comprehension of decontextualized language. They offer the following conclusion (p. 188):

> Literacy is not a dichotomous trait acquired in the first five years of primary schooling that permits the adult population of a country to be divided into literates and illiterates, but a package of cognitive and language skills which make it possible to participate in literate discourse and communication and which can improve during primary school.

Not only does primary education increase the ability to understand messages transmitted by various forms of mass media, but there is also evidence that the exposure to mass media increases with even a few years of education. The 1993-1994 Demographic and Health Survey in Bangladesh showed that 9.5 percent of women with no schooling watched television weekly, as opposed to 15.8 percent of those with incomplete primary education. Among women with no education, 28.7 percent listened to the radio weekly, as opposed to over 43 percent of those with incomplete primary education (Mitra et al., 1994), and the differential is still greater for those with completed primary education. At the same time, it should be noted that part of this effect may not be attributable to primary education increasing access to the media, but to a correlation between both education and radio and television ownership and socioeconomic status.

At the secondary level of schooling, literacy will be achieved to a relatively high standard. The individual is exposed to many forms of the written word, including information on health and family planning. For example, in the 1993-1994 Bangladesh Demographic and Health Survey, it was found that among ever-married women, 38.7 percent of those with secondary or higher education read a newspaper at least once a week, compared with 8.2 percent of those with primary education. The probability of watching television or listening to the radio once a week was also significantly higher among the former women (Mitra et al., 1994), although, as discussed above, this may in part be an effect of socioeconomic status rather than education per se. Moreover, secondary education can help develop cognitive skills needed to evaluate information and form personal opinions accordingly.

Primary education increases the information available to children not only through improved access to the media and written messages, but also through the knowledge imparted at school. For example, basic primary education generally includes some health education, although the amount and quality of the information presented varies greatly. Cleland and van Ginneken (1988:90) argue that while specific evidence is sparse, it is likely that primary schooling "imparts sufficient understanding of health matters to guide maternal behaviour in later life." Even though health education may constitute a small portion of the curriculum, the fact that it is provided means the overall concept of being biologically able to control fertility and health is likely to become apparent to the child.

In communities that have health systems and family planning programs, primary education establishes a foundation for further information received within the community, and thus can have an indirect impact through an increased ability to "hear the message" of family planning programs or through improved health for individuals or their children. As Caldwell (1994) argues for mortality, the school is the best place to inculcate a society with norms that are congruent with modern health systems.

Further, there is much evidence to show that improvements in infant and child health occur even with very low levels of maternal education (Preston, 1978). For example, in the 10-year period up to 1993-1994 in Bangladesh, infant mortality was 113/1000 among women with no education and 92/1000 among those with incomplete primary education. A number of commentators (e.g., Basu, 1994; Cleland and Streatfield, 1992; Preston, 1978) have pointed out that reduced infant and child mortality can lower fertility since it decreases the perceived need for replacement and insurance births to ensure that a certain number of children will survive to adulthood. Reduced mortality can also increase birth spacing since the death of a child truncates the period of breastfeeding, shortening the length of amenorrhea. This tendency for even small amounts of education to reduce infant and child mortality may thus represent an indirect influence of education on fertility. A caution in this regard is expressed by Basu (1994), who points out that the decline in mortality may itself be a consequence of lower fertility since there will be fewer high-risk, high-parity births to older women. This observation illustrates the complexities involved in trying to untangle the education-fertility relationship.

Formal health education in secondary schools increasingly includes family planning. For example, in some schools in East Africa, secondary school children are shown a video called "Consequences" that explores the difficulties faced by a teenage girl who becomes pregnant before she finishes her education. The effects on future fertility of childbearing at very young ages are highlighted. The aim is to discourage early marriage and childbearing, as well as premarital pregnancy, which is the focus of the film. Another important issue in the film is the negative effect of pregnancy and motherhood on employment prospects and careers, perhaps introducing to secondary school girls the idea that education is a valuable asset for improving life opportunities and offering access to a rewarding career.

In terms of cognitive skills, primary education will improve the ability to approach decision making and problem solving in a more abstract way. In terms of childbearing decisions, not only will the ability to weigh costs and benefits be more likely, but there will also be more information available with which to make such decisions. However, it should be noted that the ability to obtain and process information will reduce childbearing only where the marginal costs of childbearing at the existing level of fertility outweigh the benefits. Another condition for lower fertility is that women be able to act on their rational choices, perhaps through the increased autonomy education appears to provide (see Easterlin, 1975; Cochrane, 1979; Jejeebhoy, 1995).

It is also worth noting that childbearing is not, of course, always a planned rational decision; a large number of births are the result of unplanned or mistimed pregnancies (for example, to teenage girls). Cleland and Kaufmann (1993) observe that one way education contributes to reduced fertility is by reducing the percentage of such pregnancies. Schooling has traditionally been thought to increase children's ability to think rationally as it assists them in moving toward abstract and reasoned thought. Indeed, there is a literature from many areas of the world indicating that the incidence of unplanned pregnancy is higher among less-educated women. On the other hand, the assumption that schooling facilitates rationality is not universally accepted. Cross-cultural studies have shown that schooling does not increase rationality, but rather teaches new skills that change the way problems are approached and hence the way they are solved and decisions are made. Schooling may also emphasize the negative economic implications of large families or the health benefits of smaller/better-spaced families, or it may promote the advantages of large families. It thus alters which pieces of information and which values go into the decision, not the fact that a rational decision is made.

Social and Ideational Influences

Perhaps more important than the cognitive effects of a few years of schooling are its social and ideational influences. Through the latter influences, schooling acts as a "catalyst of modernisation" (Martin and Juarez, 1995).

Social Influences

The social values imparted in school are an important influence on the direction of the education-fertility relationship. Streatfield (1989), for example, describes how low-fertility norms were incorporated into the education system of Bali. He uses this example to argue that within a culture in which one is taught to obey and trust one's teachers and other authority figures, such as political and religious leaders and parents, even a small amount of schooling is likely to have an important influence on childbearing. Attitudes toward childbearing are likely to change in a downward direction because the perspectives promoted by schooling are generally those of the middle classes and the West, as found by Caldwell (1982) in a study of school textbooks in Kenya, Ghana, and Nigeria. The norm suggested is generally that of the nuclear family with few children.

Conversely, education is likely to influence fertility positively if the educational message is strongly traditional and pronatalist. In some societies, religious schooling provides such messages, teaching about traditional values that are inconsistent with widespread family planning. In Bangladesh, for example, particularly in rural areas, a significant number of children attend madrassas (religious schools) and schools attached to mosques, where they are unlikely to learn western or modern values (Bangladesh Task Forces, 1991). At the same time, however, religious leaders in some countries have become involved in spreading messages about family planning and the benefits of small families.

Schooling may also exert a social influence by exposing students to the outside world and the media, either while they are attending school or later, especially if schooling results in the opportunity to live away from the home and the immediate family environment, as often happens in parts of West Africa. As Cleland and van Ginneken (1988:91) suggest, "education provides a wider social network, new reference groups and authority models and a greater identification with the modern world." Thus Cleland and Kaufmann (1993) posit a process of transferred social values that differ from those of the traditional home environment. Although this transfer may begin to occur with a few years of education, it can probably be expected to increase with continued exposure.

Students in secondary school are particularly prone to identify with social groups whose norms differ from those held in the home community (see de Vries,

1992). Those norms are likely to include low fertility. Indeed, it is important to recognize that individuals play an active role in choosing a social group (see Coggans and McKellar, 1994), and secondary education may motivate women to seek peer groups in which low fertility is a norm.

Ideational Influences

Attendance at school often brings children into an environment where they are exposed to new authority figures and role models and to ideas other than those held in their home. Schooling also exposes children to different ideas, whether through the study of particular subjects, such as history, geography, or religion, or simply through the reading of storybooks. As a consequence of the increased information and exposure to new ideas and authority figures that full primary schooling brings, ideational change occurs.

An example of ideational change attributed to education has to do with the relationship between mother and child. LeVine et al. (1991) argue that the better educated the mother is, the more she will interact with her children. Verbal interaction, in particular, increases, and the child's upbringing becomes more child-centered, both factors serving to encourage greater individuality on the part of the child (though see Carter, this volume, for a critique of this point). The increased reciprocal verbal and nonverbal interaction makes childrearing more labor-intensive, with the result that the mother is likely to want fewer children.

On the other hand, not all the ideas to which children are exposed in school are conducive to lower fertility. The "modern" ideas encountered by children in school might include, for example, shorter breastfeeding durations and erosion of traditional practices such as postpartum abstinence that are particularly prevalent in sub-Saharan Africa. Shorter breastfeeding durations lead to shorter periods of postpartum amenorrhea and thus to an increase in natural fertility, and without a compensating increase in contraceptive prevalence, total marital fertility is also likely to rise. The evidence on this issue, however, is mixed. On the one hand, in Botswana (Lesetedi et al., 1989), the mean duration of breastfeeding and postpartum abstinence was found to be higher among women with incomplete primary education than among those with no education, although this finding could reflect misreporting among the group with no education. On the other hand, in the 1993-1994 Bangladesh Demographic and Health Survey (Mitra et al., 1994), the duration of full and exclusive breastfeeding was shorter among women with incomplete primary education than among those with no education, but the median duration of any breastfeeding was over 36 months for both groups. Thus at low levels of schooling, it cannot be assumed that all aspects of education will have a negative influence on fertility.

With regard to secondary education, an important influence of education on fertility comes from its close relationship to the processes of urbanization and integration into the international economy. These processes tend to be associated with reduced son preference, a rise in the opportunity costs of children, higher expectations for living standards and increased life choices as the result of better prospects and opportunities for work, and increasing acceptability of female employment.

As women achieve secondary education, the gender gap in education will narrow, and there will be an increased probability of a woman's husband being highly educated. Better-educated husbands are in turn more likely to hold ideals that are consistent with smaller families, improved health, and family planning (see also Basu, this volume). Secondary education may also delay marriage, both because it becomes more difficult for women to find a suitable husband and because women may wish to pursue cash employment. Cochrane (1979) argues that high levels of education reduce the pool of acceptable spouses, given the traditional pattern that men marry women less educated than themselves. She found that increased education reduced the probability of women entering a formal union, while it increased the probability of men doing so. Recently, similar results were found for Korea by Lee (1994) and Choe (1996). Smock and Yousseff (1977, cited in Stichter and Parpart, 1990) found that in Egypt, high levels of education or employment could jeopardize chances of a good marriage match because such women were seen as loose or immoral—another way education can make finding a spouse more difficult.

Autonomy

As noted earlier, one way in which education is posited to influence fertility negatively is by increasing women's sense of autonomy. Jejeebhoy (1995:184) believes that "the impact of women's education on their fertility is greatest when education offers women an expanded role in family decisions and control over, or access to, resources." In exposing women to new ideas and allowing them to gain cash employment, thus taking them out of the home, education may affect the autonomy of women in a number of ways. For example, it can enhance a woman's position in the community; give her increased confidence and skill, thereby enhancing her negotiating power in the household; or give her a degree of economic independence that reduces her dependence on her spouse and his family. Moreover, if education and subsequent employment have also secured the women a more-educated husband, he is likely to be more liberal in his attitudes toward women and childbearing (see Basu, this volume). Where women are more educated and autonomous, they are likely to have a greater say in their choice of husband, which has been shown to contribute to improved communication between spouses, and this in turn aids in women's control over fertility (Kabir et al., 1988).

Although this effect of increased autonomy clearly does occur in many societies, one must note that it is not universal. Cleland (1995) reports that in Bangladesh, women with schooling do not appear to have any more autonomy than their uneducated counterparts. Fertility decline in Bangladesh, he argues, has not been coupled with a change in female employment, a decline in child labor, or the evolution of alternative forms of risk insurance. Other forces, such as the decline in child mortality, are playing a more important role in the fertility transition of some South Asian nations (although education levels are, of course, a principal predictor of child mortality rates).

Moreover, greater autonomy does not guarantee that desired family size will be smaller. Where desired fertility is lower, however, women with greater autonomy are more likely to be able to implement their family-size desires and will be less influenced by other family members. The probability of ideal family size decreasing will depend to some extent on the strength of a country's family planning program. The stronger the program, the more likely educated women will be to adopt contraceptive methods—and the more quickly—in order to realize their desires for a small family size. Education leads to greater self-confidence and interpersonal skills (Caldwell, 1986; Cleland and van Ginneken, 1988), empowering women to seek medical and family planning advice and act upon it in a way that is beneficial for them. For this to occur, however, these services must be available.

Enhanced Employment Opportunities

Both the new cognitive skills and the ideational change brought about by primary education will help increase women's chances of employment outside the home. The nature and extent of this effect will depend on the overall level of education in the society. If there is very little education, a small amount of schooling will give women a relative advantage over their peers, thus increasing their employment opportunities substantially. If, on the other hand, education is not uncommon, it will not have as great an effect in this regard. Salaff (1981) showed that in Hong Kong in the mid-1970s, young women with about 3 years of formal schooling entered employment in factories producing plastic bags, wigs, and garments. In contrast, in Sri Lanka, with high levels of education relative to the rest of South Asia, Rosa (1989) found there was an unofficial requirement of 8-10 years of education in order to enter work in garment factories. In Tanzania, primary education is adequate for entry into teacher training college, whereas in other societies, such as Taiwan or Singapore, the best job available is likely to be factory employment. Thus if one of the important ways education influences fertility is through employment, the strength of that effect will depend on the nature of the labor market and whether the individual views employment as a lifetime career or a temporary phase in the life cycle before marriage.

It is important to note that the relationship between primary education and access to cash employment is not universal. For example, in South Asia the traditional norm is for women to practice seclusion and be excluded from cash employment unless absolute economic necessity dictates otherwise (Cleland and

Kaufmann, 1993; Shaheed, in Afshar and Agarwal, 1989). For the majority of women, primary education will have little impact on their job opportunities and may well serve to reduce their market employment, since families that can afford to educate their daughters to completed primary level may not feel the economic necessity of sending them to work. Indeed, primary education may increase the possibility that a woman will gain a more traditional husband, one able to provide sufficient economic resources so that the woman will not need to work. This observation may help explain why some studies, such as that of Cleland and Rodriguez (1988), conclude that education does not work through employment to affect fertility. However, with increasing industrialization and gradual weakening or adjustment of the norms of female behavior, the degree to which South Asia appears to be an exception may be reduced.

Secondary education provides the qualifications for a fairly good job, perhaps even a career for women. Eight years of education is sufficient for a career as a teacher in many developing countries (Bellew and King, cited in King and Hill, 1993). A study of 1,923 households in metropolitan Dhaka, Bangladesh, in 1992 (Mahmud, 1995) revealed that among secondary-educated women who were working, 22 percent had managerial or professional jobs, 52 percent were in skilled labor, and only 2 percent were engaged in manual labor. Among women with 5 years or less of education, 53 percent performed manual labor, and fewer than 1 percent were in managerial or professional occupations. Thus it can be seen that secondary education can give women access to an entirely different range of employment and to jobs that are far more likely to be economically and psychologically rewarding. The fact that families invest in secondary education for girls suggests that higher-level employment is a goal to which they want girls to aspire. As de Vries (1992) argues, higher levels of education mean that employment may come to replace the home-based reproductive role as the predominant activity in women's lives.

Moreover, if teachers are women, they will serve as role models for the type of career and lifestyle pupils may hope to emulate. It has been suggested that as important or perhaps more important than the overt curriculum in schools is the hidden curriculum by which pupils interpret in differing ways the unconscious messages of their teachers. These messages may concern notions of what behavior and roles are appropriate for women and how work can interact with childbearing careers and family roles.

The effect of employment on fertility depends largely on the nature of the employment and whether it is viewed as a lifetime career or a temporary phase in the life cycle before marriage. The main ways in which employment influences fertility are by delaying marriage, increasing the opportunity costs of the woman's time within marriage, and increasing the costs of childbearing as aspirations increase. The higher costs of childrearing may also be due to the urban residence of parents if they are dependent on an income they will lose if their daughter marries and leaves the labor force. The worker herself may be reluctant to give up a lifestyle that affords her relative economic and social freedom as compared with married life (Salaff, 1981). However, evidence from factory workers in Sri Lanka shows that employment in low-paid work can accelerate marriage if women are eager to leave a life of tedious factory work at low pay (Rosa, 1989).

Access to cash employment changes consumption patterns or aspirations through increased choice. Easterlin (1978, 1980) argues that as education levels in a society rise so, too, do the opportunity costs of large families. Children essentially become an "old good" as education, cash employment, and the mass media offer new consumption patterns and lifestyles. As aspirations for higher living standards come to predominate, large families become increasingly less attractive. Not only are there alternative demands on family resources, such as improved housing and leisure activities, but also the cost of each child will rise as preferences shift from "quantity" of children to "quality." For example, the more educated a couple are, the more likely they may be to want their children to be educated, generally to a higher level than they themselves were (see, e.g., Shah, 1986). Education, particularly secondary education, is expensive, and parents with such ambitions for their children may thus have fewer children.

However, employment opportunities may not exert a negative influence on marital fertility in some settings. Where the only opportunities are in low-paid, low-status jobs for young women, the only effect may be to delay marriage, after which fertility may be no different from that of women who had never worked.

Moreover, as with primary education, secondary education does not necessarily work to affect fertility through employment since a significant proportion of educated women may not work. In Bangladesh, where norms opposed to women's cash employment mean that women often work only out of economic necessity, Mahmud (1995) found that 47 percent of secondary-educated women were nonmarket workers (i.e., confined to a reproductive and productive role in their home), and their labor force participation was only 21 percent. Thus the importance of education for employment clearly is not the same in all countries, and care should be taken before assuming that secondary-educated women will enter a career. In economic terms, some women will have invested in cultural rather than economic capital through their secondary education.

SUMMARY AND CONCLUSIONS

In general, the influence of education on fertility varies greatly between countries with different levels of schooling. Yet it is fair to say that the relationship between education at all levels and fertility has in recent years been, on the whole, negative. Societies in which there is a positive relationship, particularly with small amounts of education, are now relatively rare and confined largely to specific social contexts.

The context in which education is received and in which the woman subsequently lives is fundamental in mediating the effects of education on fertility.

Three aspects of the national context have been hypothesized to be important: the presence or absence of mass education, the strength of the family planning program, and employment opportunities for women. In addition to these, the extent to which education is valued within a society and the extent to which the social structure prevents women from achieving the full economic and social benefits of their schooling should not be overlooked. It is also essential to recognize that all effects of education are influenced by such factors as insufficient opportunities for employment and the quality of the schooling (see Glewwe, this volume).

The importance of the national context applies particularly to the influence on fertility of just a few years of education. The influence is most likely to be negative when there is mass education, which typically means that broad social norms are shifting toward smaller family size. Similarly, if the country has a strong family planning program, it will be relatively easy for women to hear messages about contraception and obtain the means to control their fertility. A few years of education can also influence fertility downward where it gives access to a job that may offer an alternative to early marriage and childbearing. The influence of a few years of education on fertility may be attributable to two primary factors. First, the basic literacy skills that are conferred bring the concept of the written word into the realm of consciousness and enable the individual at the very least, to hear the message about family planning or health practices. Second, basic primary education exposes the individual to new authority figures and ideas. In situations in which there is mass education and societal norms toward low fertility, these new ideas are likely to be consistent with smaller families.

Differences in the influence on fertility of 1 or 2 years of education versus completed primary education depend heavily on context. Where there is mass education, a strong family planning program, and prospects for cash employment as a result of very basic education—for example, in Brazil—2 to 3 years of education can be associated with lower fertility as much as, or more than, completed primary education in countries where these contextual factors do not exist, such as Pakistan. Between these two extremes are countries with varying levels of these contextual factors. For example, in the Middle East, mass education is relatively prevalent, but women's opportunities for cash employment are very poor; in Bangladesh, there is a strong family planning program, but a relative absence of mass female education. Generally, however, completed primary education appears to have a stronger negative relationship with fertility than does incomplete primary education. Furthermore, the relationship between completed primary education and fertility is less dependent on mass education than is that between partial primary education and fertility because completed primary education can act to reduce fertility by making women educational pioneers within their communities. Other effects of primary education on fertility include increased likelihood of employment that may delay marriage and increase the opportunity costs of childbearing. Another effect of women's education, directly and through employment and urban living, is to increase aspirations for their own children, which in turn increases the costs of childbearing. The result is an incentive for lower fertility and a shift in childbearing aspirations from quantity to quality of children.

The effects of secondary and higher education are probably more universally generalizable since it appears that context is less important at these levels. As a result of skills and knowledge gained from secondary and higher education and the greater prospects that result, women may be better able to make independent decisions and to implement fertility control even in the absence of a family planning program. In addition, women with secondary and tertiary education usually belong to social groups with less traditional norms that generally favor lower fertility. Such women may also belong to a different social group with regard to marriage prospects. In countries with low levels of secondary and higher education, those prospects may be relatively limited because of the tradition that men marry women less educated than themselves and the perception that educated women are too westernized and independent minded. Marriage is therefore delayed, and in some cases may even be foregone.

Employment opportunities for women with secondary education—and the associated influences on fertility, such as later age at marriage—do vary among countries and appear to be closely related to cultural traditions. In South Asia, only a minority of secondary-educated women work for cash, while in Latin America and Southeast Asia, many women work. In the latter cases, secondary education is likely to provide access to more rewarding white-collar employment, such as teaching or a wide range of clerical or semiprofessional occupations that are not particularly compatible with childbearing and perhaps offer an attractive alternative to early marriage and childbearing.

In most developing countries, the number of women with higher education is very small. Therefore, the influence of higher education on national fertility is significant mainly in terms of the extent to which highly educated women act as role models for their less-educated peers and thus contribute to changing social norms with regard to childbearing.

Cleland and Rodriguez (1988:442) argue that "a recognition that fertility behaviour is strongly conditioned by culture, albeit crudely labelled by region or language is an essential first step towards future elucidation." This chapter has shown that context is extremely important in explaining the effects of education on fertility. For women with little education, the social policy and employment context (which is conditioned by culture) is of most importance; for women with higher levels of education, culture and its effects on employment opportunities continue to be important, though to a lesser extent. With low levels of education, a woman's behavior is still very much dependent on community norms, and thus what is important is whether those norms are shifting toward lower fertility. At higher levels of education, the woman's attitudes toward marriage and childbearing become more important, yet her behavior will also be affected by the norms of the social groups to which she belongs. No individual's behavior can ever be divorced from the social, economic, and cultural context in which she is situated, but as educational attainment rises, the individual moves away from community-based childbearing norms toward a more individual set of beliefs and behaviors and, perhaps, into social networks with lower fertility norms.

ACKNOWLEDGMENTS

The contributions of Sarah Varle and Margaret Newby were funded by United Kingdom Economic and Social Research Council studentships. The authors are grateful to Caroline Bledsoe, Jenna Johnson-Kuhn, and two anonymous referees for extremely helpful comments on the first draft of this chapter.

REFERENCES

Afshar, H., and B. Agarwal
1989 *Women, Poverty and Ideology in Asia: Contradictory Pressures, Uneasy Resolutions.* London: Macmillan.

Amin, S.
1996 Female education and fertility in Bangladesh: The influence of marriage and family. Pp. 184-204 in R. Jeffery and A. Basu, eds., *Girls' Schooling, Women's Autonomy and Fertility Change in South Asia.* New Delhi: Sage Publications.

Bangladesh Task Forces
1991 *Report of the Bangladesh Task Forces, Volume 3, Developing the Infrastructure.* Dhaka, Bangladesh: Dhaka University Press Ltd.

Basu, A.
1994 Maternal education, fertility and child mortality: Disentangling verbal relationships. *Health Transition Review* 4:207-215.

Caldwell, J.
1982 *Theory of Fertility Decline.* London: Academic Press.
1986 Routes to low mortality in poor countries. *Population and Development Review* 12:171-220.
1994 How is greater maternal education translated into lower child mortality? *Health Transition Review* 4:224-229.

Castro Martín, T.
1995 Women's education and fertility: Results from 26 Demographic and Health Surveys. *Studies in Family Planning* 26(4)187-202.

Castro Martín, T., and F. Juárez
1995 The impact of women's education on fertility in Latin America: Searching for explanations. *International Family Planning Perspectives* 21(2):52-57.

Choe, M.K.
1996 Changing marriage patterns in Korea with reference to Japan and the United States. Paper presented at the Nihon University International Symposium on Life and the Earth in the 21st Century. Tokyo, Japan. March 4-7.

Cleland, J.
1995 Fertility transition in South Asia. Paper presented at British Society for Population Studies Fertility Transition Meeting. London School of Hygiene and Tropical Medicine. July 1995.

Cleland, J., and G. Kaufmann

1993 Education, fertility and child survival: Unravelling the links. Paper prepared for the International Union for the Scientific Study of Population Committee on Anthropology and Demography Seminar. Barcelona, Spain. November 10-14.

Cleland, J., and G. Rodriguez

1988 The effect of parental education on marital fertility in developing countries. *Population Studies* 42:419-442.

Cleland, J., and K. Streatfield

1992 *The Demographic Transition: Bangladesh.* Staff Reference Series: 1/92. UNICEF Dhaka Programme Planning Unit.

Cleland, J., and J. van Ginneken

1988 Maternal education and child survival in developing countries: The search for pathways of influence. *Social Science and Medicine* 27:1357-1368.

Coggans, N., and S. McKellar

1994 Drug use amongst peers: Peer pressure or peer preference? *Drugs: Education, Prevention and Policy* 1:15-26.

Cochrane, S.H.

1979 *Fertility and Education: What Do We Really Know?* Baltimore, Md.: The John Hopkins University Press.

de Vries, R.F.

1992 *The Importance of Education for Differences in Female Labour Force Participation and Fertility Behaviour.* Postdoctorale Onderzoekersopleiding Demografie [PDOD] Paper No. 13. Amsterdam, Netherlands. University of Amsterdam.

Easterlin, R.

1975 An economic framework for fertility analysis. *Studies in Family Planning* 6:54-63.

1978 The economics and sociology of fertility: A synthesis. In C. Tilly, ed., *Historical Studies of Changing Fertility.* Princeton, N.J.: Princeton University Press.

1980 *Population and Economic Change in Developing Countries.* Chicago, Ill.: National Bureau of Economic Research.

Entwisle, B., and W. Mason

1985 Multilevel effects of socioeconomic development and family planning programs on children ever born. *American Journal of Sociology* 91(3):616-649.

Jeffery, R., and A. Basu

1996 Schooling as contraception? Pp. 15-47 in R. Jeffery and A. Basu, eds., *Girls' Schooling, Women's Autonomy and Fertility Change in South Asia.* New Delhi: Sage Publications.

Jejeebhoy, S.J.

1995 *Women's Education, Autonomy and Reproductive Behaviour: Experience from Developing Countries.* Oxford: Clarendon Press.

Kabir, M., M. Moslehuddin, and A.A. Howlader

1988 Husband-wife communication and status of women as a determinant of contraceptive use in rural Bangladesh. *Bangladesh Development Studies* 16(1):85-97.

Kiernan, K., and I. Diamond

1983 The age at first birth in the United Kingdom. *Population Studies* 34:363-380.

King, E.M., and M.A. Hill, eds.

1993 *Women's Education in Developing Countries: Barriers, Benefits and Policies.* Baltimore, Md.: The John Hopkins University Press.

Lee, Y.J.

1994 Education, employment and residential independence among young adults in Korea 1970-1990. Paper presented at the Conference on Women's Status in Korea. Vancouver, Canada. July 7-10.

Lesetedi, L.T., G.D. Mompati, P. Khulumani, G.N. Lesetedi, and N. Rutenberg
1989 *Botswana Family Health Survey II 1988*. Gaborone, Botswana: Central Statistics Office and Ministry of Health; and Columbia, Md.: IRD/Macro Systems, Inc.

LeVine, R.A., S.E. LeVine, A. Richman, F.M. Tapia Uribe, C. Sunderland Correa, and P.M. Miller
1991 Women's schooling and child care in the demographic transition: A Mexican case study. *Population and Development Review* 17:459-496.

LeVine, R.A., E. Dexter, P. Velasco, S. LeVine, A.R. Joshi, K.W. Stuebing, and F.M. Tapia Uribe
1994 Maternal literacy and health care in three countries: A preliminary report. *Health Transition Review* 4:186-191.

Mahmud, S.
1995 *The Context of Women's Work in Urban Bangladesh: The Need to Move Beyond Purdah.* Bangladesh: Bangladesh Institute of Development Studies (mimeographed).

Mason, K.O.
1984 *The Status of Women: A Review of Its Relationship to Fertility and Mortality.* New York: The Rockefeller Foundation.

Martin, T.C., and F. Juarez
1995 The impact of women's education on fertility in Latin America: Searching for explanations. *International Family Planning Perspectives* 21:52-57.

Mauldin, W.P., and J.A. Ross
1991 Family planning programs: Efforts and results, 1982-1989. *Studies in Family Planning* 22:350-367.

Mitra, S.N., M.N. Ali, S. Islam, A.R. Cross, and T. Saha
1994 *Bangladesh Demographic and Health Survey 1993-4.* Dhaka, Bangladesh: National Institute of Population Research and Training.

Muhuri, P.K., A. Blanc, and S. Rutstein
1994 *Socio-economic Differentials in Fertility. Demographic and Health Surveys Comparative Studies 13.* Calverton, Md.: Macro International Inc.

National Council for Population and Development and IRD/Macro Systems Inc.
1993 *Kenya Demographic and Health Survey 1993.* Columbia, Md.: National Council for Population and Development and IRD/Macro Systems Inc.

Preston, S., ed.
1978 *The Effects of Infant and Child Mortality on Fertility.* New York: Academic Press.

Rodriguez, G., and R. Aravena
1991 Socio-economic factors and the transition to low fertility in less developed countries: A comparative analysis. Paper presented at the Demographic and Health Surveys World Conference: Washington D.C. August 5-7.

Rodriguez, G., and J. Cleland
1980 Socio-economic determinants of marital fertility in twenty countries: A multivariate analysis. *WFS Conference Proceedings* 2:325-414.

Rosa, K.
1989 Export-oriented industries and women workers in Sri Lanka. Pp. 196-211 in H. Afshar and B. Agarwal, eds., *Women, Poverty and Ideology in Asia.* Basingstoke, England: Macmillan.

Salaff, J.W.
1981 *Working Daughters of Hong Kong: Filial Power or Power in the Family?* Asa Rose Monograph Series. Cambridge, England: Cambridge University Press.

Sathar, Z.
1996 Women's schooling and autonomy as factors in fertility change in Pakistan: Some empirical evidence. Pp. 133-149 in R. Jeffery and A. Basu, eds., *Girls' Schooling, Women's Autonomy and Fertility Change in South Asia.* New Delhi: Sage Publications.

Shah, N.M.
1986 *Pakistani Women: A Socioeconomic and Demographic Profile*. Honolulu, Hawaii: East-West Center.

Singh, S., and J. Casterline
1985 Socio-economic determinants. Pp. 199-222 in J. Cleland and J. Hobcraft, eds., *Reproductive Change in Developing Countries*. Oxford: Oxford University Press.

Steele, F., I. Diamond, and S. Amin
1996 Immunisation in rural Bangladesh: A multilevel analysis. *Journal of the Royal Statistical Society Series A* 159:289-299.

Streatfield, K.
1989 *Fertility Decline in a Traditional Society: The Case of Bali*. Canberra, Australia: Australian National University Press.

Stichter, S., and J.L. Parpart, eds.
1990 *Women, Employment and the Family in the International Division of Labour*. Macmillan International Political Economy Series. Basingstoke, England: Macmillan.

United Nations
1995 *Women's Education and Fertility Behavior: Recent Evidence from the Demographic and Health Surveys*. New York: United Nations.
1987 *Fertility Behaviour in the Context of Development: Evidence from the World Fertility Survey*. New York: United Nations.

Westoff, C.F., A.K. Blanc, and L. Nyblade
1994 *Marriage and Entry into Parenthood. Demographic and Health Surveys Comparative Studies No. 10*. Calverton, Md.: Macro International.

3

What Is Meant, and Measured, by "Education"?

Anthony T. Carter

INTRODUCTION

In recent years, as fertility declines have been observed to follow or accompany large expansions of education in societies that "have not experienced marked economic growth or industrialization" (Singh and Casterline, 1985:201), education, particularly the education of women, increasingly has been singled out as a prime determinant of fertility decline. That education should have such consequences comes as no surprise to those of us who read and write academic papers. Products of a powerful education system and now mostly educators ourselves, we "know" that education is a wonderful thing. At our worst, we may do little more than pour or hammer a few facts into our students, but, like Dickens' Thomas Gradgrind, we are prone to think that fact is always preferable to fancy. At our best, we like to think, we draw our students into the practice of critical thinking, helping them to replace unreflecting acceptance of traditional beliefs with proven knowledge and the capacity to make reasoned choices. Nevertheless, the source of education's efficacy remains mysterious. As the LeVines have noted, there is "scant information" on the precise mechanisms through which "the formal education of women affects their reproductive and health behaviors" (LeVine et al., 1991:459).

This chapter is a critical discussion of selected literature in demography, anthropology, and cognate disciplines on the nature and consequences of education. It begins by outlining two sharply contrasting views of education. In one, education is seen as a single autonomous process of internalization. In the other, education is regarded as a diverse collection of socially situated practices. In the second and third sections of the paper, I argue, first, that the autonomous concept of education pervades the literature on education and fertility change and, second, that it is unsatisfactory. In the fourth section of the paper, I sketch some of the implications of the alternative concept of education as socially situated practices for further research on fertility change. The final section presents some final reflections on the relationship between education and fertility from the anthropological point of view.

Though this volume is concerned with the demographic consequences of education in the developing world, I do not confine myself to examples from developing societies. To ignore the many critical discussions of education in the United States and other industrial societies is to leave unexamined what appears to be a highly optimistic if not ideologically loaded view of the universal effects of education.

TWO CONCEPTS OF EDUCATION

Education as an Autonomous Process of Internalization

According to a view that is widespread in the social sciences, formal education or schooling may be conceived of as an autonomous process of intellectual internalization (see Table 3-1). Knowledge, cognitive skills, and values that are originally external to students are made part of their internal mental apparatus. The agents of education are teachers; schools; the already-educated middle class; and, especially when education is being introduced into the developing world, "the West." Students, the objects of education, are passive vessels to be filled. Formal education is accomplished through the decontextualized use of language in schools that are removed from the contexts and values of everyday life. In this it is radically unlike apprenticeship and other forms of informal education in which what is learned is conditioned by and cannot readily be carried outside of specific settings. The longer one spends in school, the more information, ideas, and values are transferred or the more firmly they are inculcated. Education ends when schooling is completed. After one leaves school, passively internalized knowledge is put to use. The products of education are modern individuals. Education operates on and, indeed, makes individuals. This process is universal. Autonomous with respect to its social and cultural environment, education makes individuals and thus transforms society in the same way without regard to the historical situation in which it occurs.

Education as Socially Situated Practices

In the past two decades, a sharply contrasting view of education has been

TABLE 3-1 Two Contrasting Concepts of Education

Education as an Autonomous Process of Internalization	Education as Socially Situated Practices
• The transfer or internalization of given information, ideas, and values	• ". . . social process[es] involved in instructing, acquiring and transforming knowledge" (Pelissier, 1991:75)
• Learners are passive recipients	• Learners are coparticipants in pedagogical practices
• Accomplished by means of decontextualized language in the value-neutral, context-free setting of the school	• Accomplished by means of activities that are embedded in a local context and vary from one locale to another
• Formal education is radically unlike apprenticeship and other kinds of informal education	• Formal and informal education are differently situated, but not more or less situated
• After school, what is learned is put to use	• The trajectories of learners from peripheral to full participation in communities of practice extend beyond the school
• Education operates on and, indeed, makes individuals	• Education operates on relationships
• The effects of education are universal	• The effects of education are contingent on the historical and sociocultural situation in which it occurs

developed (again, see Table 3-1).[1] According to this view, formal education may be conceived of as situated practices of interaction among teachers and students in school settings. Attention must be given to the agency of learners as well as to

[1]Precisely parallel developments occur in studies of literacy. See especially Street's (1984, 1990) critique of what he calls the "autonomous" model, the idea developed by Goody and Watt (1962; see also Greenfield, 1972, and Hildyard and Olson, 1978) that the acquisition of literacy promotes "'abstract context-free thought', 'rationality', 'critical thought', . . . , 'detachment', and the kinds of logical process exemplified by syllogisms, formal language, elaborated code etc." (Street, 1984:2, 1993; see also Barton and Ivanic, 1991). This work is relevant here because education and literacy are tightly linked in theories of the role of education in declining fertility. Where education is conceived of as the transfer of knowledge and skills into new receptacles, years of schooling completed and literacy status—the ability to read and/or to sign one's name—are treated as equivalent measures of the amount of education an individual has received. Where education is conceived of in terms of the mastery of decontextualized language, reading and writing also are thought to be among the primary means through which education achieves its effects. More broadly, literacy is closely linked to the growth of mass media through which educated persons continue to have access to new values and information. Indeed, I have borrowed the term 'autonomous' from Street's critique of literacy studies and follow the outline of his critique at many points.

teachers, school systems, and bodies of knowledge. Students are not mere passive recipients of education, but are active participants in the construction of pedagogical relations and of knowledge. Education is accomplished by means of communicative practices and other activities that are embedded in local contexts and vary from one locale to another. Learning is not confined to the classroom. It continues after schooling is completed. Education operates on relationships among persons and may or may not produce individuals. Education is not an autonomous process producing uniform results. Instead, its effects are contingent on the historical and sociocultural situations in which it occurs.

The origins of the conception of education as socially situated practices lie in a series of movements, in anthropological and psychological studies of teaching, learning, and language, across a major theoretical divide.[2] On one side of the divide are positions that share a deterministic view of cognitive skills, knowledge, and teaching. On the other side, there is a convergence on a position that emphasizes practice, activity, and agency. In cross-cultural studies of cognition, the shift is from "a concern with cognitive properties as static phenomena that people do or do not have in their heads" to an interest in "the embeddedness of cognitive skills in particular interactive contexts rather than in isolated minds" (Pelissier, 1991:80). In studies of socialization, the parallel shift is from concern with the passive internalization of "given" cultural norms, values, beliefs, and behaviors to interest in how the "recipient[s] of sociocultural knowledge" are "active contributor[s] to the meaning and outcome of interactions with other members of a social group" (Pelissier, 1991:83-84, quoting Schieffelin and Ochs, 1986:165).

Work along these lines has two foci. One focus is the interactions of students and teachers inside classrooms. The other is the ways in which schools are embedded in and permeated by the wider society in which they are located. Both foci figure prominently in the work of the anthropologist Jean Lave, which, because it takes us out of the classroom, along the life course, and into the worlds of persons who are old enough to form families, I describe in some detail.

Lave's first major work on education and learning, *Cognition in Practice* (1988), is a study of arithmetic problem solving among grocery shoppers and participants in the Weight Watchers diet program in California. It begins with, and is organized around, a critique of transfer theory in psychology. Developed in the early years of this century, transfer theory is at the core of the concept of education as an autonomous process of internalization. It holds that knowledge may be conceived of as a set of tools for thinking learned in the value-neutral, context-free setting of the school and then transferred to the activities of everyday life (Lave, 1988:37).

Some of Lave's findings are consistent with transfer theory. The participants

[2]Here I follow Pelissier (1991). For a similar account of these developments see Gumperz (1986).

in her Adult Math Project averaged just 59 percent on standardized tests of arithmetic skills. Since "years of schooling is a good predictor of [test] performance," these research subjects might be regarded as poorly schooled and numerically incompetent. However, other findings point to a very different conclusion. The same research subjects performed similar calculations nearly flawlessly during the course of supermarket shopping (98 percent) or in simulated "best-buy" problems at home (93 percent) (Lave, 1988:52-56). Such results, Lave observes, confound the presuppositions of transfer theory.

> Math is the central ongoing activity in the test situation and should command resources of attention and memory greater than those available in the supermarket where math competes for attention with a number of other concerns. School algorithms should be more powerful and accurate than quick, informal procedures (that's why they are taught in school). Finally, 98% accuracy in the supermarket is practically error-free arithmetic, and belies the image of hapless [just plain folks] failing cognitive challenges in an everyday world. (1988:58-59)

To explain these paradoxial observations, Lave (1988:97) offers the concept of "activity-in-setting." Against the standard view of cognition, decision making, and agency as intramental processes, this concept holds that agency is socially distributed. "'Cognition' observed in everyday practice is distributed—stretched over, not divided among—mind, body, activity and culturally organized settings (which include other actors)" (Lave, 1988:1).

Lave's next major contribution is the concept of legitimate peripheral participation (see Lave, 1989, 1991; Lave and Wenger, 1991). This concept continues her concern with practice and adds a concern with the life course or what she calls "trajectories" along which persons move from legitimate peripheral to full participation in communities of practice. Legitimate peripheral participation directs attention to the changing practices through which newcomers and old-timers engage with one another. No longer entirely intramental, "learning, thinking, and knowing are" conceived of as located in "relations among people engaged in activity in, with, and arising from the socially and culturally constructed world" (Lave, 1991:67, emphasis removed).

The concept of learning as legitimate peripheral participation was constructed around the literature on apprenticeship, but it is intended to apply to formal schooling as well. The special character of formal schooling rests on the claim that knowledge can be decontextualized and that learning opportunities can be separated from legitimate peripheral participation. However, Lave and Wenger argue that schooling always involves a "learning curriculum" as well as "teaching curriculum."

> A learning curriculum consists of situated opportunities... for the improvisational development of new practice (Lave, 1989). A learning curriculum is a field of learning resources in everyday practice *viewed from the perspective of learners*. A teaching curriculum, by contrast, is constructed for the instruction

> of newcomers. When a teaching curriculum supplies—and thereby limits—structuring resources for learning, the meaning of what is learned (and control of access to it . . .) is mediated through an instructor's participation, by an external view of what knowing is about. The learning curriculum in didactic situations, then, evolves out of participation in a specific community of practice engendered by pedagogical relations and by a prescriptive view of the target practice as a subject matter, as well as out of the many and various relations that tie participants to their own and other communities. (Lave and Wenger, 1991:97)

The learning curriculum in schools thus remains a form of legitimate peripheral participation.

EDUCATION IN ANALYSES OF FERTILITY CHANGE

Analyses of the relationship between education and fertility appear to revolve around a series of disagreements. The areas of disagreement include the salience of microeconomic and macrosociological perspectives, the generation through which education affects fertility,[3] the character of the socioeconomic conditions that facilitate or impede the effects of education, and the question of whether education alters fertility by changing family-size preferences or the implementation of preferences within marriage.[4] The great majority of such studies rely on statistical analyses of census and survey data. At least one is based on ethnographic research. For all its surface disagreement, however, this literature is permeated by the view of education as an autonomous process of internalization.

Micro and Macro Perspectives

Consider, for example, the difference between, on the one hand, Easterlin's (1978) "The Economics and Sociology of Fertility: A Synthesis," Cochrane's (1979) *Fertility and Education: What Do We Really Know*?, and Kasarda et al.'s (1986) monograph on *Status Enhancement and Fertility* and, on the other hand, Caldwell's (1980) essay on "Mass Education as a Determinant of the Timing of Fertility Decline."[5] The microeconomic approaches of Easterlin and Cochrane

---

[3]Caldwell (1980) sees the fertility choices of parents as influenced by the experience of educating their children. Other authors stress the effects of parental education.

[4]Cleland and Kaufmann (1998) stress the effects of education on the implementation of desired fertility. Other authors give at least equal weight to the effects of education on the demand for children.

[5]All are widely cited. Easterlin's paper demands attention, in particular, because it is the lead essay in the interdisciplinary volume on *Historical Studies of Changing Fertility* (Tilly, 1978) and provides the conceptual framework for the report of the National Research Council's Committee on Population and Demography on *The Determinants of Fertility in Developing Countries* (Bulatao and Lee, 1983).

and the microsociological approach of *Status Enhancement* all emphasize the ways individuals, or couples treated as if they were individuals, respond to the changing parameters of economic calculation. In response to the microeconomic theories of fertility change that came to prominence in the 1960s and 1970s, Caldwell restates the classic macrosociological version of demographic transition theory, now emphasizing the role of formal education. In Caldwell's view, an account of "the onset of fertility transition" is logically prior to and different in kind from microeconomic and other explanations of fertility differentials that occur after the demographic transition is under way or when it has been completed. "The onset of fertility transition" per se is a consequence of mass involvement in formal schooling. The effects of mass education on the onset of fertility decline are macrosociological in that they involve changes in values or conventions rather than in the parameters of economic calculation. Mass schooling does not simply produce changes in the costs and benefits of children at the margins. Rather, it causes traditional "family moralities" to be replaced by "a new, community morality that is eventually necessary for fully developed non-family production (whether described as capitalist or socialist), and that is taught, explicitly and implicitly, by national education systems" (Caldwell, 1980:226-229).

Despite their theoretical differences, the authors of all of these studies are content to define education by the ways in which it is conventionally measured. These measures include "literacy status, years of school attended, years of school completed, [and] the possession of certain levels of certification" (Cochrane, 1979:29; see also Kasarda et al., 1986:105-106, and Caldwell, 1980:233).[6]

The micro theorists, Cochrane, Easterlin, and Kasarda et al., agree that education is one of several features of the process of modernization that reduce fertility by increasing the supply of children, decreasing the demand for them, and decreasing the costs of fertility regulation. Together with the related growth of the mass media, the expansion of formal education increases the supply of children by raising natural fertility and lowering infant mortality. It accomplishes the former by "break[ing] down traditional beliefs and customs and thus undermin[ing] cultural practices, such as an intercourse taboo, which have had the latent function of limiting reproduction." It "improve[s] health conditions"

---

[6]Cochrane (1979) observes that education has community- as well as individual-level effects. It should be noted, however, that both levels of effects pertain to individuals. What Cochrane terms individual-level effects have to do with the individual who is the focus of analysis. What she terms community-level effects have to do with other individuals with whom that individual has interactions or whose behavior may have consequences for that individual. For example, if one person obtains information about contraception through education, he or she may pass that information on to other persons who are not themselves educated. "Alternatively, when one person's education increases, their market opportunities improve, but other people's opportunities may be made slightly worse" (p. 30).

and thus lowers infant mortality "by diffusing improved knowledge with regard to personal hygiene, food care, environmental dangers, and so on." Formal education and mass media reduce the demand for children through both a "taste" and a cost effect. The taste effect comes about in two ways. Educated persons increasingly value "a 'liberated' life style for women, involving greater market work and less family activity." "Children, and the life style associated with them," come to be seen as an "'old' good." Education and exposure to mass media also may shift tastes from numbers of children to children of higher "'quality.'" The cost effect is a function of the fact that education improves women's income-earning opportunities and thus increases the cost of the time they spend in childrearing. Education and mass media lower "the subjective costs of fertility regulation by challenging traditional beliefs and encouraging a problem-solving approach to life." They decrease the costs of contraception in both money and time by providing better information.[7] (Easterlin, 1978:110-12; Cochrane, 1979: 143-44; see also Kasarda et al., 1986:98-103).

To return to Caldwell, his macrosociological analysis is constructed around five mechanisms through which mass education affects fertility:

> First, it reduces the child's potential for work inside and outside the home. . . . Second, education increases the cost of children far beyond the fees, uniforms, and stationery demanded by the school. . . . Third, schooling creates dependency, both within the family and within the society. . . . Fourth, schooling speeds up cultural change and creates new cultures. . . . Fifth, in the contemporary developing world, the school serves as a major instrument—probably the major instrument—for propagating the values, not of the local middle class, but of the Western middle class (Caldwell, 1980:227-28).

Of these mechanisms, Caldwell regards the last three as the most important. As he notes, this emphasis distinguishes his work from that of the microeconomists. It permits him to shift the generational impact of education, stressing the effects on parents of the education of their children rather than the effects on childbearing of the education of parents. It also permits him to downplay the economic costs and benefits of education. Nevertheless, his emphasis on new family moralities remains perfectly consistent with the microeconomists' inculcation of new social values and consequent abandonment of tradition.

---

[7]Cochrane adds several qualifications. Against the overall trend, education, especially husband's education, may make having children seem more affordable. Education is more likely to be inversely related to fertility in urban areas and in countries where literacy rates are above 40 percent. Fertility is more likely to be affected by female education than by male education. (Cochrane, 1979:143-44)

An Anthropological Contribution

A critical reading of the LeVine et al. (1991) paper on "Women's Schooling and Child Care in the Demographic Transition: A Mexican Case Study" confirms the preceding analysis. This important paper might be expected to offer a novel approach to the relation between education and fertility. It represents an excursion into demography by anthropologists whose major work has been concerned with childrearing and education. It is based on extensive direct observations as well as surveys designed explicitly to identify the missing links through which education influences fertility. In an earlier paper on the relation between culture and fertility, LeVine and Scrimshaw (1983) outline an approach that is sharply critical of conventional microeconomic accounts of fertility change.[8] Nevertheless, in the end, LeVine et al. fall back on the conventional view.

Much of the LeVines' work is familiar. As in other demographic studies, education is measured and, in effect, defined by years of schooling. The effects of schooling on fertility conform to the classic pattern. In rural Tilzapotla, the expected number of children ever born falls sharply with increasing maternal school attainment. Women who never attended school are expected to have an average of 3.83 children. Those who completed 9 years at school are expected to have an average of 2.62 children, nearly a third fewer. In urban Cuernavaca, however, increased maternal schooling is not associated with large declines in the expected number of children ever born. Women with 2 years of schooling are expected to have an average of 2.47 children. This number falls to 2.24 for women with 9 years of schooling. These results are consistent with the observation that current practice of contraception is strongly correlated with mother's education in Tilzapotla, rising from 17.5 percent of women with no schooling to 57.4 percent of women with 7-9 years of schooling, but not in Cuernavaca, where the range is only from 88 to 92 percent. Curiously, years of schooling is strongly associated with length of engagement in the urban sample. Women with 1-5 years of education are engaged for an average of 11.6 months, while those with 7-9 years of schooling are engaged for an average of 21.6 months.

Following Caldwell (1980), Easterlin (1983), and Kasarda et al. (1986), the LeVine study hypothesizes that schooling disseminates a modern ideology of Western individualism, "marital egalitarianism and domestic independence" (LeVine et al., 1991:473). Such an ideology breaks down the dominance of the elders in the domestic group, promotes the autonomy of the nuclear family, and increases women's motivation to enhance the status of themselves and their children. These changes tend to reduce fertility in several ways. Women who are no longer under the domestic control of elder relatives and who have a more

[8]See Carter (1998) for a critical discussion of the Bulatao and Lee volumes in which this paper appears.

egalitarian relationship with their husbands are more likely to be able to pursue their own goals and to seek and use information on child survival and family planning. Women who value education for their children find that the costs of rearing children are increased, while the economic returns are decreased. The authors suggest that these hypotheses are confirmed by their survey results. In the more nuanced Cuernavaca survey, women with more schooling reported more joint marital decisions, increased discussion of family planning with their husbands, higher aspirations for their children, and reduced expectations of help from and coresidence with children. In Tilzapotla, women with more years of schooling are more likely to read and to watch television on a regular basis, thus exposing themselves to information about family planning (LeVine et al., 1991: 482-84, 489-490).

The novel aspect of the LeVine study derives from Robert LeVine's own work "on the classroom as a source of new models of adult-child interpersonal relationships and communication for schoolgirls from agrarian communities" (LeVine et al., 1991:486). The authors propose that "schooling leads women to reconceptualize child care as a labor-intensive task requiring a great deal of her own attention throughout the preschool years and that this concept ultimately reduces her willingness to bear more than a few children." This hypothesis rests on a broad contrast between agrarian and modern industrial societies. Agrarian societies are characterized by a "protective style" of childrearing "which emphasizes physical nurturance and comfort" and by systems of apprenticeship in which learning takes place through "graduated participation." Modern industrial societies, on the other hand, are characterized by systems of formal education in which learning takes place through decontextualized verbal instruction in the classroom. In such settings, children achieve widely varying levels of competence. As a consequence, the school "introduces considerations of long-term competitive advantage into childhood." The core of the LeVines' hypothesis runs as follows:

> As schooling becomes institutionalized, mothers who have acquired this model in the classroom increasingly prepare their children for school, engaging them in pedagogical interaction at younger and younger ages. This means verbal responsiveness to the child during infancy, which has the effect of producing a verbally active toddler who frequently initiates demands for maternal attention during the post-infancy years. Such children are on the average less compliant and more 'difficult' and 'exhausting' to raise, reinforcing the mother's assumption that child care is a labor-intensive task—requiring more of her time and energy than it did for her own mother (prior to female schooling in an agrarian community) and inducing her to bear fewer children (LeVine et al., 1991:486-88).[9]

[9]This part of the LeVines' argument also rests on LeVine (1983, 1987), LeVine and White (1986), Bornstein (1989), and Rogoff (1990).

To test this hypothesis, 72 Cuernavaca women were observed interacting with their infants at home. Observers noted (1) the proportion of infant vocalizations followed by maternal speech, (2) the proportion of infant looks followed by maternal speech, (3) the proportion of infant looks followed by maternal looks, (4) the proportion of infant motor acts followed by maternal speech, and (5) the proportion of time mother held infant. Significant positive correlations with maternal education were found for (1) and (4) at all infant ages, for (2) at 10 and 15 months and for (3) at 15 months. Significant negative correlations with maternal education were found for (5) at 15 months. The authors conclude "that women who attend school longer acquire a conception of child care as a labor-intensive task requiring more attention for a longer period of time—a conception that may contribute to child survival and impede fertility" (LeVine et al., 1991:488).

The LeVines did not do home observations in rural Tilzapotla, but in their view several components of their Tilzapotla survey provide insights into the same processes. One of the survey questions asked about arrangements made for childcare when the mother left the home. As mother's education increases, the percentage of children cared for by the oldest child or left alone in these circumstances declines, while the percentage of mothers taking their child with them increases. The percentage of mothers reporting that they leave their child with another adult does not vary significantly with mother's education. This last is also the preferred arrangement, ranging from 57 to 60 percent. LeVine et al. argue that this finding "supports the hypothesis that schooling enhances a woman's concept of child care as a labor-intensive task to be carried out by the mother herself or by another adult" (pp. 488-89).

Another part of the survey tested mastery of abstract or decontextualized language by asking respondents to define nouns and complete simple syllogisms. Following Snow (1990), LeVine et al. (1991:489-90) argue that exposure to formal schooling increases mastery of abstract or decontextualized uses of language in which the speaker/hearer must be able "to assume the perspective of someone who does not know the contextual background taken for granted in conversation" in order to communicate effectively. "This skill . . . is notably absent from normal conversation in small face-to-face communities, where people can safely assume that hearers share their contextual perspective." "Transmitted in the classroom," decontextualized language becomes a "pathway to the increased use of medical and contraceptive services. Specifically, women with more schooling are likely to be more conversant with the decontextualized language that is standard in health bureaucracies. . . ."[10]

[10]It should be noted that these arguments suffer from several technical weaknesses. LeVine et al. offer no data on household composition. However, their qualitative observations on the link between education and length of engagement in Cuernavaca suggests that women with more schooling are

LeVine et al. (1991:492) regard these as the primary effects of education:

> Formal education everywhere, regardless of its quality, entails the presence of an adult whose role is entirely instructional, talking to children, often in a formal language they have to learn to understand. For girls in rural areas of countries where mass schooling is still a relatively recent innovation, this model of social interaction between an adult and children stands in contrast to their previous experience, and over time it reshapes their skills and preferences in social communication. They acquire in school and retain in adulthood skills of literacy and decontextualized language providing access to distant sources of information and institutionalized health care. Identifying with the role of pupil, they continue to seek useful knowledge wherever they can find it; identifying with the role of teacher, they are verbally responsive to their children during infancy and after. A new kind of mother-child relationship is built around reciprocal verbal interaction, one which helps mothers monitor the needs of their preschool children but which also demands so much of their attention that fertility control becomes imperative.

This conclusion carries Levine et al. some distance from an economic analysis of the consequences of education. However, its emphasis on the ways in which education promotes new values and enhances cognitive skills places it squarely within the conventional approach. The agency of young women in participating in the construction of classroom talk or in creatively applying what is learned in the classroom to the home is given short shrift. Like knowledge of abstract noun definitions, knowledge of the pedagogical style of childrearing is produced at school in a process in which the objects of education are passive recipients.

FORMAL SCHOOLING AND DECONTEXTUALIZED LANGUAGE: AN ETHNOGRAPHIC TEST

With its pioneering attempt to trace connections between the experience of formal schooling and subsequent routine activities involved in fertility, the work of LeVine et al. (1991) provides an opportunity to test some of the central ideas

---

more likely to establish nuclear family households immediately following their weddings. If this is true generally, the observations of LeVine et al. on mother-child interactions and childcare arrangements must be reconsidered. A number of other studies, most carried out in North America, report that mothers often expand "the child's vocalization into a sentence which is in turn responded to by the mother in a conversational frame of alternating turns at talking," but careful reviews of this literature point out that most are "of first-born children reared in homes in which mother and child have only each other as a communicative partner for a large portion of the day" (Heath, 1983:374, note 7; see also Snow, 1977). Subsequent children or children born into extended family households may be reared differently. Similarly, the fact that more-educated Tilzapotlan women are more likely to take their children with them when they leave the house may simply be a function of the fact that there are no other adults or older children in their households or that the work is agricultural. On methods of observation, see note 11 below.

of the education-fertility literature against the ethnographic record. As noted above, LeVine et al. put particular emphasis on the peculiar features of classroom talk. They adopt the widely held view that classroom teaching universally includes the use of formal or decontextualized language. Mothers who have been to school are more likely to use a version of such language in caring for their own children. This transforms the care of children into a time-consuming activity and shifts more of the burden to mothers.

The Situated Character of Pedagogical Discourse

The work of Heath (1983) and Minick (1993) is prominent among the ethnographic studies relevant to this view of education and its consequences. Both Heath and Minick describe instructional speech practices in which routine contexts are suspended, and participants attempt to "construct close relationships between what is meant and what is said, between what is made known through an utterance and what is explicitly represented in language" (Minick, 1993:346). Such speech practices are what the LeVines and others call "formal" or "decontextualized" speech; Minick writes of "representational speech." To this extent, the positions of Heath and Minick are similar to the one adopted in the LeVine study, but the agreement ends there.

In the primary classrooms observed by Minick, representational speech often took the form of directives. Minick argues that the seemingly decontextualized character of representational directives is more accurately seen as a contextually defined accomplishment. The evidence for this argument consists of two sets of observations. The first concerns the fact that "formal training" in the representational directives genre "is a recognized part of the school curriculum, beginning with the introduction of what are commonly referred to as 'listening exercises' at the kindergarten level" (Minick, 1993:358). In these exercises, the students' task is limited to following the teacher's directions. Any "'situational sense' that might create an interpretation of intended meaning that would go beyond what is represented in a particular sentence or phrase" is excluded by the invocation of the listening exercise context. The invocation of this context is precarious; other, more routine contexts continually threaten to intrude. This is a consequence of the fact that the teacher utterances of which such exercises are composed are ambiguous. Teachers attempt to render their directives unambiguous and to protect the listening exercise context by increasing "the amount of 'information' actually represented in language. Rather than say 'point to' the teacher says 'put your finger on'" (Minick, 1993:360).

The second set of observations turns on the fact that in other kinds of classroom activities, it is often unclear that teachers intend their utterances to be understood as representational directives at the time they are made. In these instances, a representational interpretation of an utterance may be constructed after the fact in response to the actions of students. In one episode discussed by Minick, a second-grade teacher working with four children in a "reading group"

> . . . attempts to shift from a discussion of library books that are on the table in front of the children to work on a story in the basal readers that are under the children's chairs. The teacher initiates this shift by clearing away several notebooks that lie atop her copy of the reader while saying, "Now. We are going to read a story. Please put your books under your chair. And, we are going to read a story which you are going to enjoy."

One boy, Todd, promptly responds by putting his library book under his chair and putting his reader on the table. When the teacher begins to page through her reader, Todd looks through his.

> Framed by the suggestion that "we are going to read a story" and the teacher's subsequent actions, Todd has apparently taken the teacher's directive as a [non-representational directive] indicating that they are to prepare to do that reading. This task begins with putting the library books away, but also includes taking the reader out and locating the new story.

Another boy puts his library book away under his chair and sits back up, but when he sees "Todd looking through his reader, he begins to look nervously back and forth from Todd to the teacher." Two girls in the reading group put their library books away but then remain bent over, also looking from Todd to the teacher. When the teacher pays no attention to what Todd is doing, they, too, take "their readers out from under their chairs and begin to look through them." At this point the teacher takes note of the children's actions, saying in an irritated tone, "Todd, did Mrs. W. say, 'Open your book to…' Did she?" [Todd shakes his head, "No."] "No, she did not." In response to this reinterpretation of the teacher's initial utterance as a representational directive, all of the children put their readers back under their seats. The teacher begins "to review new vocabulary before beginning to read," but several of the children again looked "furtively" at their readers. Now the teacher lowers the representational boom, emphatically invoking the listening exercise context:

> "Excuse me. I have not good listeners today. Now, put your hands on your books." [The "guilty" three immediately place their hands on their books.] "Put your books under your chairs." [The three immediately put their books under their chairs.] Here, the teacher makes several nested moves that make it clear that she is demanding a representational interpretation of directives. First, she begins with a directive that has a clear representational meaning but a rather opaque situational significance (i.e., "put your hands on your books"), encouraging a shift to representational interpretation. She follows this with a directive that is identical to that which initiated the episode, returning them to the position they would have been in had they followed a representational interpretation of her first directive (i.e., "put your books under your chairs"). (pp. 355-56)

In addition to representational directives, Heath (1983:279-83) describes a distinct genre of classroom talk connected with reading aloud and discussing the content of books. This genre is distinct from talk about "contextualized first-hand experiences." Like play, reading aloud and talking about reading "suspends reality, and is so framed, either through verbal or prop-type cues, that everyone knows immediately that it is not normal conversation." Reading involves "decontextualized representations of experience" insofar as it suspends the conventions in which first-hand experiences are discussed, but, as in the case of representational directives, this is a matter of reframing or recontextualization, rather than the removal of all contexts. The reframing is achieved in part through the use of "a particular kind of prosody which is different from regular conversational prosody."[11]

Both Minick and Heath link the use of representational directives to classroom control. Minick (1993:361) found that teachers most often use representational directives to negotiate "comparatively mechanical task[s] that [have] little immediate pedagogical significance," tasks such as putting one book away and getting another out. Implicit in the use of the representational frame are differences in power. "The ubiquity of representational directives in the classroom," Minick suggests, "stems from the fact that the activities that are to be carried out there are defined by social realities such as curriculum, standardized testing, and teaching materials that have their roots in social systems that extend substantially beyond the classroom walls" (pp. 370-71).

That the exercise of power in the teacher/student relation cannot be reduced to the teaching curriculum or to differences in age is suggested by the fact that not all teachers manage their classrooms in the same way. A teacher who used representational directives less often also differed from others in Minick's sample in that

> . . . she delegate[d] to her pupils much of the responsibility for defining 'situational sense.' Because she [did] not assume 'ownership of meaning' in organizing classroom activities, this teacher [was] not constantly faced with the task of conveying *her definition* of situational sense to her class, a task that demands either a nonrepresentational communication of this definition or a resort to the use of representational directives. (p. 370)

In the primary classrooms observed by Heath, issues of classroom control are linked to cultural diversity as well as power. Her study (1983) was designed to explain how children from two culturally distinctive groups in the Carolina

---

[11]See also Cook-Gumperz (1977), Michaels and Cook-Gumperz (1979), Michaels (1981), and Scollon and Scollon (1979, 1981). For the relevant linguistic theory, see Hanks (1996). The methodological differences between Minick's research and the LeVine study also deserve comment. In their study of mother-child interactions, the LeVines counted occurrences of decontextualized variables. Minick attends to ongoing interactions.

Piedmont responded to "mainstream" schools. Roadville was inhabited by whites, fairly recent immigrants from the Appalachians, most of whom worked in the textile mills. Trackton was inhabited by African-Americans. The "mainstream" was composed of white townspeople, many of whose "norms of conduct and bases for forming judgments about their own and others' behavior [had] much in common with the national mainstream middle class generally presented in the public media as the American client or customer" (Heath, 1983:236). In the decade 1969 to 1978, when Heath worked in the area, the residents of Roadville and Trackton were new to mainstream Piedmont schools, the first as a result of immigration and the second as a result of integration.

Heath (1983:279-83) notes that mainstream teachers expected their students to follow classroom rules. Lists of the rules were posted on bulletin boards, but in the first few months of school they were seldom stated explicitly or explained.

> [Instead teachers used] indirect instruction and modeling for the children. They used familiar verbal formulae from their own home experiences: Is this where the scissors belong? . . . Someone else is talking now; we'll all have to wait. We have visitors coming to the school this afternoon; we want our school to look nice.

That is to say, they used contextualized language. This had the desired effect with children from the same mainstream background as the teacher, children who had learned these forms of contextualized language at home. But "Roadville and Trackton children had difficulty interpreting these indirect requests for adherence to an unstated set of rules." The teachers perceived these children as impolite.

> Many teachers learned to deal with this by expressing directives as directly as possible. Instead of 'Can we get ready on time?' as an indirect directive to tell children to put their toys away and begin lining up for snack time, teachers tried to say: 'put your toys back where you took them from. We have to line up for lunch. Table three will wash hands first.'

The Acquisition of Pedagogical Discourse

These observations cast doubt on the universal validity of the distinction between informal, contextualized language and formal, decontextualized language on which the distinctiveness of schooling rests. Heath's work also undermines the LeVines' argument that women who have attended school model their interactions with young children on the interactions between teachers and children in school. Heath was concerned with the effects on school success of prior participation in speech practices that differed from those used in the school, but it appears that her material can be read the other way around as well.[12] The young

[12]For critical discussion of this aspect of Heath's work see Rosen (1985), Erickson (1987), DeCastell and Walker (1991), and Heath (1993).

mothers Heath studied could read and write and certainly had attended school. Most likely, all remained in school until they were at least 16 years old. Most likely, too, given that Heath's research was carried out from 1969 to 1978, most attended mainstream schools for at least part of their educational careers. Nevertheless, it would appear that the principal influence on their childrearing practices was their position as legitimate peripheral participants in their residential communities and family networks.

Of the two kinds of distinctively contextualized speech practices observed by Heath, those involved in reading aloud and talking about reading were found in "mainstream" homes as well as in the newly integrated "mainstream" Piedmont schools. Representational directives appear to have occurred mostly in the school setting. Heath suggests that this is a consequence of the fact that they served as a technology of control where the participants in education did not have a shared sense of the rules. Though some "mainstream" childrearing practices were consonant with the practices of formal schooling, there is no evidence that schooling was the source of these practices.

Trackton and Roadville parents had culturally variable ways of interacting with and rearing children that were little affected by formal schooling. A brief discussion of one case will suggest the magnitude of the variation. African-Americans in Trackton speak of "children 'comin up'" (Heath, 1983:144). A new baby need not be taken home to a nuclear family household consisting of its parents and siblings. For example,

> Annie Mae's daughter, Marcy, became pregnant at fifteen after a one-time liaison with Miner Baine, a boy of sixteen. . . . When the child—a boy—was born, Miner came around to visit infrequently, and brought milk and diapers occasionally in the first few months. Soon after he went into the service and left the area. Miner's family, however, enjoyed the baby, Larry Lee, and they took the child every weekend, and Miner's sister and parents lavished attention on the baby. Annie Mae became the baby's 'mamma,' taking major responsibility for the child. Larry Lee learned to call his biological mother by her given name, and Annie Mae was 'mamma.' Marcy, after the birth of the child, went back to school at night, then on to a technical college, working steadily at various jobs and helping her mother pay the expenses for Larry Lee. Mr. and Mrs. Smith, the old couple near the railroad tracks, became co-parents with Annie Mae of Larry Lee, keeping him a good part of the time. (Heath, 1983:69-70)

Regardless of its domestic arrangements, much of a child's time is spent outdoors, where it interacts with the wider community.

During the first year of life, Trackton babies are constantly in the midst of family and community life, often "carried astride the hip or nestled in the cradle of an arm" so that "they can see the face of their caregiver or the person the caregiver is talking to."

> [They] are in the midst of nearly constant human communication, verbal and nonverbal. They literally feel the body signals of shifts in emotion of those who

> hold them; they are never excluded from verbal interactions. They are listeners and observers in a stream of communication which flows about them, but is not especially channeled or modified for them. Everyone talks *about* the baby, but rarely *to* the baby." (Heath, 1983:75)

Adults regard the early vocalizations of children as noise.

> [They] respond incredulously to queries such as 'Did you hear him say *milk*?' They believe they should not have to depend on their babies to tell them what they need or when they are uncomfortable. Adults are the knowing participants; children only 'come to know.' Thus, if asked, community members explain away their lack of responses to children's early utterances; they do not repeat the utterance, announce it as a label for an item or event, or place the 'word' in an expanded phrase or sentence. To them, the response carries no meaning which can be directly linked to an object or event; it is just 'noise'. (Heath, 1983:76)

VARIETIES OF EDUCATIONAL EXPERIENCE: NEW DIRECTIONS FOR RESEARCH

As Kasarda et al. (1986:106) observe, "cross-national comparisons of [quantitative] research findings" on the association of increased education with reduced fertility rest on the assumption "that educational experience is equivalent from country to country (in terms of economic value and opportunities availed) or that the standardized measures we use to summarize educational experience have the same meaning in all cultural settings." The core of this assumption is the idea, integral to the concept of education as internalization, that education is autonomous with respect to its social and cultural environment and that its effects are therefore universal.

The alternative view of education as situated processes of interaction abandons the search for universals. It directs attention instead to the ways in which schooling and its consequences vary with the practices of which it is composed and the social and cultural context in which it is embedded. This view opens up new ways of investigating the links between education and fertility.

Ideologies of Education

It is helpful to keep in mind that many of our ideas about the nature and value of education are themselves situated and contested. According to the conventional view of education employed in the literature on its demographic effects, education is liberating and empowering. In Easterlin's (1978:111) formulation, it "encourag[es] a problem-solving approach to life" by breaking down tradition, giving people access to information and "improved knowledge," and inculcating reasoning skills. This view is by no means universal. Advocates of formal schooling for working-class communities in nineteenth-century England (Vincent,

1989) and France (Furet and Ozouf, 1982) and twentieth-century South Carolina (Heath, 1983) all saw it as providing new channels through which the emerging class of industrial workers could be disciplined. Both views of education—that which equates it with liberation and empowerment and that which equates it with discipline—reflect the concerns of middle- and upper-class interests. They fail to recognize that schools

> exist as a site of struggle between and among interests of the state, capital, labor, educators, community representatives, advocates, students, and parents. Schools distribute skills and opportunities in ways textured by class, race, and gender asymmetries. Privileged are notions of individualism, competition, mobility, meritocracy, and marriage, and silenced are discussions of social class, race, gender, and sexual arrangements. Finally, the presentation of public schools as 'public' obscures the vastly differential educations and outcomes made available to students by virtue of their social class, race/ethnicity, gender, sexual orientation, disability, and geography, and undercuts the creation of spaces which nurture democracy, difference, critique, and movements for social change. (Fine, 1991:199-200)

Educational Histories

Conventional accounts of the relation between education and fertility erase educational histories, replacing them with years of schooling completed as a measure of education. No doubt this is in part simply a matter of research convenience, but it also is consistent with the concept of education as an autonomous process of internalization. Such a measure assumes that formal education is additive. The more years are spent in school, the more the individual is transformed. It is recognized that educational achievement may be affected by economic factors and the events in a woman's reproductive history (see, e.g., Kasarda et al., 1986:106), but schools also are assumed to provide the same sorts of opportunities to all categories of students. Within broad limits, therefore, the number of years of schooling completed can also be treated as an indication of the student's inherent capacity to benefit from education. In contrast, the concept of education as situated practices, with its emphasis on the active participation of students in educational processes and the trajectories of interaction described by learners as they move from peripheral to full participation in communities of practice, places educational histories in the foreground.

The available data on educational histories are fragmentary and incomplete, the byproducts of studies directed to other concerns. They are sufficient, nevertheless, to suggest that this would be a fruitful area for further research.

Harbison and Hanushek (1992) provide a rare glimpse of the educational histories of primary school children in rural northeast Brazil in the 1980s. The data are derived from a series of surveys designed to evaluate the effects of the Northeast Brazil Basic Education Project (EDURURAL) on access to primary schooling, progress through the primary grades, and educational achievement.

This study was "the most comprehensive survey of rural education ever attempted in a developing country" (Harbison and Hanushek, 1992:37). Nevertheless, as regards educational histories per se, the EDURURAL data have major limitations. The surveys were designed to sample schools, rather than to track individual students. It was expected that many of the second graders who were studied during one round of the survey would reappear as fourth graders 2 years later. However, this expectation was not met. Schools themselves led a precarious existence, often disappearing from one survey to the next. Students in schools that did survive had high rates of retention in grade and dropout (p. 41). The final, 1987, round of data collection was changed to compensate for these difficulties. Abandoning any attempt to produce a representative sample, this round concentrated on a local subset of schools and incorporated special efforts to locate second graders surveyed in 1985. Because the surveys were collected at 2-year intervals, the educational histories derived from them are discontinuous. The survey data themselves are limited in at least two respects. The investigators were unable to obtain "reliable direct measures of attendance" (pp. 97, 42). They measured student work with a crude "dummy variable reflecting employment status," thus setting aside "wide variations in time commitments, in strenuousness of the activity, or in effects on attendance or homework" (p. 326, note 110). No observations were made in classrooms.

Figure 3-1 is Harbison and Hanushek's (1992:60) representation of the "possible paths for a student initially observed in second grade." If they followed the standard course, the educational histories of all primary students would carry them along the path on the extreme left of Figure 3-1. That a great many students in rural northeastern Brazil deviated from this standard path is only partly a consequence of high rates of school demise, the inability of many schools to provide a full set of primary grades, and the geographical mobility of students' families. Progress through this fragile school system also was affected by gender; age; performance on initial standardized tests; and characteristics of the student's family, school, and region.

Additional complexity is introduced by the interaction between the student's experience in school and his or her role in rural agrarian households. The families of students in counties with higher agricultural productivity were less likely to migrate. Students who belonged to families in which the father was a farmer were more likely to drop out. Boys and older students were more likely to drop out than girls and younger students. Harbison and Hanushek (1992:70) suggest that the difference between boys and girls "reflects a lower opportunity cost of school attendance for girls; their value on the farms is less, so they are less likely to quit school to work." Since the work done "by second graders typically involves lesser time commitments and therefore is less intrusive on schooling" (p. 98), opportunity costs also may have been involved in the differences between older and younger students. Among students who remained in school and were promoted from second to fourth grade on time, work had a negative effect on

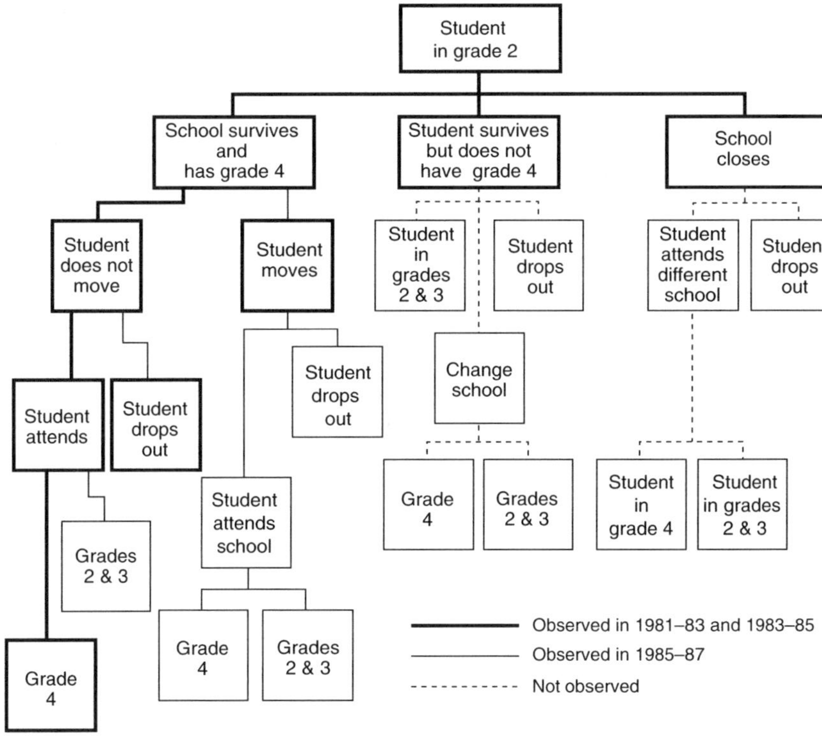

FIGURE 3-1 Educational histories in rural northeastern Brazil: "Possible Paths for a Student Initially Observed in Second Grade." SOURCE: Reprinted from Harbison and Hanushek (1992:60) with permission of Oxford University Press.

achievement as measured by changes in scores on standardized tests of Portuguese and mathematics. Underlying these findings is the undoubted but also unobserved fact that the educational histories of "many students [consist of] on-and-off attendance over extended periods of time" (p. 97).

Harbison and Hanushek (1992:100-103) also explore the factors contributing to achievement among students who remained in school and were promoted from one grade to another on time. Their findings can be read to suggest that students' experiences of classroom interaction also are a significant feature of educational histories. The EDURURAL data provide no support for the idea that the achievement of individual students is affected by the gender composition of their classes. Though the statistical results are not robust, data from the 1985 survey do suggest that a student's achievement is affected by the gender of his or her teacher. Achievement also is affected by the socioeconomic status of students in the classroom, especially the proportion of families not farming.

For additional material on educational histories one must turn to the United States and Europe. Fine's (1991) study of dropping out in a public high school in New York City is a particularly valuable study of a much-discussed problem (see also Cicourel and Kitsue, 1963; Willis, 1977). As Fine observes, dropping out is a majority phenomenon. Something like 80 percent of ninth graders drop out before graduating. Fine (1991:14) argues that this cannot be accounted for by the poor quality of the students. "When students drop out of a high school in majority proportions, their exit must be read as a structural, if not self-conscious critique."

A key element of Fine's argument is the claim that educational achievement is not well correlated with ability.

> [It is true that] students who read and compute at or above the ninth-grade level are more likely to be promoted than retained, and that students who read and compute below the ninth-grade level are more likely to be retained than promoted. However, it is also clear that almost half of those students who have been retained in ninth grade are reading and computing at or above grade level. (p. 240)

Retaining students in grade level in turn increases the chances that they will drop out. Conversely, enrollment in bilingual education programs results in a small increase in the probability of persisting to graduation, even though "students in bilingual education are allegedly most at risk" and were more likely to be retained in ninth grade (Fine, 1991:236).

The EDURURAL research and Fine's study of dropping out in effect look backward. They show that students can arrive at a given number of years of education completed by very diverse routes. Furstenberg et al.'s (1987) study of *Adolescent Mothers in Later Life* looks forward, cautioning that the apparent end of formal education may not mark a real completion.

Furstenberg et al. report on a follow-up study, 16 to 17 years after delivery, of an initial cohort of 403 adolescent mothers and their firstborn children, mostly black, who participated in a program for pregnant adolescents at Sinai Hospital in Baltimore, Maryland. The researchers expected that "premature" childbearing would have a negative effect on educational attainment. These expectations were confirmed by the first phase of the study. Most of the adolescent mothers in the Baltimore study left school "before or soon after their child was born." Five years later, slightly fewer than half had returned to school and finished high school. ". . . [O]nly 8% of the women who had not graduated were currently enrolled (along with 9% of the high school graduates)" (Furstenberg et al., 1987:25).

Reinterviewing these women 16 to 17 years after the birth of their first child, Furstenberg and his colleagues were surprised to find that many of them had continued their educations beyond this apparent end.

> *Of all the educational attainment that occurred following the birth of the first child, more than half took place in the second segment of the study.* High school graduates, pursuing higher education, accounted for a significant proportion of the further schooling. But one woman in six completed high school in the second segment of the study or a third of the young mothers who had not graduated by 1972. . . . Clearly, many women returned to school to obtain a diploma, or more often a GED, when they were well into their twenties. This often occurred when their youngest child entered school. (Furstenberg et al., 1987:25-26)

Beyond the Classroom

More ambitiously, anthropologists (and others) can pursue the LeVines' lead, attempting to produce detailed ethnographic accounts of the culturally and historically specific connections between forms of education and literacy and subsequent practices involved in fertility. One study that allows us to imagine what such ethnographic accounts might look like is Brodie's (1994) *Contraception and Abortion in 19th-Century America.* McLaren (1978) and Gordon (1977) have written extensively about the lively public debates concerning population and family planning that have taken place in England and the United States. Nevertheless, Brodie's work is unusual in the degree to which it traces the ways in which ordinary persons consumed or made something of the representations with which the debates are filled, putting them to use in their own lives (see also Seccombe, 1992). Her rich material allows us to explore the links between literacy practices and fertility in the lives of ordinary men and women, well after they have left school.

In brief, Brodie argues that during the course of the nineteenth century, more American women used contraception. They also used new forms of contraception, shifting from coitus interruptus, abortion, and breastfeeding to postcoital douching, a variety of rhythm methods, condoms, pessaries, and sponges. The evidence for this comes from Clelia Duel Mosher's small turn-of-the-century survey of reproductive control and sexual practices among her women patients, an extensive body of personal letters, and a few private diaries. Brodie also traces some of the connections between changing contraceptive practices and a wide range of features of nineteenth-century American popular culture and economic organization. Among these are overlapping groups of participants in the debate over birth control, authors of self-help manuals, physicians, providers of water-cure therapy, concepts of personal hygiene, lecture circuits, organizations devoted to free thought, and publishers of newspapers and other periodical literature. The developing postal system and network of railroads also were important.

As regards the relationship between education and fertility, Brodie's work demonstrates that it is not enough to say that new discoveries were circulated in printed mass media and passively absorbed by women and their partners. The spread of new contraceptive practices cannot be accounted for simply by arguing that the members of an increasingly educated population gained access to already existing scientific knowledge because they could now read and write.

The changing nineteenth-century American "culture of contraception" (Gillis et al., 1992:5) depended on at least three kinds of reading and writing. There was an enormous genre of self-help or advice manuals. These included Robert Owen's *Moral Physiology*, a staple work in histories of the birth control debate; Charles Knowlton's *Fruits of Philosophy; or, The Private Companion of Young Married People*; Russell Thacher Trall's *The Hydropathic Encyclopedia . . . with an Appendix on Conception*; and A. M. Mauriceau's (pseudonym for Ann Trow Lohman, Charles Lohman, and/or Joseph Trow) *The Married Woman's Private Medical Companion* (Brodie, 1994:357-65). Many of the advice manuals were privately published. Their distribution depended on a network of commercial agents, the postal system, the railroads, halls of science and other organizations of freethinkers, organizations of medical sectarians, and so on. They also were offered for sale by their authors at public lectures. In some cases, written advice manuals could convey information in ways that oral communication could not.

> . . . [T]he first three editions of [Knowlton's] *Fruits of Philosophy* were almost miniature books, only about three inches by two and half inches in size. It was designed for private perusal and passing on to friends, not for public display. (Brodie, 1994:105)

More speculatively, Brodie (1994:162) suggests that "it may have [been] easier for Knowlton to leave copies of his pamphlet with his patients than for him or them to circle the topic in conversation with embarrassed euphemisms."

Advertising also was critical. Advertisements were included in many advice manuals.

> The water-cure publication the *Herald of Health*, with one of the largest circulations of any nineteenth-century medical journal, publicized douching syringes, promoted "voluntary motherhood," and argued the need for controlled reproduction.

Racy tabloids "aimed at an urban class of stable boys, maids, day laborers, upwardly mobile young clerks, and salespeople" carried advertisements for condoms and diaphragms. "In the 1830s and 1840s abortion drugs, condoms, cures for venereal disease, aphrodisiacs, and abortions were advertised in major urban newspapers in New England and the Middle Atlantic states." Opponents of birth control noted that advertisers could obtain the names of prospective customers from newspaper announcements of marriages. John Todd, a Congregational minister, complained:

> No young lady in New England (and probably in the United States) can have a marriage announced in the papers without receiving in the mail within a week a printed circular offering information and instrumentalities and all needed facilities. (Brodie, 1994:190-93)

The whole circulation of contraceptive information depended, finally, on the personal letter. Until the passage of the Comstock Law in 1873, this was a mail order business.

> The advertising pamphlet put out by the Beach Company in the 1860s, Habits of a Well-Organized Life, explained how to cope with the intricate process of a mail transaction. The circular gave detailed directions about how to order and pay for the products, how to contact the nearest express company office or post office to place an order through the mail, how to use a C.O.D. express, how to get a money order, how to endorse it so that no one would know to whom it was sent, how to involve a third person in the transaction. (Brodie, 1994:232)

A great many purveyors of advice conducted all or part of their business by mail. Following the publication of his popular manual *The Marriage Guide; or, Natural History of Generation*, Frederick Hollick was able to give up lecturing and "devote himself to writing popular medical books and to his growing private practice, conducted almost entirely by correspondence. About fifty letters arrived daily at his post office box in Manhattan" (Brodie, 1994:117). In at least some social classes, people used personal letters to share contraceptive information with others in their personal networks of acquaintances.

> In 1885, Rose Williams wrote from the Dakota Territory to answer a question put to her by an Ohio friend, Allettie Mosher: how to prevent pregnancy. "You want to know of a sure prevenative [sic]. Well plague take it. The best way is for you to sleep in one bed and your Man in another & bet you will laugh and say 'You goose you think I am going to do that' no and I bet you would for I don't see any one that does. Well now the thing we [use] (when I say *we* I mean us girls) is a thing: but it hasn't always been *sure* as you know but that was our own carelessness for it is we have been sure. I do not know whether you can get them out there. They are called Pessairre [sic] or female prevenative. They cost one dollar when Sis got hers it was before any of us went to Dak. She paid five dollars for it. The Directions are with it." (Brodie, 1994:212)

As Lave and Wenger (1991) suggest, it is communities of practice that learn. As a result of their use of culturally specific literacy practices, women were legitimate participants in these communities. Rather than being passed from the knowledgeable to the ignorant, information was generated out of the interactions among participants. In the 1852 edition of his popular *The Hydropathic Encyclopedia*, Russell Thacher Trall wrote:

> [The fertile period generally] occurred from the 'commencement of menstruation through twelve days' after. By 1867, however, he added the warning that the mid-menstrual period, though generally safe, was not infallibly infertile. He therefore advised waiting ten to twelve days after menstruation. In 1867 he cited statistics collected from 'several hundred' patients to prove that for none of the women had an ovum passed into the uterus before the third day after menstruation or after the fourteenth. The satisfaction Trall's patients appear to have found with the sterile period probably did not come from his timetables as

> much as from his careful instructions to women about how to discern their own ovulation. He recommended: 'By noticing the time for two or three successive periods at which the egg or clot passes off she will ascertain her menstrual habit.' (Brodie, 1994:84)

One imagines that the basis of Trall's instructions was the prior experience of women. Certainly the results of women's noticings were passed back to medical "professionals" of one stripe or another, sometimes in writing. Brodie (1994:161) reports that

> Knowlton asked the female attendants at a birth for their opinions about treatments and about their own histories of conception and pregnancy. These discussions of women's earlier reproductive histories were sometimes carried on in writing—an important point, for the fact that a brash and direct doctor like Knowlton communicated in written notes with his female patients suggests a shift to greater reliance on the written word.

REFLECTIONS

Kasarda et al. (1986) are correct. Research on classroom language and its very circumscribed acquisition suggests the assumption that the experience of formal education in one country is broadly equivalent to the experience of formal education in another is untenable. It seems likely that education always is socially situated. There is no satisfactory culture-free definition of education as an autonomous process of internalization.

Where are we, then, if our notions of the universal cognitive consequences of education are ill-founded while the statistical support for the idea that education is a powerful indirect determinant of mortality and fertility change remains? In her 1997 presidential address to the Population Association of America, Mason (1997:446,449) observes that explanations of fertility transition have been "set . . . up for failure" by "the tendency to assume that there is only one 'master' cause of all fertility transitions." To the contrary, she argues:

> Fertility transitions occur under a variety of institutional, cultural, and environmental conditions; they occur when *combinations* of conditions are sufficient to motivate or enable a substantial portion of the population to adopt birth prevention measures on a parity-specific basis.

Similarly, it seems likely that education influences fertility (and mortality) through a variety of combinations of links, not just one.

The consequences of education, including its links with fertility, may be expected to vary from one sort of student to another within national populations, as well as from one national population to another. Most research on the consequences of education appears to assume that those consequences are consistent and additive. A person who leaves school after three completed years gets three doses of something, a person who leaves school after seven years gets seven doses, and a person who leaves school as a college graduate after seventeen years gets seventeen doses, but the something is always the same. Not surprisingly, however, the classroom experiences of children in particular grades appear to be conditioned by aspects of their ascribed identities and their experiences prior to entering that grade. In the Carolina Piedmont, Trackton and Roadville children experience teachers who feel they, the children, are rude. Harbison and Hanushek's (1992) data from Northeast Brazil suggest that teachers respond differently to male and female students and that classes composed largely of children from farming families operate differently from classes composed largely of children from nonfarming families. Rather more sharply, Fine's New York research suggests that students from poor urban neighborhoods, largely racial and ethnic minorities, also receive differential treatment and leave school in disproportionate numbers, in part precisely because they reject that treatment. This and a great deal more evidence concerning what Fine (1991:200) calls "the vastly differential educations and outcomes made available to students by virtue of their social class, race/ethnicity, gender, sexual orientation, disability, and geography" suggests that schooling has different kinds of consequences for different kinds of people.

At a minimum, in large-scale quantitative studies it would be helpful to qualify measures of educational attainment such as years of education completed with some sense of the variety of individual educational histories and of the ways these weave through reproductive histories. Relatively simple measures of this variety might include years behind standard grade for individual students or the distribution by age of students in various grades. Because education is "a process with components rather than a cumulative trait" that interacts with fertility over the life course in complex ways, it may be necessary "to obtain educational histories with the same rigor as we obtain pregnancy histories" (Kasarda et al., 1986:106). This would follow the lead, especially, of Furstenberg et al. (1987).

At a maximum, it would be helpful to carry out much more intensive studies of single societies or groups of connected societies. This would follow the paths opened by the LeVines (1991) and Brodie (1994). Research along these lines would bring developments in the anthropology of education and literacy to bear on the recent upsurge of demographic interest in social interaction and "diffusion." Where they are produced by schooling, literacy and other educated practices are likely to be an important element in at least some of the "networks and other structures of social relationships" in which individuals "are embedded" and through which they exercise mutual influence (Montgomery and Casterline, 1996:152; see also Bongaarts and Watkins, 1997). Because they are unlikely to be the simple reflex of school practices and years of exposure to them, the educated practices of adults must be studied independently, in all their cultural specificity and historical contingency. Searching for multiple links between education and fertility may require new research strategies.

REFERENCES

Barton, D., and R. Ivanic
1991 *Writing in the Community*. Newbury Park: Sage Publications.

Bongaarts, J., and S. Watkins
1997 Social interactions and contemporary fertility transitions. *Population and Development Review* 22(4):639-682.

Bornstein, M.H., ed.
1989 *Maternal Responsiveness: Characteristics and Consequences*. San Francisco, Calif.: Jossey-Bass.

Brodie, J.F.
1994 *Contraception and Abortion in 19th-Century America*. Ithaca, N.Y.: Cornell University Press.

Bulatao, R., and R. Lee, eds.
1983 *Determinants of Fertility in Developing Countries*. New York: Academic Press.

Caldwell, J.
1980 Mass education as a determinant of the timing of fertility decline. *Population and Development Review* 6(2):225-255.

Carter, A.T.
1998 Cultural models and reproductive behavior. In A. Basu and P. Aaby, eds., *The Methods and Uses of Anthropological Demography*. Oxford: Oxford University Press.

Cicourel, A.V., and J.I. Kitsue
1963 *The Educational Decision-Makers*. Indianapolis, Ind.: Bobbs-Merrill.

Cleland, J., and G. Kaufmann
1998 Education, fertility and child survival: Unraveling the links. In A. Basu and P. Aaby, eds., *The Methods and Uses of Anthropological Demography*. Oxford: Oxford University Press.

Cochrane, S.H.
1979 *Fertility and Education: What Do We Really Know?* Baltimore, Md.: The Johns Hopkins University Press.

Cook-Gumperz, J.
1977 Situated instructions: Language socialization of school-age children. In S. Ervin-Tripp and C. Mitchell-Kernana, eds., *Child Discourse*. New York: Academic Press.

DeCastell, S., and T. Walker
1991 Identity, metamorphosis, and ethnographic research: What kind of story is ways with words? *Anthropology and Education Quarterly* 22:3-20.

Easterlin, R.A.
1978 The economics and sociology of fertility: A synthesis. In C. Tilly, ed., *Historical Studies of Changing Fertility*. Princeton, N.J.: Princeton University Press.
1983 Modernization and fertility: A critical essay. Pp. 562-586 in R. Bulatao and R. Lee, eds., *Determinants of Fertility in Developing Countries*. Volume 2. New York: Academic Press.

Erickson, F.D.
1987 Transformation and school success: The politics and culture of educational achievement. *Anthropology and Education Quarterly* 18:335-355.

Fine, M.
1991 *Framing Dropouts: Notes on the Politics of an Urban Public High School*. Albany, N.Y.: State University of New York Press.

Furet, F., and J. Ozouf
1982 *Reading and Writing: Literacy in France from Calvin to Jules Ferry*. Cambridge: Cambridge University Press.

Furstenberg, F.F., Jr., J. Brooks-Gunn, and S.P. Morgan
1987 *Adolescent Mothers in Later Life.* Cambridge: Cambridge University Press.

Gillis, J.R., L.A. Tilly, and D. Levine
1992 The quiet revolution. In J.R. Gillis, L.A. Tilly, and D. Levine, eds., *The European Experience of Declining Fertility.* Cambridge, Mass.: Blackwell Publishers.

Goody, J., and I. Watt
1962 The consequences of literacy. *Comparative Studies in Society and History* 5:304-345.

Gordon, L.
1977 *Woman's Body, Woman's Right: Birth Control in America.* New York: Penguin Books.

Greenfield, P.M.
1972 Oral or written language: The consequences for cognitive development in Africa, U.S. and England. *Language and Speech* 15(2):169-178.

Gumperz, J.J.
1986 Interactional sociolinguistics in the study of schooling. In J. Cook-Gumperz, ed., *The Social Construction of Literacy.* Cambridge: Cambridge University Press.

Hanks, W.F.
1996 *Language and Communicative Practices.* Boulder, Colo.: Westview Press.

Harbison, R.W., and E.A. Hanushek
1992 *Educational Performance of the Poor: Lessons from Rural Northeast Brazil.* New York: Oxford University Press.

Heath, S.B.
1983 *Ways with Words: Language, Life, and Work in Communities and Classrooms.* Cambridge: Cambridge University Press.
1993 The madness(es) of reading and writing ethnography. *Anthropology and Education Quarterly* 24:256-268.

Hildyard, A., and D. Olson
1978 *Literacy and the Specialisation of Language.* Toronto: Ontario Institute for Studies in Education (mimeographed).

Kasarda, J.D., J. Billy, and K. West
1986 *Status Enhancement and Fertility: Reproductive Responses to Social Mobility and Educational Opportunity.* Orlando, Fla.: Academic Press.

Lave, J.
1988 *Cognition in Practice.* Cambridge: Cambridge University Press.
1989 The acquisition of culture and the practice of understanding. In J. Stigler, R. Shweder, and G. Herdt, eds., *The Chicago Symposia on Human Development.* Cambridge: Cambridge University Press.
1991 Situated learning in communities of practice. In L.B. Resnick, J.M. Levine, and S.D. Teasley, eds., *Perspectives on Socially Shared Cognition.* Washington, D.C.: American Psychological Association.

Lave, J., and E. Wenger
1991 *Situated Learning: Legitimate Peripheral Participation.* Cambridge: Cambridge University Press.

LeVine, R.A.
1983 Fertility and child development: An anthropological view. In D. Wagner, ed., *Child Development and International Development: Research-Policy Interfaces.* San Francisco, Calif.: Jossey-Bass.
1987 Women's schooling, patterns of fertility and child survival. *Educational Researcher* 16:21-27.

LeVine, R.A., S.E. LeVine, A. Richman, F.M. Tapia Uribe, C. Sunderland Correa, and P.M. Miller
1991 Women's schooling and child care in the demographic transition: A Mexican case study. *Population and Development Review* 17(3):459-496.

LeVine, R.A., and S.C.M. Scrimshaw
1983 Effects of culture on fertility: Anthropological contributions. Pp. 666-695 in R. Bulatao and R. Lee, eds., *Determinants of Fertility in Developing Countries.* Volume 2. New York: Academic Press.
LeVine, R.A., and M.I. White
1986 *Human Conditions: The Cognitive Basis of Educational Development.* New York: Routledge and Kegan Paul.
Mason, K.O.
1997 Explaining fertility transitions. *Demography* 34(4):443-454.
McLaren, A.
1978 *Birth Control in Nineteenth-Century England.* London: Croom Helm.
Michaels, S.
1981 'Sharing time': Children's narrative styles and differential access to literacy. *Language in Society* 10(3):423-442.
Michaels, S., and J. Cook-Gumperz
1979 A study of sharing time with first-grade students: Discourse narratives in the classroom. Proceedings of the Fifth Annual Meetings of the Berkeley Linguistics Society. Berkeley, Calif.: University of California.
Minick, N.
1993 Teacher's directives: The social construction of 'literal meanings' and 'real worlds' in classroom discourse. In S. Chaiklin and J. Lave, eds., *Understanding Practice: Perspectives on Activity and Context.* Cambridge: Cambridge University Press.
Montgomery, M., and J. Casterline
1996 Social learning, social influence, and new models of fertility. *Population and Development Review* 22(Suppl.):151-175.
Pelissier, C.
1991 The anthropology of teaching and learning. *Annual Review of Anthropology* 20:75-95.
Rogoff, B.
1990 *Apprenticeship in Thinking: Cognitive Development in Social Context.* New York: Oxford University Press.
Rosen, H.
1985 The voices of communities and language in classrooms. *Harvard Educational Review* 55:448-456.
Schieffelin, B.B., and E. Ochs
1986 Language socialization. *Annual Review of Anthropology* 15:163-191.
Scollon, R., and S. Scollon
1979 *Linguistic Convergence: An Ethnography of Speaking at Fort Chipawyan, Alberta.* New York: Academic Press.
1981 *Narrative, Literacy, and Face in Interethnic Communication.* Norwood, N.J.: Ablex.
Seccombe, W.
1992 Men's 'marital rights' and women's 'wifely duties': Changing conjugal relations in the fertility decline. In J.R. Gillis, L.A. Tilly, and D. Levine, eds., *The European Experience of Declining Fertility.* Cambridge, Mass.: Blackwell Publishers.
Singh, S., and J. Casterline
1985 The socio-economic determinants of fertility. Pp. 199-222 in J. Cleland and J. Hobcraft, eds., *Reproductive Change in Developing Countries.* Oxford: Oxford University Press.
Snow, C.E.
1977 Mother's speech research: From input to interaction. In C.E. Snow and C.A. Ferguson, eds., *Talking to Children.* Cambridge: Cambridge University Press.

1990 The development of definitional skill. *Journal of Child Language* 17:697-710.
Street, B.V.
1984 *Literacy in Theory and Practice*. Cambridge: Cambridge University Press.
Street, B.V., ed.
1990 *Cross-cultural Approaches to Literacy*. Cambridge: Cambridge University Press.
Tilly, C., ed.
1978 *Historical Studies of Changing Fertility*. Princeton, N.J.: Princeton University Press.
Vincent, D.
1989 *Literacy and Popular Culture: England 1750-1914*. Cambridge: Cambridge University Press.
Willis, P.E.
1977 *Learning to Labour*. Westmead: Saxon House.

4
Implications of Formal Schooling for Girls' Transitions to Adulthood in Developing Countries

Cynthia B. Lloyd and Barbara Mensch

The main interest of demographers in the relationship between education and childbearing has been the negative association between years of schooling and achieved fertility among adult women, an interest that has spawned an extensive empirical literature on fertility differentials. The experience of being in school, however, occurs prior to adulthood, during childhood and adolescence, and involves much more than years of exposure to school. It is therefore surprising that demographers have paid little attention to the process and content of formal schooling and its more immediate implications for the maturation of girls. Specifically, there has been no investigation of the determinants of schooling duration and its attendant implications for the timing of entry into adulthood—a life cycle phase that, for females in most societies is synonymous with marriage or motherhood, whichever comes first. The timing of girls' entry into adulthood takes on particular demographic significance among most populations of the South, where rapid population growth is explained largely by the size of the population under 20 and the space between generations. However, no demographic study of which we are aware has attempted to open the schoolhouse door to see what happens inside and how this might affect the timing of girls' transitions to adulthood.

This chapter draws on insights from two literatures on education in developing countries in order to place the traditional demographic literature on education and fertility into a larger conceptual framework that focuses on successful transitions to adulthood. In reviewing these literatures, we take a particular interest in what they can tell us about how school provides different experiences for girls and for boys, as well as the role of formal schooling in gender role socialization.

We define a successful transition to adulthood not only as a delayed transition, but also one in which a young person is allowed to grow to develop her/his full potential physically, intellectually, and emotionally before taking on adult responsibilities such as bearing and rearing children or providing for their material support (or the support of other family members). Furthermore for girls, a successful transition to adulthood in a world in which adult men continue to hold greater power requires, in our view, not only the development of their human capital, but also the acquisition of a sense of self-esteem and personal mastery that will be necessary if they are to realize that potential in their public and private life.

The first education literature we review relates to school quality (or school effectiveness) and academic achievement in low-income countries. It is primarily an economic literature prepared from a Western perspective. Here, schooling is viewed as a production process. The goal is to identify critical inputs to formal schooling that contribute positively to the development of students' cognitive competencies as reflected in various standardized test scores. Few insights can be found in these studies about the nature or context of adolescents' daily lives in school, nor do they address how schooling might reinforce or change adolescents' learning and socialization, with consequences for their continuation in school or the timing of their entry into reproductive roles. However, much can be learned from this literature about elements of school quality that potentially have implications for school retention and transitions to adulthood.

The second literature relates to the role of formal schooling in the socialization process in traditional societies undergoing development. This literature is less easily characterized than the first and draws from anthropological studies as well as comparative education studies emerging from schools of education. It is particularly rich in African materials from which we draw many of our examples. From these studies one can develop a culturally oriented understanding of formal Western school as an institution situated within the larger society and of its role in the socialization of boys and girls. While this body of research offers a more textured description of schools than that provided by the schooling effectiveness literature, systematic comparative assessment of the schooling experience is rare, and rigorous empirical analysis linking life within the school to outcomes other than test scores has not, to our knowledge, been undertaken. However, as with the economic literature on education, much can be learned from this literature about potential characteristics of school that might be important in encouraging girls to remain in school into their late teens.

This chapter begins with some background on what is known from the demographic literature about the relationship between years of schooling and the subsequent demographic behavior of adolescents. This is followed by a discussion of the more immediate linkages between teenage pregnancy and continuation in school. From this background on the demographic importance of years of formal schooling, we shift our focus to the potential demographic implications of school quality and school experiences by reviewing in turn the literature on school effectiveness and that on schooling and socialization. Key points are illustrated with recent data on the primary schooling experience of adolescents collected in 3 of Kenya's 50 districts—Kilifi, Nakuru, and Nyeri—expressly to bring some empirical content to the many hypotheses that emerge from these literatures (Ajayi et al., 1997).[1] We conclude the discussion by proposing a broadened approach to the study of schooling that includes various dimensions of successful transitions to adulthood as the outcomes of schooling, and that extends the range of inputs traditionally used to capture school quality to include inputs having implications for other aspects of maturation beyond the development of cognitive competencies.

SCHOOLING AND THE SUBSEQUENT DEMOGRAPHIC BEHAVIOR OF ADOLESCENTS

The literature on schooling and the subsequent demographic behavior of adolescents focuses largely on the relationship between years of formal schooling and critical demographic events in girls' transition to adulthood. The duration of schooling or the achievement of critical levels is seen as a factor that can influence the timing of these events, a view that is based primarily on extensive empirical evidence of strong statistical associations. Evidence consistently shows that women with no or less than primary schooling tend to have earlier ages at marriage or first birth and higher subsequent fertility than those who have completed primary schooling (United Nations, 1995; Jejeebhoy, 1995; Ainsworth et al., 1996). The ages at marriage of secondary school graduates are usually higher still, with completed fertility being sharply lower. At the same time, the age at marriage and fertility of women with equal levels of schooling vary greatly among different societies, as does the relationship between years of schooling and age at marriage and fertility. For example, the extensive survey data assembled by Jejeebhoy (1995) show age at marriage among women with no schooling ranging from lows of 14.4 and 14.5, respectively, in Uttar Pradesh and

[1]Because the majority of adolescents who attend school in Africa are at the primary level and because performance in primary school is crucial in determining chances for further education, we draw on data collected from 36 primary schools in the three districts. These districts were selected to reflect the range of school experience in Kenya. Although data were also collected from 15 secondary schools in these districts, the secondary school sample is somewhat problematic. Note that in addition to visiting schools, interviewers also met with adolescents and their parents at their homes. In selecting sampling clusters and schools, the goal was to maximize the overlap between adolescents and schools. Indeed, 78 percent of adolescents interviewed in our household-based sample attended the primary schools that were visited in our school sample. Because secondary schools draw from a much larger area, the overlap is much smaller; thus the small sample of these schools cannot be considered fully representative of the secondary schools that young people in the sample would attend.

Maharashtra, India (1992-1993), to a high of 24 years in the Philippines (1978) and Costa Rica (1976). Small percentage differences (less than 10 percent) in age at marriage between women with no schooling and those with completed primary schooling can be observed in countries with both high and low ages at marriage.[2] Larger percentage differences in age at marriage (more than 25 percent) between women with no education and those with more than primary schooling are more typical and tend to be associated with lower ages at marriage among the unschooled (below 18); there are, however, numerous exceptions to this finding as well. While these findings clearly point to the importance of culture in explaining cross-country variations in the relationship between years of schooling and timing of marriage, they might also suggest the potential importance of variations in the content and quality of schooling.

In most developing countries, marriage or childbearing and continued schooling are typically incompatible; girls who become pregnant or marry are asked to leave school as a matter of policy. Such policies create the potential for a direct link between age at leaving school and age at entry into marriage and childbearing. In most societies, however, there is a gap between age at leaving school and age at marriage, so that many girls experience at least a few of their premarriage years of adolescence out of school. Therefore, the relationship between years of schooling and the timing of demographic events cannot be understood as a purely mechanistic one.

While it is clear that schools play an active role in the education and socialization of the next generation, little progress has been made to date in identifying what aspects of education are transforming in ways that ultimately matter for the timing of marriage and childbearing. Several recent studies hypothesize that education delays marriage and childbirth by enhancing the autonomy of women (Jejeebhoy, 1995), giving them more influence in marriage decisions and, through employment prior to marriage, greater control over resources (Jejeebhoy, 1995; see also Diamond et al., this volume). Using the same logic, these gains in autonomy should also give girls a greater say with their parents in prolonging their schooling, thus increasing their exposure to those aspects of schooling that affect these demographic processes.

Other researchers are more skeptical of the autonomy-enhancing effects of schooling for girls, given the strong gender role messages conveyed by teachers and textbooks and the fundamentally conservative nature of schooling. "The content of the curriculum and the way it is taught hold up an image of docility and modesty rather than self-assertion and reward girls who conform to it" (Jeffery and Basu, 1996:20). Moreover, education may reduce women's value in the

---

[2]Jejeebhoy (1995) made comparisons among those with no education, 1-3 years, 4-6 years, and 7+ years. Because most education systems have 5-6 years of primary school, individuals with 4-6 years cannot be assumed to have completed primary schooling. Therefore, we focus here on a comparison between those with 7+ and those with 0 years of schooling.

marriage market as a result of the universal tendency for women to marry "up." For example, in Bangladesh there is a "strong cultural preference for very young brides reflected in the common Bengali adage kuri te buri ('old at twenty'). . . . A girl who is married late requires a great amount of dowry to compensate for her reduced value to that groom's family" (Amin, 1996:197; see also Basu, this volume).

Possible outcomes of schooling other than enhanced autonomy may be more important determinants of demographic behavior (see also Diamond et al., this volume). For example, education leads to greater earning capacity, thereby increasing the opportunity cost of women's time. Other salient effects of schooling relate to the acquisition of specific bodies of knowledge or particular skills. The literature on maternal education and child mortality has struggled with identifying and documenting the mechanisms through which schooling of women improves the health outcomes of their offspring (see, for example, Cleland and van Ginneken, 1988; Kaufman and Cleland, 1994); some of the same pathways that are hypothesized in this literature may operate in the linkage with marriage and fertility. Even if schooling does not always produce literacy, time in a classroom may improve literacy skills, giving women the ability to understand decontextualized language, which in turn alters behavior (LeVine et al., 1994). Such language is used in health and family planning messages broadcast over the radio; it is also the means of discourse in clinics and pharmacies. Still another possibility is that education broadens one's outlook, "making citizens of those whose horizons had been largely confined to the family" (Caldwell, 1980:235). In exposing women to Western middle-class values and norms, education may challenge preconceived notions about the importance of early marriage and childbearing.

TEENAGE PREGNANCY AND CONTINUATION IN SCHOOL

In general, as noted earlier, continued attendance in school is possible only for young women who can avoid pregnancy or childbirth while in school—even while still in primary school, where most girls are when they reach adolescence because of delayed entry and/or grade repetition (Mensch and Lloyd, 1998). At the same time, the risks of pregnancy for unmarried adolescent girls may be affected both positively and negatively by schooling. For example, the availability of family-life education may provide girls with information about sexuality and contraception that would help them avoid pregnancy. On the other hand, schools may provide an environment that fosters sexual harassment of girls by both teachers and fellow students, thus increasing their pregnancy risk. In focus groups involving young people in Kenya, conducted as a prelude to our broader examination of schooling and the experience of adolescents, girls revealed how they were sexually harassed in school, while boys discussed how they harassed girls (Mensch and Lloyd, 1998). Recent reports of a mass rape of schoolgirls in

Kenya, by no means the first to be publicized (Mwati and Munyiri, 1996), reveal symptoms of a larger social problem.

In Africa, as elsewhere in the developing world, there is concern about the growing percentage of teenage births among the unmarried. Furthermore, the rapid expansion of education in the region has led to an increasing focus in the literature on the link between premarital childbearing and girls' dropping out of school, particularly out of secondary schools, where adolescents are assumed primarily to be enrolled (Ferguson, 1988; Meekers et al., 1995). However, there is no evidence that pregnancy is the principal reason for African girls' early withdrawal from school. The only study of which we are aware that has attempted to quantify dropouts directly attributable to pregnancy focused primarily on secondary schools in Kenya and did not collect data on dropouts for other reasons; thus comparisons with other causes of dropout were not possible (Ferguson, 1988). Yet this study did show reported dropouts due to pregnancy affecting only about 1 percent of girls in school each year (Ferguson, 1988), so that pregnancy is unlikely to be a leading proximate cause of dropping out despite the concern raised by the author of this report.

Furthermore, the literature on schoolgirl pregnancy in developing countries implicitly assumes that girls who are forced to withdraw from school because of pregnancy would have continued in school if they had not become pregnant. Yet there are many other reasons a girl might withdraw from school during her adolescence. Moreover, for those girls who do become pregnant, a nonsupportive school environment may increase the chances that they will give birth instead of seeking an abortion and continuing in school. Indeed, rather than pregnancy causing girls to drop out, the lack of social and economic opportunities for girls and women and the domestic demands placed on them, coupled with the gender inequities of the education system, may result in unsatisfactory school experiences, poor academic performance, and acquiescence in or endorsement of early motherhood.

In marked contrast to the absence of studies from developing-country settings, there is a considerable literature on the consequences of teenage childbearing for school completion (as well as other socioeconomic outcomes) in the United States. Early U.S. studies concluded that childbearing disrupts the educational careers of adolescents, and, as in current reports from Kenya, identified pregnancy as the primary reason for dropping out among females (Furstenberg, 1976; Trussell, 1976; Mott and Marsiglio, 1985). While these studies attempted to control for confounding factors, they did not consider the possibility that teenage reproductive behavior may be endogenous to school completion, leading to inflated estimates of the effect of early fertility (Ribar, 1994; Hoffman et al., 1993; Geronimus and Korenman, 1992; Ahn, 1994). The question is whether the association between adolescent childbearing and dropping out of school is due at least in part to the birth itself interrupting education, or whether it is due to some underlying set of attributes—measurable or unobserved—that induce both early birth and early dropping out. Such issues led us to explore the other literatures on education noted earlier for what they can tell us about the association between the quality of the schooling experience—as regards both cognitive competencies and gender equity—and schooling outcomes.

SCHOOL QUALITY AND ACADEMIC ACHIEVEMENT

In the economic literature on the effects of school quality in developing countries, researchers have focused primarily on the direct relationship between school quality (variously defined) and academic achievement as measured by student performance on standardized tests (Fuller and Clarke, 1994; Harbison and Hanushek, 1992; Lockheed et al., 1991; Fuller, 1987; Heyneman and Loxley, 1983; Tan et al., 1997) and only secondarily on unraveling the links among school inputs, enrollment and retention, and ultimate achievement (Card and Krueger, 1996). These production-function studies conclude that school quality matters for immediately measurable school outcomes (Hanushek, 1995), but there is little consensus about how to define school quality or about what dimensions of quality actually make a difference. Indeed, quality is often measured in terms not of specific inputs such as the number of desks, the credentials of the teachers, or the availability of laboratory equipment, but of correlates such as financial resources per student or class size.

Furthermore, this literature gives little attention to teacher attitudes or classroom dynamics as elements of school quality or to those aspects of the school and classroom environment that may result in different experiences for boys and girls. One notable exception of which we are aware from our comprehensive review of the African literature is Appleton (1995), who studied gender differences in performance on exams in Kenya and found both parents' and teachers' attitudes about the natural ability of boys and girls to be significantly correlated with differentials in performance. At the same time, it may be noted that the concern with regard to including attitudinal variables in a production function of school inputs and outputs is that they may be jointly determined, in that gender differences in actual performance may be a factor in shaping teachers' attitudes.

The benefit an adolescent derives from a good school is directly related to the amount of time he or she spends there. In studying the links between school quality and adolescent educational achievement, it is necessary to understand not only the various elements of good schooling, but also which elements in particular encourage enrollment, attendance, and continuation. Studies of the determinants of school enrollment and attainment, however, have focused primarily on the measurement and assessment of family factors because of their clear importance (e.g., Hill and King, 1993; Lloyd and Blanc, 1996) and have paid little attention, beyond the anecdotal, to school characteristics. The relationship between school characteristics and the length of time adolescents spend in school is rarely explored directly (for two exceptions see Glewwe and Jacoby, 1994, and

Hanushek and Lavy, 1994; see also Glewwe, this volume); the evidence cited, even from the U.S. literature, is primarily indirect and suggestive, rather than conclusive (Card and Krueger, 1996). Indeed, it was with that research gap in mind that we designed a study in Kenya to systematically collect data on the school environment, as well as to collect data from a sample of adolescents and parents in the same communities (see Ajayi et al., 1997).[3]

Adapting the framework developed by Lockheed et al. (1991) to assess school effectiveness, we concentrate on evidence related to three broad elements of the educational process that have some independent support in the literature as being salient for academic achievement: (1) time to learn, such as hours spent in class and time spent using available facilities; (2) material inputs, such as books, desks, libraries, laboratories, and playing fields; and (3) effective teaching, including pedagogical practices and teacher competency. Our interest is in identifying which elements might have different effects on boys and girls and as a consequence might have implications for school retention.

Time to Learn

There is broad consensus in the education literature that the amount of time effectively dedicated to learning in school is directly related to positive educational outcomes (Lockheed et al., 1991). Many factors can detract from learning time, and some can affect boys and girls differently. School-based factors include disruptions due to teacher absence, ceremonial events, and time out of class for domestic chores or punishment. Anthropological evidence from West Africa suggests that girls are sometimes asked to do more domestic chores than boys, with the consequence that their learning time is reduced relative to boys (Biraimah, 1980; Anderson-Levitt et al., 1998). In our Kenyan survey, we collected data on various aspects of learning time. From our primary school data, based on a sample of mainly mixed schools where boys and girls can be compared within the same school settings, we found that a slightly higher percentage of girls than boys performed chores during the day prior to the survey (72 versus 64 percent in Kilifi, 79 versus 71 percent in Nakuru, and 77 versus 64 percent in Nyeri), and on average, girls performed slightly more chores than boys (.95 versus .80 in Kilifi, .96 versus .83 in Nakuru, and 1.02 versus .80 in Nyeri). However, these differences are not large. Rates of punishment for girls varied by district, being highest in Kilifi, where overall exam scores are lowest, and lowest

[3]It must be recognized that schools are not necessarily distributed randomly, but their placement and quality may be influenced by national political forces, as well as community and family factors. For example, poorer districts may be allocated more resources by the government or, alternatively, less if the wealthy are politically influential. Furthermore, for communities with school choice, parents can chose the school that most embodies their values and tastes in education, or they can move to a community with preferable schools, thus complicating the empirical distinction between school effects and community or household effects.

in Nyeri, where school performance is much higher. On the other hand, rates of punishment for boys did not vary systematically by district. As for sex differences in punishment, girls were slightly more likely to be punished in Kilifi and Nakuru and boys more likely in Nyeri. That girls in any of the three districts were more likely to be punished came as a surprise, given that girls are generally thought to be better behaved than boys. However, in Kenya punishment in school is often the result of poor performance, and girls in Kenya do worse than boys academically. On balance, there does not appear to be strong evidence that boys and girls in Kenya differ in quantitatively important ways with regard to the time available for learning within mixed school environments (Ajayi et al., 1997).

One additional factor that is sometimes seen to increase learning time, particularly for girls, is sex-segregated classes or single-sex schools. Studies in Nigeria and Thailand have shown higher math achievement for girls in single-sex relative to mixed schools, but lower achievement for boys when schools with similar resources are compared. One factor identified is the greater amount of time spent on instruction in all-girl relative to mixed schools. A problem that plagues these studies, however, is the high-income elasticity of demand for single-sex schooling for girls, making it difficult to disentangle the role of the school from the role of family factors in determining these outcomes. In our Kenyan study, we found that the educational background of parents of girls in single-sex secondary schools (such schools are rare at the primary level) was significantly higher than that of parents of boys in single-sex secondary schools, which was higher again than that of parents of boys and girls in mixed secondary schools. Furthermore, we found no evidence of differences in the length of the school day in all-boy versus all-girl schools.

Other dimensions of school quality can affect time to learn indirectly to the extent that they influence daily attendance rates. For example, inadequate toilet facilities could deter girls from attending on days when they are menstruating. We found no evidence that this was the case in Kenya, however, where less than 3 percent of adolescent girls currently enrolled in school who had reached menarche reported staying home when menstruating. This pattern exists despite descriptions of appallingly dirty toilets with little privacy even in high-performing schools (Mensch and Lloyd, 1998). Another dimension of time to learn is the degree of participation in teacher-student classroom interaction. The literature indicates that girls participate in such interaction less frequently than boys and thus have fewer opportunities to be engaged in active learning (e.g., Grisay, 1984). Our own Kenyan data show fewer teacher-student interactions for girls than for boys in a standard-sized class of normal duration (20.2 versus 16.7 in Kilifi, 16.7 versus 14.7 in Nakuru, and 16.7 versus 15.6 in Nyeri).[4]

[4]In each school visited, math and English classes were observed, and the interactions between teachers and students were counted. The numbers reported are the average for a standard class lasting 40 minutes and containing 20 boys and 20 girls (see Ajayi et al., 1997).

Material Inputs

Various material inputs affect school quality, including (1) the availability of instructional materials (e.g., textbooks, desks, library, science laboratory), (2) the condition of and access to basic facilities (classrooms, toilets, and playing fields), (3) the availability of certain amenities (water, electricity, transport), and (4) school-specific elements of the curriculum that go beyond the core (such as sports, clubs, and family-life education). Over the past decade, researchers have found that the availability of textbooks and other instructional materials has a consistently positive effect on student achievement in developing countries (Heyneman and Loxley, 1983). For example, girls' schools have been found to have inferior science equipment relative to boys' schools, which may undermine the content of the science curriculum and contribute to girls' poorer performance on examinations (Herz et al., 1991; Kinyanjui, 1993).[5]

A recent study evaluated the impact on average test scores of increasing the supply of textbooks in poor schools in Kenya (Kremer et al., 1997). The study found that the program stimulated such an increase in enrollment in the experimental schools that the positive effects of additional textbooks on test scores were negated by the negative consequences of the increased enrollment. This study provides direct evidence of the potential responsiveness of enrollment to changes in school inputs and underscores the importance of disentangling the effects of school quality on cognitive competencies from its effects on enrollment and retention.

There has been less attention in the literature to other material inputs to schooling, which, while less directly linked to academic learning, may have important implications for gender differences in the quality of the school experience and may affect girls' continuation in school. We have already mentioned the potential consequences of inadequate toilet facilities for opportunities to learn. Lack of privacy in toilets can also provide opportunities for sexual harassment, a further discouragement to girls (see Anderson-Levitt et al., 1998, for recent evidence from Guinea). In our Kenyan sample, witnesses observed harassment of girls by boys around the toilets in 62 percent of the schools visited in Nyeri, 20 percent in Nakuru, but none in Kilifi, suggesting that the problem arises only in certain settings (Ajayi et al., 1997).

Family-life education, even if provided to both sexes, can have differential benefits for girls given their greater vulnerability and the risks they face in terms

[5]Ironically, the literature on gender equity in education argues for the establishment of more girls' schools because of the better performance on exams of girls who have attended single-sex schools (Herz et al., 1991). Yet this finding may have less to do with the inherent superiority of single-sex education than it has to do with the fact that where there is an option of mixed or single-sex schools, the latter attract the elite. (See the earlier discussion of time to learn.)

of pregnancy and school continuation. In our Kenyan survey, we found that topics such as sexuality and family planning were rarely taught as part of family-life education, and even where they were taught, appeared to have no effect on the students' knowledge or understanding of pregnancy risks (Ajayi et al., 1997). Only about a third of students in primary schools were able to give correct answers to questions on pregnancy risk.

Other material inputs with a potential gender dimension include sports facilities for girls. Even the casual traveler in developing-country settings is struck by the common sight of groups of boys kicking a ball around during their free time after school or on weekends. Girls are rarely seen in similar circumstances. The question arises as to whether these differences are reinforced within the school environment through the sports curriculum and facilities provided for boys and girls. Evidence from developed countries suggests that sports are important for adolescents in developing a sense of teamwork, goal setting, competition, and the pursuit of excellence in performance, as well in improving health (Brady, 1998). A particular benefit of sports for girls that is hypothesized in the literature is the development of self-esteem. While we found no evidence from our Kenyan data that sports facilities within the school environment were less available for girls than for boys, we expect this finding is atypical of most developing-country settings, where athletic facilities for girls are generally inferior, and their use is often discouraged. Indeed, in Pakistan "from grade 1 onwards public school girls are taught to cover their heads and refrain from participating in sports" (Shaheed and Mumtaz, 1993:70-71). Our Kenyan findings can probably be explained by the widespread availability in schools of netball, a sport played only by girls that is common in Britain and its former colonies and requires less space than other sports.

Effective Teaching

The most consistent finding with respect to teacher credentials and effective teaching is the importance of teachers' knowledge of the subject matter and their verbal proficiency (Cleghorn et al., 1989; Fuller and Clarke, 1994). There is no consistent evidence that girls perform better with female than with male teachers (Abraha et al., 1991; Fuller et al., 1994; Appleton, 1995), except possibly in single-sex schools, where female teachers deal exclusively with female students (Lee and Lockheed, 1990). In the case of Kenya, where better schools (at least insofar as performance on the primary school leaving exam is concerned) appear to have a higher ratio of female-to-male teachers than is found in the weaker schools, there appear to be no differences between male and female teachers in either credentials or attitudes. This finding suggests that any positive effects female teachers may have on girls may be explained largely in terms of serving as a role model of a professional woman, rather than providing any special encouragement.

Summary

The production function approach to the study of school effectiveness in developing countries has led to many frustrations. School inputs that appear statistically important in one context are unimportant in others. Furthermore, gender differences that appear potentially important in one context do not bear out systematically. In a recent review of the literature, Fuller and Clarke (1994) make a strong appeal for the recognition of culture and context in the linking of inputs to outputs. They also draw attention to another group of education researchers whom they classify as "classroom culturalists":

> These observers of schools focus on the normative socialization that occurs within classrooms: the value children come to place on individualistic versus cooperative work, legitimated forms of adult authority and power and acquired attitudes toward achievement and modern forms of status. (p. 120)

In the discussion that follows, we seek guidance from this second body of literature relating to the role of formal schooling in the socialization process in traditional societies undergoing development.

SCHOOLING, GENDER, AND SOCIALIZATION

In a modernizing society, formal Western-style schooling provides a new context within which socialization takes place. While there is strong evidence that the formal school curriculum is becoming increasingly homogeneous across societies, reflecting the emergence of a global culture (Meyer et al., 1992), school administrators and teachers can be creative in finding ways to adapt, reinterpret, and transmit traditional gender systems and modes of learning in this new educational context. Bledsoe (1992) uses Sierra Leone to illustrate how Western education has been transformed to reflect the traditional culture. In traditional Mende society, knowledge is power; the elders within the community, who have special knowledge, control access to that knowledge and seek gain in exchange for sharing it. Knowledge does not have value in itself unless it is imparted in the appropriate way. Through an exchange, the recipient is properly "blessed," and the giver is recompensed. "Since blessings legitimate rights to certain domains of knowledge, how children learn is as important as what they actually learn" (Bledsoe, 1992:192). In a village study conducted in rural Madagascar, Bloch (1993) found that the uncritical acceptance of knowledge acquired in school could be explained in terms of its association with the wisdom of elders in the community. The knowledge of elders is seen to be absolute and morally true because it emanates from ancestors and beyond, but at the same time it is seen as irrelevant for practical day-to-day activities. The "chalk and talk" (Fuller and Snyder, 1991) approach to teaching in most classrooms, where the teacher is vocal, dominant, and often punitive, takes on new meaning when one understands the link between traditional authority structures and the transmission of knowledge in different cultural contexts.

This approach to the transmission of knowledge in traditional societies gives school principals and teachers special power and authority and potentially makes girls, particularly during their adolescence, especially vulnerable. School principals, teachers, and students bring their knowledge and experience with gender systems in the traditional culture into the school and into the classroom. These systems are adapted and reinforced through the daily interactions between teacher and students and among students, as well as through the formal curriculum; the content of required texts; and formal administrative rules and regulations, which operate through the distribution of rewards, punishments, and duties. In states that were formerly colonies, some of the values and educational goals of the early missionaries and colonial administrators may also be reflected in administrative and teaching practices (Yates, 1982).

Administrative Practices

Certain school policies and administrative practices convey strong messages to boys and girls about their respective roles and social status. Policies requiring the expulsion of girls who are found to be pregnant (but not of the boys who are equally responsible) and preventing their readmission to the same school suggest to both boys and girls that society values the education of boys more than that of girls and gives girls a disproportionate responsibility for pregnancy prevention in a context of unequal power in sexual relations. In Malawi, for example, there are school policies that either differ for girls and boys or are differentially enforced. To illustrate, children are traditionally supposed to kneel when speaking to their parents, a courtesy that is also extended to teachers. However, while girls are compelled to do so, "male students were seldom observed kneeling when they spoke to teachers and even those who did were more likely to crouch than actually kneel" (Hyde, 1994:19). As another example, to "protect" girls at boarding schools (where about half of girls attending secondary school in Malawi are enrolled) there are rules confining them to crowded dorms in the evening and early morning, whereas boys are allowed to use classrooms and other rooms to study (Hyde, 1994). Other practices that embody messages to boys and girls may include uniform policies, the assignment of different types of school duties to boys and girls, the provision of different extracurricular activities, or the differential assignment of honors and awards. In our Kenyan study, we found evidence that boys receive twice as many of the academic prizes as girls on average, but this is in a context in which boys outperform girls in most subjects (Mensch and Lloyd, 1998). Nevertheless, while awards may have been given fairly to the top students, who are typically boys, the practice of giving awards in mixed schools in such a context conveys strong and discouraging messages to girls, who may already suffer from low self-esteem.

Curriculum

Messages conveyed through school policies and administrative and teacher practices are heavily reinforced by centrally designed teaching materials, which rigidly reinforce cultural notions of appropriate gender roles. "In developing countries, textbooks transmit heavily stereotyped images of men and women, with women adopting low profiles and having traits of passivity, dependence on men, low intelligence and [a lack of] leadership" (Stromquist, 1994:2409). An analysis of the gender content of Kenyan textbooks found images of women appearing much less frequently than those of men; when women are depicted, they typically are in a position subordinate to men and are portrayed in fewer types of roles, and their physical appearance is assigned more importance than their achievement (Obura, 1991). A survey from the Middle East found that females were most frequently depicted as mothers and little girls in Arabic textbooks (El-Sanabary, 1993). Latin American textbooks also portray women as housewives and mothers; "when working women are shown, they hold jobs traditionally associated with female nurturing (teaching, nursing, and domestic service)" (Bustillo, 1993:193). Sometimes the stereotyped images of females go beyond the traditional and are quite negative, particularly by comparison with the images of men. In Pakistan, while "attributes such as bravery, rationality, respectability and humaneness are all associated with males, . . . women, especially in Urdu textbooks, are quite prominently portrayed as cunning, careless, noncooperative, and repentant" (Shaheed and Mumtaz, 1993:69).

While textbooks reinforce traditional images of women, the curriculum available to girls has been said to limit their options (see, for example, Hyde, 1993, and El-Sanabary, 1993). Unfortunately, however, the literature on the content of education has failed to investigate systematically whether girls and boys actually take different courses or are discouraged by teachers from pursuing specific academic subjects. For example, Benavot and Kamens (1989) conducted an exhaustive review of the curriculum policies of primary schools in developing countries, but did not address the issue of gender differences in curricular content. It has been asserted—although not documented—that in technical schools in Africa, the curriculum for girls is restricted to secretarial and home economics courses, while boys have the option of pursuing carpentry, welding, mechanical drawing, electronics, and the like (Njeuma, 1993). In some countries, a "home science" curriculum is designed exclusively for girls for the express purpose of reinforcing gender stereotypes by preparing girls for their socially prescribed roles (Herrera, 1992).

Family-life education, discussed earlier in the context of school quality, has the potential to convey empowering messages to adolescent girls and boys. Moreover, the content of the material presented is of great importance for the reproductive health and well-being of adolescents. A lack of information about sex and contraception may not only increase the risk of sexually transmitted diseases for both boys and girls, but also, if it leads to pregnancy, jeopardize girls' continued enrollment in school (Mensch and Lloyd, 1998). While there has been no exhaustive survey of family-life education programs in schools, the United Nations Population Fund reports it has supported such programs in 79 countries. Most of these programs are didactic in nature and "focus on helping young people plan productive lives" (McCauley et al., 1995:23). Although systematic evaluation of the content and efficacy of family-life education in developing-country settings has not been undertaken,[6] there is suspicion that sensitive issues, including gender-power dynamics and sexual relations, are ignored. Thus one observer has asserted that "when sex education evolved into family life education, much of the key sexuality content was removed" (Senderowitz, 1995:30). Perhaps expectations about the efficacy of family-life education programs are unrealistically high. A review of such programs in several African countries is quite pessimistic about their ability to affect attitudes and behavior, arguing that the solution to early and unprotected adolescent sex is not to be found "in the education of the young" because "male promiscuity and, by extension, female availability has remained unchallenged in most of our societies" (Hyde, 1997:22).

Teacher Attitudes

To the extent that there are empirical studies of teacher attitudes toward girls, they tend to be purely descriptive in nature, lacking analytical links to outcomes such as performance and retention. The picture that emerges from this body of research is not particularly complimentary. School-based studies often report negative expectations and attitudes toward girls on the part of both male and female teachers. In Togo, for example, teachers disparaged their female students, characterizing them as "disruptive" or as "lack[ing] interest in school," whereas they described male students as "responsible," "hardworking," and "scholarly" (Biraimah, 1980). Positive attributes for girls related mainly to their appearance. In Malawi, teachers depicted girls as less "serious" and capable (Davidson and Kanyuka, 1992), less interested in their schoolwork, and sometimes lazy (Hyde, 1997). In Guinea, teachers described boys as able to learn lessons well, more likely to participate in class and provide "good" responses to teachers' questions, and "ambitious," whereas girls were typically described as well behaved but timid and not as hardworking as boys (Anderson-Levitt et al., 1998).

---

[6]School-based programs have been extensively evaluated in the United States. The initial goal was to respond to the concern that sex education programs may actually hasten the onset of intercourse by encouraging experimentation. None of the 26 studies investigated found an increase in the age of sexual initiation. Examination of the efficacy of such programs in reducing the frequency of sex and the number of sexual partners and increasing contraceptive use produced mixed findings (Kirby, 1995).

The reasons teachers give for boys' better academic performance often relate to negative attributes of girls rather than positive attributes of boys (Davidson and Kanyuka, 1992). Of particular interest in this regard are the responses of Kenyan primary school teachers in Appleton's (1995) study to the question: "Girls tend to do less well in the primary leaving exam. Why do you think this is?" The largest number of responses were related to the effects of adolescence on girls, who become disturbed by their bodily changes, lose interest in school, become more interested in boys and in their own appearance, and suffer from mood swings. Other responses were related to sexuality, immorality, and pregnancy. Male and female teachers gave similar responses, although female teachers were slightly more likely to mention adolescence, whereas male teachers were more likely to mention girls' interest in boys. It may be noted that Appleton was careful to use general terms in phrasing questions to teachers and parents that applied to men and women or boys and girls in order to identify attitudes formed outside the immediate context of the study.

In our Kenyan study, the most striking findings about teacher attitudes emerged from questions about teachers' preference for the teaching of boys or girls (Ajayi et al., 1997). Of those primary school teachers who said they preferred teaching one sex over the other, the overwhelming preference was for boys. Overall, an average of 22 percent of primary school teachers said they preferred teaching boys, while only 5 percent said they preferred teaching girls. This discrepancy was most marked in Nyeri (one of the best-performing districts in Kenya as measured by school exam scores), where 33 percent preferred boys and 6 percent girls, and least marked in Kilifi. Overall, an average of 39 percent of Nyeri teachers expressed a preference for one sex over the other, while only 10 percent of Kilifi teachers did so; on the other hand, 63 percent of Nyeri teachers felt students learn better in mixed classes, while only 38 percent of Kilifi teachers held this opinion. Perhaps surprisingly, female teachers in every district expressed a stronger preference for boys than did their male counterparts.

We also investigated teachers' gender role attitudes by asking about the importance of various subjects for girls and boys and the relative ease with which boys and girls learn each subject (Ajayi et al., 1997). In general, primary school teachers believe math is somewhat more important for boys to learn than for girls and that English is about equally important for both. Teachers also appear to believe very strongly that English is easier for girls than for boys: an average of 52 percent of teachers overall hold this opinion, while just 4 percent consider English easier for boys. Opinions about gender differences in math are even stronger: 67 percent of teachers, averaged overall, said math is easier for boys, while no teacher said math is easier for girls. These relationships hold, with some variation, in each of the three districts.

School and Classroom Dynamics

How might the attitudes described above affect the interactions within the classroom between teachers and students, as well as between boys and girls? Bellew and King (1993:311), note that "empirical evidence is lacking from developing countries to support or refute the hypothesis that teachers' interactions with female students discourage girls' attendance or achievement." Yet there is some evidence in the literature that girls do indeed participate less in the classroom because they volunteer less (Biraimah, 1980; Anderson-Levitt et al., 1998). Although there is no systematic evidence that teachers are actively biased against the classroom participation of girls, in that they appear to select fairly from among those who volunteer, their passive response to the sexual differential that emerges results in uneven treatment nonetheless (Biraimah, 1989). This fair but passive behavior of teachers may be particularly powerful in reinforcing gender attitudes and expectations among students in a context where the culture prescribes different forms of knowledge and different styles of learning for boys and girls (Fuller et al., 1994). It may also explain why the introduction of teaching practices that are viewed positively in the West, such as more open-ended questioning and discussion and the use of programmed teaching and instructional materials, may sometimes appear to accentuate rather than alleviate gender differences. For example, Fuller et al. (1994) found that teachers' greater use of open-ended questioning reduced girls' advantage in learning English. Similarly, the introduction of a programmed teaching approach in Liberia resulted in improved performance on average for both boys and girls, but greater gender differentiation in favor of boys than was observed with more conventional approaches (Boothroyd and Chapman, 1987).

Inspired by the work of Sadker and Sadker (1995), who documented the subtleties of gender bias in U.S. classrooms through many hours of observation of the quality and nature of student-teacher interactions, we designed a classroom observation instrument for our Kenyan study that involved counting and assessing student-teacher interactions during a class period:

> Our goal was to assess whether teachers pay more attention to boys and provide them with more encouragement or whether they treat girls and boys equitably. In constructing variables to measure "good interaction" we tried to include all events recorded by our observers that had a positive or supportive tone—or at least those that did not have a negative one. Thus, we included instances of students reading aloud; students making presentations in front of the class, teachers instructing or explaining; teachers acknowledging, extending, amplifying or praising correct answers; teachers completing explaining or seeking responses to student questions; and teachers positively acknowledging, expanding upon or encouraging student comments. (Mensch and Lloyd, 1998:176)

Our results indicated small but systematic differences between boys and girls in the number of positively toned interactions with their teachers (in a class standardized for duration and composition, see footnote 4). Teachers had, on average, 15.4 positively toned interactions with boys and only 13.8 such interactions with girls, with consistent differences found in all three districts.

Gender relations in the larger society are also reflected in the way girls and boys interact with each other in school and what behaviors are tolerated by the school administration. We have much anecdotal evidence from the field assistants in our Kenyan study that the schools worked hard to show their best side to our observation teams despite our assurances that we were not part of a school inspection team. Nonetheless, we were able to observe systematic differences in the extent of bullying and harassment of girls by boys and of boys by girls. In the majority of schools in each district, boys were observed harassing girls. On the other hand, in only 10 percent or less of the schools in each district were girls observed to be harassing boys (Ajayi et al., 1997). In such an environment, girls may come to develop a sense of inferiority and powerlessness vis-à-vis the opposite sex.

Physical Maturation and School Attendance

Tensions between the traditional culture and formal schooling are particularly visible when children stay in school past the point of physical maturation or the onset of puberty. Parents in traditional societies exert control over their daughters' sexuality; initiation ceremonies for both boys and girls that are tied to puberty define the beginning of social adulthood. The knowledge gained during these ceremonies readies young men and women for marriage and a sexual life (Hyde and Kadzamira, 1994). In such settings, the persistence of girls in school causes social confusion; a schoolgirl is viewed as a child from a social point of view, whereas a girl who has been initiated (or circumcised) is considered a social adult. One reason many school systems in developing countries are reluctant to introduce family-life education may be that they see it as conveying privileged adult information to pupils who must remain children if they are to stay in school.

Bledsoe (1990) emphasizes the symbolic importance of the school uniform, which, like the clothes worn by girls during initiation ceremonies, conveys their status as initiates or trainees who should be recognized as belonging to a protected class. In many settings, however, wearing a uniform is not sufficient to protect girls from the sexual advances of fellow students and teachers. A schoolgirl's sexuality can be exploited by powerful teachers who are able to manipulate their position of privilege to seek recompense for their support or "blessings." At the same time, in a period of rapidly rising school fees, a schoolgirl's sexuality can become an asset, if carefully managed, to help finance her school fees. Bledsoe (1990) describes the complex symbolism of school fees in the marriage negotiations of the Mende of Sierra Leone and the simultaneous risks and opportunities conveyed to girls through their participation in school as sexually mature adolescents.

SCHOOL AS A FACTOR IN SUCCESSFUL TRANSITIONS TO ADULTHOOD

The socialization literature and the economic and demographic literatures previously reviewed appear to be saying quite different things about the benefits of schooling for girls. In the demographic literature, formal schooling is seen as uniformly positive in that it leads women to delay marriage and childbearing, and ultimately to bear fewer children and invest more in each. In the economic literature, good schools enhance cognitive competencies, with lifetime benefits in terms of higher earnings. On the other hand, in the socialization literature, schools are seen as conservative institutions that reinforce the gender inequalities present in the surrounding society. It would seem that schools are simultaneously reinforcing existing gender bias and inducing more modern forms of behavior that have the potential to help women acquire marketable skills, useful information, and a more modern and global outlook.

To understand the processes that underlie these apparently contradictory outcomes, the production-function approach needs to be broadened to allow for the assessment of a wider range of inputs and outputs. On the input side, not enough attention has been given to teacher attitudes and classroom dynamics. On the output side, not enough attention has been given to school attendance and retention on the one hand and reproductive outcomes on the other. As a first step in this direction, we have estimated the effects of various dimensions of primary school quality, including gender differences in student perceptions and experiences, on dropout rates in Kenya. We have found that, while household factors remain overwhelmingly important in explaining girls' higher dropout rates, gender differences in treatment within the school are also statistically important explanatory factors (Lloyd and Mensch, 1998).

How can formal schooling make a positive contribution to successful transitions to adulthood as defined at the beginning of this chapter? First, it can provide sufficient support and encouragement to parents and students so that students can attend formal schooling for the number of years necessary to acquire critical knowledge and skills.[7] Second, it can convey a range of academic and practical knowledge and teach both marketable and other life skills. Third, it can provide a protective environment that removes students from the risks of harassment and sexual exploitation while attending school. Fourth, it can treat boys and girls equally and teach values of fairness and equality. The first of these at-

[7]This statement assumes no compulsory schooling laws or limited enforcement—the typical situation in most developing countries.

tributes of school effectiveness becomes a prerequisite for the other three in that each additional year of exposure to school allows those other attributes to operate over a longer period of time. Thus school factors affecting retention become critical to school effectiveness. For this reason, it is surprising that the school effectiveness literature has had so little to say on factors affecting retention.

What might those factors be? Clearly the traditional three factors of time to learn, material inputs, and effective teaching play a role. Students will be encouraged to continue in school when they perform well. But within any school, there will always be students at the top of the class and others at the bottom.

What are the school factors that might encourage continued attendance among middling and lower-ranked students and continued support among their parents? Here teachers' attitudes are likely to be critical. In Kenya, where girls underperform boys in all subjects except Kiswahili and English in the primary leaving exam, girls begin to drop out of school at an earlier age than boys because of their poorer performance. Yet we know that this poorer performance cannot be explained by underlying differences between boys and girls in basic aptitude because in many other settings, girls' exam performance is equal to or better than that of boys at this level of schooling. Therefore, forces must be at work in the schools and/or in the larger society that discourage girls, leading simultaneously to poorer performance and increased dropout rates. Again the most likely culprit within the schools is the gender role attitudes of teachers, identified by Appleton (1995) as a key factor in girls' poorer performance on exams in Kenya.

Because of the strength of the association between education and both fertility and child mortality, demographers have stressed the critical role of years of schooling and hypothesized at length about the pathways of influence.[8] In contrast to demographers, economists have begun to realize the importance of opening the schoolhouse door. They increasingly recognize that inadequate attention to school quality can bias estimates of the effects of education on a range of outcomes, including cognitive competencies, school attainment, earnings, fertility, and mortality. To date, however, they have focused their energy on identifying which school inputs are most effective in raising academic achievement. This particular outcome by its very nature produces a list of inputs that is too narrow. Throughout this chapter and our previous work in this area (Mensch and Lloyd, 1998), we have argued that school is a critical institution not just because of its traditional role in expanding knowledge and cognitive skills, but also because of its more intangible role in socializing adolescents to be productive adults. If we are interested in successful transitions to adulthood, we must widen our definition of school quality and pay particular attention to the ways in which school as a social institution delays transitions to adulthood and empowers or undermines the next generation.

[8]This phrase comes from Cleland and van Ginneken (1988).

REFERENCES

Abraha, S., A. Beyene, T. Dubale, B.S. Holloway, and E. King
1991 What factors shape girls, school performance? Evidence from Ethiopia. *International Journal of Educational Development* 11(2):107-118.

Ahn, N.
1994 Teenage childbearing and high school completion: Accounting for individual heterogeneity. *Studies in Family Planning* 26(1):17-21.

Ajayi, A., W. Clark, A. Erulkar, K. Hyde, C.B. Lloyd, B.S. Mensch, C. Ndeti, and B. Ravitch
1997 *Schooling and the Experience of Adolescents in Kenya.* Nairobi, Kenya: Population Council.

Ainsworth, M., K. Beegle, and A. Nyamete
1996 The impact of women's schooling on fertility and contraceptive use: A study of fourteen SubSaharan African communities. *World Bank Economic Review* 10(1):85-122.

Amin, S.
1996 Female education and fertility in Bangladesh: The influence of marriage and the family. In R. Jeffrey and A.M. Basu, eds., *Girls' Schooling, Women's Autonomy and Fertility Change in South Asia.* New Delhi, India: Sage Publications.

Anderson-Levitt, K.M., M. Bloch, and A.M. Soumare
1998 Inside classrooms in Guinea: Girls' experiences. In M. Bloch, J. Beoku-Betts, and R. Tabachnick, eds., *Women and Education in Sub-Saharan Africa.* Boulder, Colo.: Lynne Rienner Publishers.

Appleton, S.
1995 Exam Determinants in Kenyan Primary School: Determinants and Gender Differences. Washington, D.C.: McNamara Fellowships Program, Economic Development Institute of the World Bank.

Bellew, R.T., and E.M. King
1993 Educating women: Lessons from experience. In E.M. King and A.M. Hill, eds., *Women's Education in Developing Countries: Barriers, Benefits and Policies.* Baltimore, Md.: Johns Hopkins University Press.

Benavot, A., and D. Kamens
1989 The Curricular Content of Primary Education in Developing Countries. Working Paper Series 237. Washington, D.C.: The World Bank.

Biraimah, K.C.
1980 The impact of western schools on girls expectations: A Togolese case. *Comparative Education Review* 24:S197-S209.
1989 The process and outcomes of gender bias in elementary schools: A Nigerian case. *Journal of Negro Education* 58(1):50-67.

Bledsoe, C.H.
1990 School fees and the marriage process for Mende girls in Sierra Leone. Pp. 283-309 in P.R. Sanday and R.G. Goodenough, eds., *New Directions in the Anthropology of Gender.* Philadelphia, Pa.: University of Pennsylvania.
1992 The cultural transformation of western education in Sierra Leone. *Africa* 62(2):182-202.

Bloch, M.
1993 The uses of schooling and literacy in a Zafimaniry village. Pp. 87-109 in B. Street, ed., *Cross Cultural Approaches to Literacy.* Cambridge, UK: Cambridge University Press.

Boothroyd, R.A., and D.W. Chapman
1987 Gender differences and achievement in Liberian primary school children. *International Journal of Education Development* 7(2):99-105.

Brady, M.
1998 Laying the foundation for girls' healthy futures: Can sports play a role? *Studies in Family Planning* 29(1):79-82.

Bustillo, I.
1993 Latin America and the Caribbean. In E.M. King and A.M. Hill, eds., *Women's Education in Developing Countries: Barriers, Benefits and Policies.* Baltimore, Md.: The Johns Hopkins University Press.

Caldwell, J.
1980 Mass education as a determinant of the timing of fertility decline. *Population and Development Review* 6(2):225-251.

Card, D., and A.D. Krueger
1996 School resources and student outcomes: An overview of the literature and new evidence from North and South Carolina. *Journal of Economic Perspectives* 10(4):31-50.

Cleghorn, A., M. Merritt, and J.O. Abagi
1989 Language policy and science instruction in Kenyan primary schools. *Comparative Education Review* 33(l):21-39.

Cleland, J.G., and J.K. van Ginneken
1988 Maternal education and child survival in developing countries: The search for pathways of influence. *Social Science and Medicine* 27(12):1357-1368.

Davidson, J., and M. Kanyuka
1992 Girls' participation in basic education in southern Malawi. *Comparative Education Review* 36(4):446-466.

El-Sanabary, N.
1993 Middle East and North Africa. In E.M. King and A.M. Hill, eds., *Women's Education in Developing Countries: Barriers, Benefits and Policies.* Baltimore, Md.: The Johns Hopkins University Press.

Ferguson, A.
1988 *Schoolgirl Pregnancy in Kenya: Report of a Study of Discontinuation Rates and Associated Factors.* Nairobi, Kenya: Ministry of Health, Division of Family Health.

Fuller, B.
1987 What factors raise achievement in the third world? *Review of Educational Research* 57:255-292.

Fuller, D., and P. Clarke
1994 Raising school effects while ignoring culture? Local conditions and the influence of classroom tools, rules, and pedagogy. *Review of Educational Research* 64(l):119-157.

Fuller, B., H. Hua, and C.W. Snyder
1994 When girls learn more than boys: The influence of time in school and pedagogy in Botswana. *Comparative Education Review* 38(3):347-376.

Fuller, B., and C.W. Snyder
1991 Vocal teachers, silent pupils? Life in Botswana classrooms. *Comparative Education Review* 35(2):274-294.

Furstenberg, F.
1976 The social consequences of teenage parenthood. *Family Planning Perspectives* 8(4):148-167.

Geronimus, A.T., and S. Korenman
1992 The socio-economic consequences of teen childbearing reconsidered. *Quarterly Journal of Economics* 107(4):1187-1215.

Glewwe, P., and H. Jacoby
1994 Student achievement and schooling choice in low income countries. *Journal of Human Resources* 29(3):843-864.

Grisay, A.
1984 Analyse des inegalites de rendement liees au sexe de l'eleve dans l'enseignement primaire Ivoirien. *International Review of Education* 30:25-39.
Hanushek, E.A.
1995 Interpreting recent research on schooling in developing countries. *World Bank Research Observer* 10(2):227-246.
Hanushek, E.A., and V. Lavy
1994 *School Quality, Achievement Bias, and Dropout Behavior in Egypt.* Living Standards Measurement Study Working Paper 107. Washington, D.C.: The World Bank.
Harbison, R.W., and E.A. Hanushek
1992 *Educational Performance of the Poor: Lessons from Rural Northeast Brazil.* New York: Oxford University Press.
Herrera, L.
1992 Scenes of schooling: Inside a girls' school in Cairo. *Cairo Paper in Social Science* 15(1). American University of Cairo Press.
Herz, B., K. Subbarao, M. Habib, and L. Raney
1991 *Letting Girls Learn: Promising Approaches in Primary and Secondary Education.* World Bank Discussion Papers 133. Washington, D.C.: The World Bank.
Heyneman, S.P., and W.A. Loxley
1983 The effect of primary-school quality on academic achievement across twenty-nine high- and low-income countries. *American Journal of Sociology* 88(6):1162-1194.
Hill, A.M., and E.M. King
1993 Women's education in developing countries: An overview. In E.M. King and A.M. Hill, eds., *Women's Education in Developing Countries: Barriers, Benefits and Policies.* Baltimore, Md.: The Johns Hopkins University Press.
Hoffman, S.D., E.M. Foster, and F.F. Furstenberg, Jr.
1993 Reevaluating the costs of teenage childbearing. *Demography* 30(1):1-15.
Hyde, K.
1993 Sub-Saharan Africa. In E.M. King and A.M. Hill, eds., *Women's Education in Developing Countries: Barriers, Benefits and Policies.* Baltimore, Md.: The Johns Hopkins University Press.
1994 Barriers to equality of educational opportunity in mixed sex secondary schools in Malawi. In S. Erskine and M. Wilson, eds., *Gender Issues in International Education.* Malawi: University of Malawi, Centre for Social Research.
1997 Sexuality education programmes in African schools: A review. Paper presented at National Academy of Sciences' Workshop on Adolescent Sexuality and Reproductive Health in Developing Countries. Washington, D.C., March 24-25, 1997.
Hyde, K., and E. Kadzamira
1994 *Girls' Attainment in Basic Literacy and Education Project: Knowledge, Attitudes and Practices Pilot Survey.* Final report. Malawi: Centre for Social Research, University of Malawi.
Jeffrey, R., and A.M. Basu
1996 Schooling as contraception? In R. Jeffrey and A.M. Basu, eds., *Girls' Schooling, Women's Autonomy and Fertility Change in South Asia.* New Delhi, India: Sage Publications.
Jejeebhoy, S.
1995 *Women's Education, Autonomy, and Reproductive Behaviour: Experience from Developing Countries.* Oxford: Clarendon Press.
Kaufman, G., and J. Cleland
1994 Maternal education and child survival: anthropological responses to demographic evidence. *Health Transition Review* 4(2):196-199.

Kinyanjui, K.
1993 Enhancing women's participation in the science-based curriculum: The case of Kenya. In J.K. Conway and S.C. Bourque, eds., *The Politics of Women's Education*. Ann Arbor, Mich.: The University of Michigan Press.

Kirby, D.
1995 *A Review of Educational Programs Designed to Reduce Sexual Risk-taking Behaviors Among Schoolaged Youth in the United States*. Santa Cruz, Calif.: ETR Associates.

Kremer, M., S. Moulin, D. Myatt, and R. Namunyu
1997 Textbooks, class size, and test scores: Evidence from a prospective evaluation in Kenya. Institute for Policy Reform Working Paper Series. Washington, D.C.: Institute for Policy Reform.

Lee, V.E., and M.E. Lockheed
1990 The effects of single-sex schooling on achievement and attitudes in Nigeria. *Comparative Education Review* 34(2):209-231.

LeVine, R.A., E. Dexter, P. Velasco, S. LeVine, A.R. Joshi, K.W. Stuebing, and F.M. Tapia Uribe
1994 Maternal literacy and health care in three countries: A preliminary report. *Health Transition Review* 4(2):186-192.

Lloyd, C.B., and A. Blanc
1996 Children's schooling in Sub-Saharan Africa: The role of fathers, mothers and others. *Population and Development Review* 22(2):265-298.

Lloyd, C.B., B.S. Mensch, and W. Clark
1998 The effects of school quality on the educational participation and attainment of Kenyan boys and girls. Presented at the Annual Conference of the Population Association of America. Chicago, Ill. April 2-4.

Lockheed, M.E., A.M. Verspoor, D. Bloch, P. Englebert, B. Fuller, E. King, J. Middleton, V. Paqueo, A. Rodd, R. Romain, and M. Welmond
1991 *Improving Primary Education in Developing Countries*. Oxford: Oxford University Press.

McCauley, A.P., C. Salter, K. Kiragu, and J. Senderowitz
1995 *Meeting the Needs of Young Adults*. Population Reports 41. Baltimore, Md.: Johns Hopkins School of Public Health, Population Information Program.

Meekers, D., A. Gage, and L. Zhan
1995 Preparing adolescents for adulthood: Family life education and pregnancy-related school expulsion in Kenya. *Population Research and Policy Review* 14:91-110.

Mensch, B.S., and C.B. Lloyd
1998 Gender differences in the schooling experiences of adolescents in low-income countries: The case of Kenya. *Studies in Family Planning* 29(2):167-184.

Meyer, J.W., D.H. Kamens, and A. Benavot
1992 *School Knowledge for the Masses: World Models and National Primary Curricular Categories in the Twentieth Century*. Washington, D.C.: The Falmer Press.

Mott, F.L., and W. Marsiglio
1985 Early childbearing and completion of high school. *Family Planning Perspectives* 17(5):234-238.

Mwati, M.W., and S. Munyiri
1996 Gang rapes schoolgirls. *The Nation* 40.

Njeuma, D.L.
1993 An overview of women's education in Africa. In J.K. Conway and S.C. Bourque, eds., *The Politics of Women's Education*. Ann Arbor, Mich.: University of Michigan Press.

Obura, A.P.
1991 *Changing Images: Portrayal of Girls and Women in Kenyan Textbooks.* Nairobi, Kenya: ACTS Press.

Ribar, D.C.
1994 *The Socioeconomic Consequences of Young Women's Childbearing: Reconciling Disparate Evidence.* State Park, Pa: Pennsylvania State University, Department of Economics and Population Research Institute.

Sadker, M., and D. Sadker
1995 *Failing at Fairness: How Our Schools Cheat Girls.* New York: Simon & Schuster.

Senderowitz, J.
1995 *Adolescent Health: Reassessing the Passage to Adulthood.* World Bank Discussion Papers 272. Washington, D.C.: The World Bank.

Shaheed, F., and K. Mumtaz
1993 Women's education in Pakistan. In J.K. Conway and S.C. Bourque, eds., *The Politics of Womens' Education.* Ann Arbor, Mich.: University of Michigan Press.

Stromquist, N.
1994 Gender and education. Pp. 2407-2412 in T. Husen and T.N. Postlethwaite, eds., *The International Encyclopedia of Education.* Second Edition. Tarrytown, N.Y.: Elsevier Science/Pergamon.

Tan, J., J. Lane, and P. Coustere
1997 Putting inputs to work in elementary schools: What can be done in the Philippines? *Economic Development and Cultural Change* 45(4):857-881.

Trussell, J.T.
1976 The social consequences of teenage parenthood. *Family Planning Perspectives* 8(4):184-192.

United Nations
1995 *Women's Education and Fertility Behavior: Recent Evidence from the Demographic and Health Surveys.* New York: United Nations.

Yates, B.A.
1982 Church, state, and education in Belgian Africa: Implications for contemporary third world women. Pp. 127-151 in G.P. Kelly and C.M. Elliott, eds., *Women's Education in the Third World: Comparative Perspectives.* Albany, N.Y.: State University of New York Press.

5

School Quality, Student Achievement, and Fertility in Developing Countries

Paul Glewwe

INTRODUCTION

Investments in education are increasingly viewed as essential for economic growth in developing countries (World Bank, 1990; United Nations Development Programme, 1990; Becker, 1995). Education also has nonmarket effects, such as better health and lower fertility, that may not be captured in income numbers at the national or individual level (Haveman and Wolfe, 1984). Parents' decisions regarding their children's education depend in part on the characteristics of local schools, most of which are public schools. Unfortunately, in many countries the low quality of schools severely limits households' opportunities for educating their children. Examples of countries with school-quality problems are Brazil (Harbison and Hanushek, 1992), Ghana (Glewwe, 1998), and Pakistan (World Bank, 1995). Many more developing countries also have poor school quality; these three examples simply illustrate that the problem exists in each region of the developing world.

Low school quality can take various forms; recent studies have shown that schools in developing countries suffer from many deficiencies that lead to reduced learning among students (Lockheed and Verspoor, 1991; Hanushek, 1995). While remedying these deficiencies should raise school quality and lead to substantial increases in student learning, much remains to be discovered about which policy options are most effective in achieving this goal. Moreover, evidence is incomplete concerning the likely impacts of improved school quality on fertility and other socioeconomic outcomes.

This chapter examines the relationship between school quality and fertility in developing countries. A large amount of research has shown convincingly that the quantity of schooling in those countries is associated with significant reductions in fertility (Schultz, 1993), but very little research has examined the relationship between school quality and fertility. Given the low levels of school quality in many developing countries and increasing recognition of the need for improvement, two questions arise: First, do we really know how best to improve school quality? Second, what impact will increased school quality have on fertility? To answer these questions, the chapter first provides a critical assessment of the literature on the determinants of school quality in developing countries. It then examines the likely impact of improved school quality on fertility. Particular attention is given to the role played by cognitive skills, such as literacy and numeracy, and on the need to address a host of statistical estimation problems and data inadequacies that, regrettably, often receive insufficient attention in the literature.

The chapter is organized as follows. The next section begins by presenting a simple economic model of the determinants of educational outcomes, focusing on the role of school quality, and uses this model to draw implications for empirical work. The third section provides a critical review of the current state of knowledge on the impact of school quality on learning. The following two sections address the relationship between school quality and fertility, reviewing, respectively, what economic theory says about the impact of school quality on fertility and the scant empirical evidence that is available. The final section presents concluding remarks.

A SIMPLE ECONOMIC MODEL OF EDUCATIONAL OUTCOMES

Overview of the Issues

Schooling provides children with many benefits. Most obvious are the skills taught explicitly as a part of the curriculum, such as literacy, numeracy, scientific knowledge, and advanced thinking skills. Schooling also provides social skills and values that can help children succeed in the adult world. Finally, a certain prestige may be associated with completing particular levels of education, so that one may be able to obtain better employment or a "better" spouse (see Basu, this volume). The present discussion focuses on the basic cognitive skills school curricula are designed to impart, but occasional reference is made to other benefits of schooling as well.

The cognitive skills acquired by a child per year of schooling depend on the characteristics of the child, of his or her household, and of the school attended. The variation in acquired cognitive skills that is due to school characteristics can serve as an indicator of school quality. In particular, school quality can be defined as those school (and teacher) characteristics that increase the cognitive skills children acquire per year of schooling. This concept of school quality is fairly intuitive. As discussed below, however, much remains to be learned about which school characteristics lead to the acquisition of cognitive skills.

The cognitive skills children acquire in school can play a very important role in determining their standard of living as adults. The best example is the role played by those skills in determining income, with better-educated individuals generally having higher incomes. At the same time, however, the exact relationship between cognitive skills and income is poorly understood and probably quite complex because different skills are likely to have different effects on income, and there has been very little research in either developed or developing countries on which skills are most important in this regard. Cognitive skills also affect individuals' living standards by helping to determine many other socioeconomic outcomes, such as health status, marriage prospects, and fertility. Yet almost nothing is known about which skills have the most important effect on these outcomes. Knowledge of the impact of different skills on income and on other socioeconomic outcomes could have implications for school curriculum. For example, if literacy skills were identified as much more important than, say, scientific knowledge in determining future income, it might be desirable to reduce some of the classroom time devoted to science while increasing the time devoted to language skills.

Figure 5-1 provides a visual framework for conceptualizing the relationships among school quality, school attainment, cognitive skills, and socioeconomic outcomes. At the top of the diagram, school, child, and family characteristics influence both schooling and other socioeconomic outcomes. One can think of these characteristics as exogenous (beyond the control of the child and the family), at least initially.[1] Given these exogenous characteristics, parents (perhaps considering their child's wishes) decide how long to send their child to school. School quality may influence this decision (arrow a in Figure 5-1) because higher-quality schools should provide more benefits per year of schooling, making additional years of schooling more attractive. In contrast, school costs (arrow b) will tend to reduce years of schooling. Many child characteristics can affect years of schooling (arrow c); on the positive side, more talented children are likely to go to school longer, while on the negative side, children with greater potential to contribute to household income may receive less schooling. Finally, several family characteristics can affect years of schooling (arrow d); two examples are household income and parental tastes for their children's schooling, both of which may increase educational attainment.

Once a child enters school, the acquisition of cognitive skills begins. Time spent in school should increase skill acquisition (arrow f in Figure 5-1), as should

[1] In particular, school quality may not be fixed when parents can choose from more than one school for their children. This issue is discussed in detail in the next section.

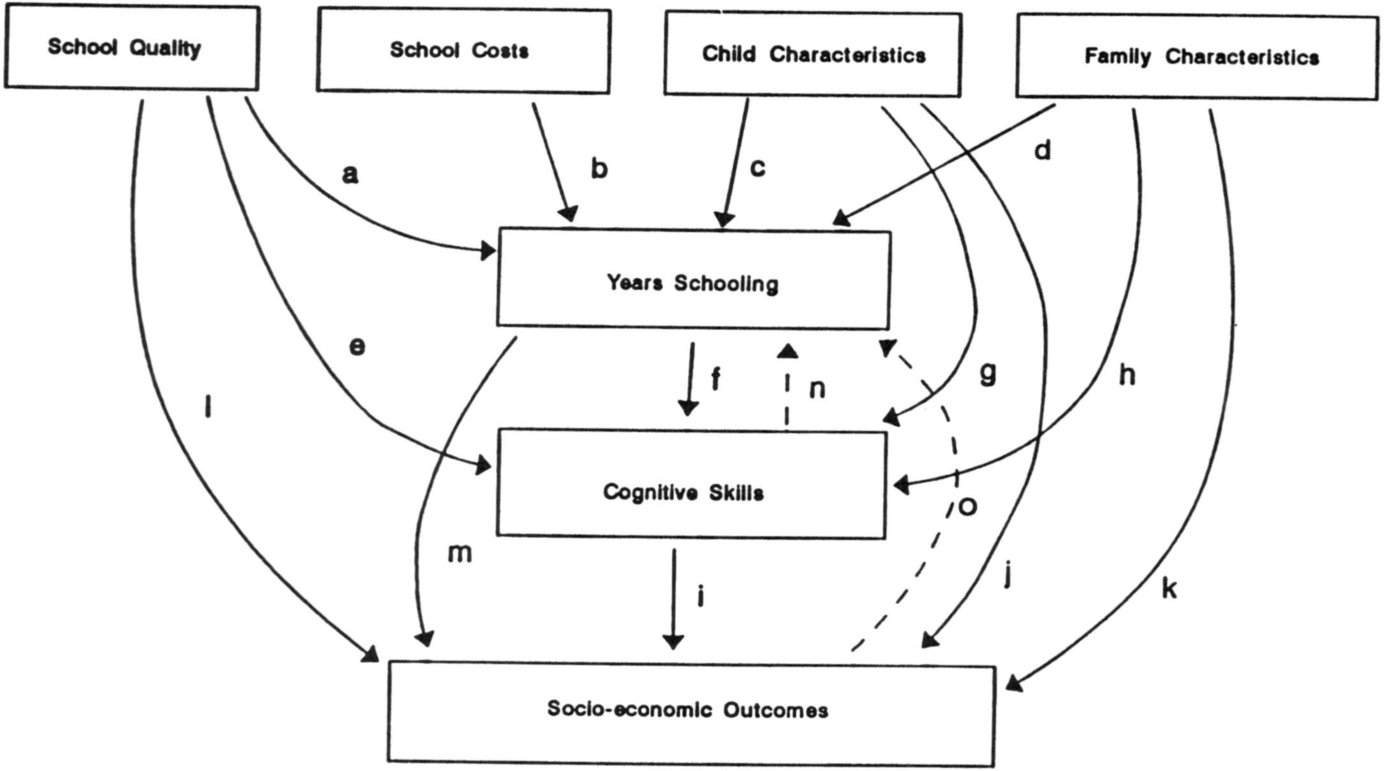

FIGURE 5-1 Relationship among school quality, school attainment, and student achievement.

school quality (arrow e). In addition, child and family characteristics can play important roles (arrows g and h, respectively); for example, child ability should increase learning, holding other factors constant, and parents' education can do the same if they help their children with schoolwork. Note that school costs have no impact on learning once years of schooling are accounted for; there is no reason that school fees paid should affect skills acquired beyond their role in determining years of schooling.[2]

The bottom of Figure 5-1 shows the impact of schooling and other factors on socioeconomic outcomes, of which fertility is one example. The cognitive skills a child acquires in school should have substantial effects on many socioeconomic outcomes (arrow i). Family and child characteristics may have separate effects (arrows j and k, respectively). For example, children with more motivation or a better work ethic may be more successful even after controlling for cognitive skills, and parents may use social connections to help their children obtain better jobs. School quality and years of schooling may also affect socioeconomic outcomes beyond the direct effect of cognitive skills (arrows l and m). For example, years of schooling may signal employers about traits they seek in workers (e.g., innate ability, motivation, work ethic) that are difficult to measure.[3] Similarly, enrollment in a higher-quality school may improve a child's socioeconomic prospects because of the prestige attached to that particular school.

Although the direction of causality in Figure 5-1 generally flows from top to bottom, some reverse causality is possible. These effects are indicated by dashed lines. For example, cognitive skills may determine years of schooling (arrow n) if schools prevent students from advancing to the next grade until they pass a standardized test; a child who fails such tests two or three times may be forced to drop out of school. As another example, one socioeconomic outcome that could affect years of schooling (arrow o) is pregnancy among female students; pregnant students may be forced to leave school because schooling is thought to be incompatible with their childcare responsibilities.

Obviously, the simple scheme presented in Figure 5-1 could be made more realistic through the addition of more detail. However, it is intended only to provide a basic framework, not a complete picture. The next subsection presents a formal economic model of the determinants of school quality, school attainment, and the acquisition of cognitive skills that will prove useful in the literature assessment presented in the next section.

---

[2]School costs can have an effect if parents spend money on extra classes or better material inputs. However, such additional inputs can be included as part of the influence of income, a family characteristic measured by arrow h.

[3]In fact, a child's motivation and work ethic may be influenced by his or her schooling. These effects can be thought of as being among the social skills and values acquired from schooling.

The Model

This chapter, while somewhat eclectic, approaches education issues from a (neoclassical) economic perspective. In particular, it takes the position that a model of rational behavior is needed to ensure that proper statistical procedures are used in attempting to estimate the impact of school characteristics and school policies on educational outcomes and of schooling and cognitive skills on socioeconomic outcomes. The argument is quite simple. Explicit models of human behavior provide significant insight into whether assumptions underlying specific statistical methods are satisfied. If a plausible theory suggests that some assumptions are not satisfied, the empirical results based on those methods may be invalid. The model may also suggest how to test to determine whether the statistical assumptions hold and what statistical procedure should be used if they fail to hold. Note that this is not intended to be the definitive model on schooling, only a plausible model that can illuminate several statistical issues.

To formulate the model, it is assumed that parents make decisions for their children and that their objective is to maximize a utility function that has two arguments: household consumption (of goods and services) and child cognitive skills. More specifically, it is assumed that there are only two time periods. In time period 1, a child may attend school, work, or both (if both, the child first goes to school and works only after schooling is completed). In time period 2, the child becomes an adult and works.[4] Whenever the child works in time period 1 or 2, part or all of the child's earnings may be given to his or her parents. The following simple utility function takes consumption in both time periods (C_1 and C_2) and child cognitive skills (A) as its arguments:

$$U = C_1 + \delta C_2 + \sigma A \tag{5.1}$$

Note that δ is effectively a discount factor for future consumption, and σ is a parameter indicating tastes for educated children (higher values indicate a greater desire for educated children). Thus parents may value educated children for two distinct reasons: (1) educating children may increase the parents' levels of consumption, and (2) educating children directly affects utility (through σ).

The next step is to explain how cognitive skills, A, are produced. The following simple production function keeps the mathematics at a relatively elementary level:

$$A = \alpha f(Q)g(S) \tag{5.2}$$

where α is the "learning efficiency" of the child, Q is school quality, and S is

[4]To keep the exposition simple, it is assumed that there is only one child per family. The possibility that the number of children is another choice variable is considered in a later section.

years of schooling. Increases in either Q or S should increase the cognitive skills produced, so f( ) and g( ) are increasing functions of Q and S, respectively. The learning efficiency of the child, α, can represent several different factors, such as innate (i.e., genetically inherited) ability, child motivation and tastes for schooling, and parents' motivation (and capacity) to help their children with their schoolwork. For simplicity, these different factors are combined into a single parameter, α.

The model is completed by specifying the relationships between consumption and child schooling and between child schooling and child income. Consumption levels in each time period are given by:

$$C_1 = Y_1 - pS + (1 - S)kY_c \quad (5.3)$$

$$C_2 = Y_2 + kY_c \quad (5.4)$$

where p is the price of schooling (e.g., annual tuition); Y_1 and Y_2 are (exogenous) parental income in periods 1 and 2, respectively; Y_c is the income of the child when he or she works in either time period; and k is the fraction of that income given to the parents.[5] The last term in equation (5.3), $(1 - S)kY_c$, requires some explanation. For convenience, S has been rescaled to represent the fraction of time spent in school by the child in time period 1. The remaining time during that period, 1 – S, is spent working. This rescaling is purely for notational convenience and has no effect on the results; however, to keep the vocabulary simple, S is still called "years of schooling."

Finally, equation (5.5) relates the child's cognitive skills to employment income in either time period:

$$Y_c = \pi A \quad (5.5)$$

where π can be thought of as the productivity of cognitive skills in the labor market.

By substituting equation (5.2) into equation (5.5), then equation (5.5) into equations (5.3) and (5.4), and finally equations (5.2), (5.3), and (5.4) into equation (5.1), parents' utility is expressed as a function of years of schooling (S):

[5]Note that it is implicitly assumed that there is no borrowing or saving; the only way to transfer income between periods 1 and 2 is to invest in children's education. This assumption is made for simplicity. Allowing for other possibilities would complicate the mathematics and is not pursued here. In general, allowing for borrowing or saving would reduce the need for parents to invest in their children's education. However, it would not completely eliminate the investment motive for educating one's children because almost all investments are risky, and thus it is prudent to diversify one's investments among several different alternatives, including children's education.

$$U = Y_1 - pS + \delta Y_2 + ((1 - S + \delta)k\pi + \sigma)\alpha f(Q)g(S) \tag{5.6}$$

One can show (see the appendix) how the optimal (utility-maximizing) value of years of schooling is affected by changes in the model's various parameters. The findings are all intuitively plausible. Years of schooling increases when the following increase: (1) children's learning efficiency (α), (2) school quality (Q), (3) the weight (δ) parents give to future relative to current consumption, and (4) parents' tastes for schooling (σ). Years of schooling decreases when the price of schooling (p) rises. Finally, years of schooling is likely, though not certain, to rise when parents expect to receive a larger proportion (k) of their children's income from working and when the value of cognitive skills in the labor market (π) is higher.

Sometimes parents can choose not only years of school, but also school quality. The model can easily be extended to the case in which both years in school (S) and school quality (Q) are choice variables. To make the model more realistic, assume that the price of a school depends on its quality[6]:

$$p = p_o Q \tag{5.7}$$

where p_o is the "base" price of schooling. Thus high-quality schools have higher costs (p rises as Q increases). Equation (5.7) may at first seem to have an arbitrary functional form: If one school has a level of quality twice as high as that of another, why should the price be exactly twice as high, as opposed to less or more than twice as high? In fact, equation (5.7) is simply a normalization; Q should be interpreted as an index of expenditures on quality. Whether or not, say, doubling expenditures doubles the impact of school quality on learning (i.e., doubles f(Q)) depends on the functional form of f(Q).

After replacing p with p_oQ in equation (5.6), one obtains the following expression, which is to be maximized with respect to both S and Q:

$$U = Y_1 - p_o QS + \delta Y_2 + \alpha f(Q)g(S)((1 - S+\delta)k\pi + \sigma) \tag{5.8}$$

Without further assumptions about the functional forms of f( ) and g( ), one cannot determine how changes in the various parameters, such as p_o, α, δ, and σ, affect S and Q. For ease of exposition, assume that $f(Q) = Q^\beta$, where $\beta > 0$, and $g(S) = S^\gamma$, where $\gamma > 0$. Differing values of β and γ allow for a wide range of the shapes of both f( ) and g( ). Both β and γ must be greater than zero to guarantee that f( ) and g( ) increase as Q and S, respectively, increase. Using these func-

[6]Making this assumption is not only more realistic, but also necessary for the model to make sense. If higher quality could be obtained at no additional cost, all households would choose the highest quality possible.

tional forms, one can show (see the appendix) that parents' utility as given in equation (5.8) is maximized by setting S and Q as follows:

$$S^* = (\gamma - \beta)(1 + \delta + \sigma/k\pi)/(1 + \gamma - \beta) \tag{5.9}$$

$$Q^* = (\alpha\beta k\pi/p_o)(\gamma - \beta)^{\gamma-1}((1 + \delta + \sigma/k\pi)/(1 + \gamma - \beta))^{\gamma} \tag{5.10}$$

where the asterisk indicates the utility-maximizing (optimal) level for each variable. The optimal level of cognitive skills (A) is obtained by inserting equations (5.9) and (5.10) into equation (5.2).

Note that the optimal levels of S and Q in equations (5.9) and (5.10) are intuitively reasonable. Both years of schooling (S) and school quality (Q) are higher when parents give higher weight (δ) to future relative to current consumption, and parents have higher tastes for schooling (σ). School quality (Q) increases as learning efficiency (α) increases, but decreases as the base price of schooling (p_o) increases. A less plausible result is that years of schooling depends on neither the base price of schooling nor the innate ability of the child. This result admittedly is due to the functional forms used for f( ) and g( ), but it is not as unreasonable as it may first appear to be. What happens is that parents, in response to a lower base price or higher child learning efficiency, shift to higher quality, which raises their children's cognitive skills without changing years of schooling. By opting for higher quality instead of more years of schooling, parents avoid a cost associated with the latter—a reduction in the length of time a child works during time period 1 (see equation (5.3)). If school quality were not a choice variable, greater learning efficiency (α) or a lower price would lead to increased years of schooling, as explained above.

A final result that also appears counterintuitive is that an increase in the propensity of children to give money to their parents (k) or in the market return to cognitive skills (π) decreases years of schooling. Here again intuition suggests that the best response to such changes is to increase school quality and reduce time spent in school, which will increase the time the child spends working in time period 1.[7]

Implications of the Model for Statistical Analysis

The model presented above is useful for discussing several statistical issues involved in measuring the impact of school quality on learning. Most empirical studies of the impact of school characteristics on the acquisition of cognitive

---

[7]School quality is likely to increase when k or π increases, but it may decrease. In the event of a decrease, total cognitive skills attained must decline, but this loss in income to the parents is outweighed by the increase in income due to the child's working longer in the first time period.

skills are based on linear statistical models, an approach that simplifies estimation. Taking the logarithm of both sides of equation (5.2) and assuming exponential functional forms for f( ) and g( ) yields an equation that is linear in the logarithms of the variables.[8] For ease of exposition, assume this latter equation is linear in the original variables; this assumption can be made because the following line of reasoning also applies to the linear-in-logarithms case. Thus the equation of interest is:

$$A = \mu_0 + \mu_1 S + \mu_2 \alpha + \mu_3 Q + e \qquad (5.2')$$

where the μ coefficients are unknown parameters to be estimated. The residual term e is added to account for the fact that in empirical work, no data fit the model perfectly.

Equation (5.2′) can be estimated using simple statistical methods, but its specification of school quality is oversimplified. It is more realistic, and more useful for policy analysis, to decompose school quality into a function or index of the different school characteristics that promote learning. Doing so yields:

$$A = \mu_0 + \mu_1 S + \mu_2 \alpha + \tau_1 Q_1 + \tau_2 Q_2 + \ldots + \tau_n Q_n + e \qquad (5.2'')$$

In equation (5.2″), Q has been replaced by an index of n different school characteristics (Q_1, Q_2, etc.) that affect the acquisition of cognitive skills. What policy makers want to know, and analysts need to estimate, is the magnitude of the various τ's. These estimates can be combined with data on the costs of the different school characteristics to assess the cost-effectiveness of each characteristic in promoting learning.

Equation (2″) implicitly assumes that learning efficiency, α, can be observed. In fact, there are often few data on the factors determining learning efficiency, so equation (5.2") must be rewritten as:

$$A = \mu_0 + \mu_1 S + \tau_1 Q_1 + \tau_2 Q_2 + \ldots + \tau_n Q_n + u \qquad (5.11)$$

where α (and its coefficient) is combined with e to produce u, a residual term that represents both random "noise" from imperfectly fitting data and the impact of unobserved aspects of learning efficiency (α) on cognitive skill acquisition (A). Examples of learning efficiency variables that are difficult to observe are the child's innate ability and motivation and the parents' motivation (and ability) to help children with schoolwork.[9]

---

[8]In particular, assuming that $f(Q) = \Theta Q^{\beta}$ and $g(S) = \Phi S^{\gamma}$ for some parameters Θ, β, Φ, and γ.

[9]While some of these factors may be measured (e.g., using an IQ test to measure innate ability and using parental schooling to indicate parents' ability to assist their children), it is highly unlikely that

Equation (5.11) is commonly estimated using ordinary least squares (OLS) regression. OLS provides unbiased estimates of all parameters (the μ's and τ's) in equation (5.11) only if the residual term, u, is uncorrelated with S and the various Q's. However, the simple model presented earlier shows that such correlation is very likely; in equation (5.10), higher learning efficiency (α) increases school quality (Q), implying that u, which represents (in part) variation in α, is positively correlated with the various Q's. The result in general will be overestimation of the associated parameters (τ's). Few empirical studies do anything to avoid this statistical problem.

If school quality is not a choice variable, the estimation problem discussed above can be avoided. In rural areas of many developing countries, school quality may well be exogenous because each village has only one school, and villages are too far apart for children to attend school in a neighboring village. In such cases, the Q variables in equation (5.11) may not be correlated with the error term, u. Yet even under this scenario, parents may still be able to influence school quality. First, they may directly affect quality at the sole local school by participating in the parent-teacher association (PTA) or using political connections to obtain better educational services. Second, they may send their children to live with relatives or at a boarding school, thus allowing them to attend a nonlocal school.[10] Third, families with higher tastes for educated children may migrate to areas with better schools, a common occurrence in the United States.

Since parents may affect school quality even in rural areas, then, overestimation is possible. Yet it is also possible that endogenous school quality leads to underestimation. Even if parents cannot affect school quality, it could be correlated with the error term because governments may provide better schools to areas with unobserved education problems (Pitt et al., 1993). These unmeasured problems would again be relegated to u in equation (5.11), producing negative correlation between the error term and the school quality variables (Q's) and thus underestimating the impact of school quality.

Even when school quality is completely uncorrelated with the error term in equation (5.11), years of schooling (S) may be correlated. Note that in equation (5.9), parents with higher tastes for schooling (σ) send their children to school longer. These tastes are rarely measured, and any effect they have on learning efficiency (e.g., such parents help children more with schoolwork) would be reflected in the error term u, leading to positive correlation with S. This in turn

---

one can measure all of them. Indeed, it is not even clear that innate ability can be measured; any test that purports to do so (in the sense of genetic endowment) is likely to reflect environmental factors (American Psychological Association, 1995). One possible way to get around this problem is to use data on twins (see Behrman et al., 1994). However, such data are very rare in developing countries.

[10]About 19 percent of secondary students in rural Peru live away from their families (Gertler and Glewwe, 1990), and the same applies to 27 percent of middle school students in Ghana (Glewwe and Jacoby, 1994).

would lead to biased estimates of the coefficient on S, as well as of the other estimated coefficients, both μ's and τ's. Instrumental variable techniques, such as two-stage least squares, may correct this problem. One possible instrument for years of schooling is the price of schooling, which should affect learning only by affecting years of schooling. Another approach is to estimate equation (5.11) for a single grade to remove variation in S.

Three additional problems merit attention. First, if some children in the relevant age range are not in school, the remaining children (whether in one or several grades) are not a random sample of the population. Intuitively, communities with high-quality schools will keep children in school longer, leading to a student population with lower average learning efficiency (because more "less-efficient" children stay in school). This implies that u in equation (5.11) will be negatively correlated with school quality, resulting in underestimation of the impact of school quality on learning. Second, no data set includes every determinant of school quality, and observed aspects of quality may be positively correlated with unobserved aspects (because "good" schools are often good in many ways, only some of which are measured). Again, unmeasured aspects of school quality are, by default, part of the residual term in equation (5.11), causing u to be positively correlated with observed school quality variables and causing the τ parameters to be overestimated. A final difficulty in empirical work is measurement error in the explanatory variables, both S and the various Q variables. If these variables are not measured precisely, random measurement error will cause underestimation of the impact of both S and Q on the acquisition of skills. Nonrandom measurement error could lead to either underestimation or overestimation.

In summary, there are at least six ways in which uncritical application of common statistical methods can lead to biased estimates of the impact of school quality on learning. Some lead to underestimation and others to overestimation, while still others could go either way. These potential problems must be considered in assessing the findings of existing research, which are addressed in the next section.

WHAT IS KNOWN ABOUT THE IMPACT OF SCHOOL QUALITY ON LEARNING AND YEARS OF SCHOOLING?

The simple model presented in the previous section suggests that the impact of school quality on students' cognitive skills operates in two ways—raising years of schooling attained and increasing learning per year of schooling. Building on the preceding discussion, this section assesses the literature on the determinants of cognitive skill attainment in developing countries, focusing on the role of school quality. It is argued that much remains to be learned, and several suggestions for future research are made.

Assessment of the Recent Literature

There is a large literature for developed countries and a growing literature for developing countries on the determinants of educational attainment and cognitive skill acquisition. The discussion here focuses on the developing-country literature; for recent reviews of the developed-country literature, see Hanushek (1986) and Hanushek et al. (1994).

Most of the literature on the determinants of learning in developing countries has focused on the impact of school quality on skills learned per year of schooling. Less work has addressed the impact of school quality on educational attainment. Comprehensive reviews of the literature since 1990 include Lockheed and Verspoor (1991), Harbison and Hanushek (1992), Velez et al. (1993), Fuller and Clarke (1994), Strauss and Thomas (1995), and Hanushek (1995). These reviews usually assemble a large number of studies and then tally, for many different school and teacher characteristics (or policies), (1) the number of studies that examined a particular characteristic and (2) the number of those studies that found a statistically significant effect of that characteristic on achievement test scores. Only one review, Strauss and Thomas (1995), seriously criticizes the statistical methods used. The others tend to accept results at face value even though, as Hanushek (1995:231-32) points out, "the standards of data collection and analysis are so variable that the results . . . are subject to considerable uncertainty."

Table 5-1 summarizes the findings of four reviews that follow the "typical" approach.[11] The Strauss and Thomas study is excluded because it examines only five studies and draws few specific conclusions (see pp. 1956-59), and the later Hanushek study is excluded because it is based on Harbison and Hanushek (1992). Table 5-1 reveals three consistent findings: (1) class size has no effect, (2) teacher salaries have no effect, and (3) textbooks have a positive effect. A few other school or teacher characteristics look promising, but their effect is less certain because it is based on only two of the four reviews (radio instruction, school library, nutrition and feeding program, teacher's cognitive skills) or because the results for that characteristic are mixed (teacher education, physical facilities). However, meta-analysis techniques can be used to form judgments on many, if not most, of the ambiguous cases; for example, Kremer (1995) shows how the apparently ambiguous results in Harbison and Hanushek (1992), as reported in Hanushek (1995), can provide definitive answers.[12]

[11]Table 5-1 does not include all the findings presented in each literature review. In particular, it excludes findings unrelated to school quality or considered by only one of the four reviews. Note that the table sometimes imputes values of "yes," "no," or "maybe" when the authors were reluctant to be so explicit.

[12]See Hedges et al. (1994) for an application of meta-analysis techniques to U.S. data, and Hanushek (1995) for a somewhat skeptical interpretation of the results.

TABLE 5-1 Summary of Findings on Determinants of Cognitive Achievement from Four Recent Literature Reviews

Characteristic	Lockheed and Verspoor (1991)	Harbison and Hanushek (1992)	Velez et al. (1993)	Fuller and Clarke (1994)
Class Size	No	No	No	No
Expenditure per Pupil	—	Maybe	—	Yes
Teacher Salaries	—	No	No	No
Textbooks	Yes	Yes	Yes	Yes
Radio Instruction	Yes	—	—	Yes
School Library	—	Yes	—	Yes
Nutrition/Feeding Program	Yes	—	—	Yes
Teacher Training	Yes	Maybe	No	Yes
Teacher Skills (test scores)	—	—	Yes	Yes
Teacher Education	—	Yes/Maybe	Yes	Maybe
Teacher Experience	—	No	Yes	Maybe
Physical Facilities	—	Yes	Maybe	Yes
Number of Studies Analyzed	Large number, but not specified	96	18	Over 100

Unfortunately, the greater clarity offered by meta-analysis techniques must be balanced against the fact that most of the results discussed in these literature reviews should not be taken at face value. In particular, it is not clear whether the regularities found indicate real phenomena or simply reflect inappropriate use and interpretation of commonly employed statistical methods. The statistical problems raised at the end of the previous section are rarely considered in the literature.[13] Moreover, even with a rich set of data and careful use of sophisticated statistical methods, it is almost impossible to eliminate completely all potential sources of bias. In principle, the best method for overcoming almost all sources of bias is randomized trials of specific educational interventions. Such trials randomly divide a set of schools into a treatment group that receives a particular educational input or enacts a particular policy and a control group that receives no inputs and enacts no new policy. Very few such studies have been done in developing countries,[14] though some new studies are under way at the

[13]A few studies, mostly by economists, attempt to address at least some of these problems. Examples are Alderman et al. (1995), Cox and Jimenez (1991), Glewwe and Jacoby (1994), Harbison and Hanushek (1992), and Jimenez et al. (1988, 1991). Yet Strauss and Thomas (1995) point out that many problems remain.

[14]The only ones identified for this review are Heyneman et al. (1984), Jamison et al. (1981), Kagitcibasi et al. (1993), Kremer et al. (1997), and Glewwe et al. (1998).

World Bank. Such studies are rare because they are very expensive and because they can examine only one or two policy changes at a time.

Finally, two other gaps remain in the literature. First, as noted by Fuller and Clarke (1994), cost-effectiveness calculations are rarely done. Improvements in cognitive achievement per dollar spent is the ultimate concern of policy makers. For example, consider the use of computers; Lockheed and Verspoor (1991) point out that although computers increase learning in developing countries, they are much more expensive (in terms of learning per dollar spent) than several other policies to the same end. Unfortunately, some school policies, such as changes in instructional techniques, are difficult to price. The study by Glewwe et al. (1995) was explicitly designed for cost-effectiveness calculations, but in the end could not achieve this purpose because almost no effective school policies could easily be priced. A second gap in the literature is that studies rarely examine the impact of school quality on learning through its effect on years of schooling.[15] This may be an important pathway for increasing human capital in developing countries. Glewwe and Jacoby (1994) show that it can account for a third, or even more, of the total impact of particular school quality improvements on learning.

In summary, the existing literature on the impact of school quality on learning in developing countries suffers from many deficiencies. Some results are found so consistently that one can probably subscribe to them, but many more have less solid support. Even the findings with apparently solid support can be questioned because they are based on uncritical use of statistical methods. The most serious statistical problems are (1) omission of many important school and teacher variables from analyses because of data limitations and (2) measurement error in school quality variables. Problems of endogeneity and sample selectivity are less salient because studies that attempt to address them rarely find that the main results change.[16] Recall that omitted-variable bias generally leads to overestimation, while random measurement error generally leads to underestimation. Given these effects in opposite directions, it is unclear how much confidence one can have in the existing literature. Yet in fairness to the literature, one must recognize that education is a highly complex process and that the data for analyzing it have typically been inadequate. A final complication is that the true determinants of learning may vary widely across developing countries. Nothing can be done about this, and sizeable variation should be expected given the vast differences in the school systems in developing countries.

---

[15]Of course, as any economist could point out, raising years of schooling entails opportunity costs of time, which must be balanced against the benefits of increased cognitive skills.

[16]Studies in which the results do not change after statistical methods are used to account for endogeneity and selectivity are Cox and Jimenez (1991), Glewwe and Jacoby (1994), and Glewwe et al. (1995). One study in which selectivity does make a difference is Jimenez et al. (1988). Of course, the identifying assumptions underlying the use of these methods could be questioned.

Recommendations for Future Research

The pessimistic assessment of the current literature given above raises the question of what can be done to improve the state of knowledge in this area. Three broad recommendations are offered here.

First, statistical and econometric techniques need to be used more cautiously, with more rigorous testing of the underlying assumptions. In the econometric literature, this is known as specification testing (see Godfrey, 1988). Economists have only recently begun to do rigorous specification tests, and such tests are even rarer in research on education in developing (and developed) countries. The need to examine statistical methods critically also applies to literature reviews. There is an urgent need for a literature review that separates insufficiently rigorous findings (which may predominate in the literature) from findings based on careful statistical analysis and then applies meta-analysis techniques to the latter to assess what really works.

Second, much better data need to be collected. Education researchers often use school-based data that include little information on students' home characteristics. Moreover, in countries without universal school enrollment, school-based samples are nonrandom samples of the population. Other researchers use household survey data that provide little information on school and teacher characteristics. Future data collection should combine household surveys with detailed data on schools and teachers, and should also include more collection of panel data, which may avoid several estimation problems. Regrettably, panel data are rare in the developing-country education literature. Finally, many developing countries do not regularly collect data on student performance (Lockheed, 1995). These countries urgently need national testing of cognitive skills to see what students are really learning. These assessments can also lower the cost of collecting data for research purposes, since testing children is a major cost of such research.

Third, more randomized trials of educational interventions are needed. Such trials are one way to address the statistical problems that cast serious doubt on most existing studies. In addition, their results are fairly easy to explain to policy makers. Major multilateral and bilateral agencies that fund educational interventions should incorporate randomized trials in all major projects to assess project effectiveness and build a better information base on what really works. Of particular interest are comparisons of results from randomized trials with results produced by more conventional studies, which may indicate when the latter results are reliable. At the same time, it should be borne in mind that despite these advantages, randomized trials are no panacea; they can suffer from a variety of design and implementation problems, as pointed out by Heckman and Smith (1995).

POSSIBLE IMPACT OF IMPROVEMENTS IN SCHOOL QUALITY ON FERTILITY

This and the next section focus on the impact of school quality on fertility. As noted earlier, while a fair amount of work has been done on the impact of school *quantity* on fertility, there is almost no theoretical or empirical work that specifically addresses the impact of improvements in school *quality*. However, what little work there is on the latter does provide some insights. This section reviews what economic theory can say about the likely impact of improvements in school quality on fertility, while the following section reviews the limited empirical literature that addresses this issue.

Changes in school quality can affect fertility in two distinct ways. First, when today's parents are making current childbearing decisions, they may take into account the quality of local schools. If school quality changes, parents may revise their childbearing plans, and if they do so, there will be an immediate effect of school quality on fertility. Second, even if today's parents make no significant changes in their childbearing plans, improved school quality will probably lead them to provide more education to each of their children, as was shown in the model presented earlier. When children, particularly daughters, reach childbearing age, their increased levels of schooling and higher cognitive skills per year of schooling may well lead them to have fewer children (see also Chapter 2). This effect of school quality on fertility will not manifest itself until many years after school quality changes. The following subsections address each of these pathways in turn.

Impact of School Quality on Current Fertility Decisions of Today's Parents

The standard reference for economic models of fertility is Becker (1981), particularly Chapter 5. The basic model is not presented here, but its essence is quite simple. Parents' utility is determined by three factors: (1) consumption of goods and services; (2) the number (quantity) of children they have; and (3) the average quality of their children, as measured by cognitive skills and schooling. All three factors have associated prices; note in particular that the price of child quality is primarily the cost of a year of schooling. This utility function is a generalization of the parental utility function presented earlier in equation (5.1), in which utility depends on consumption and child quality, but not on the number of children (which is assumed to be exogenous).

In virtually all discussions of Becker's model, it is assumed that the price of schooling refers to the quantity of schooling. However, there is no reason price cannot also be interpreted as referring to school quality. In particular, recall equation (5.7), and note how it enters the utility function in equation (5.8). The expression p_0QS rises if either Q or S rises; it can be interpreted as the price of S

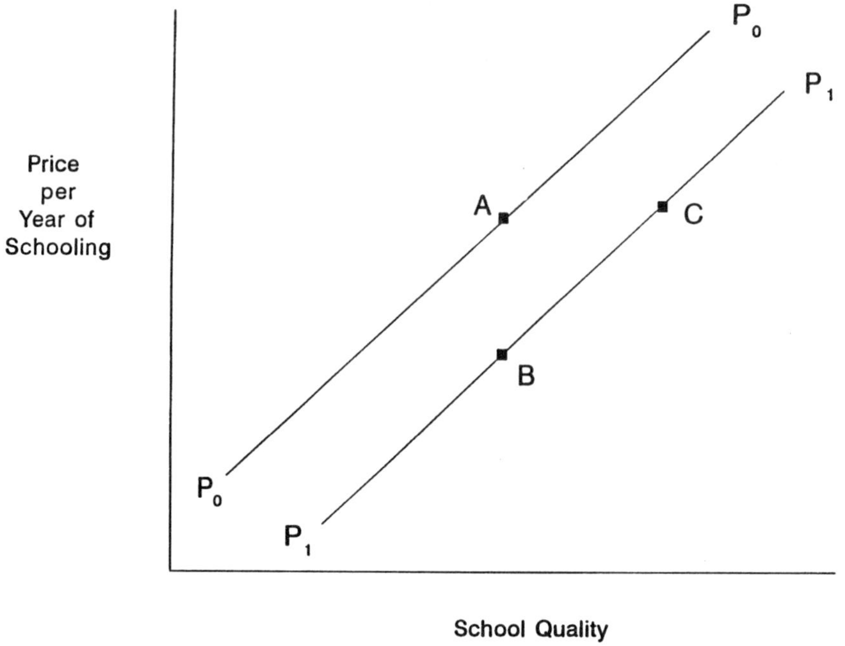

FIGURE 5-2 Price per year of schooling and school quality.

when Q is fixed or the price of Q when S is fixed.[17] This point is made more intuitively by Figure 5-2, which shows the price of a year of schooling as a function of school quality. The line P_0P_0 shows the initial set of prices for different levels of school quality, and the line P_1P_1 shows a reduction in that price that is equivalent to a reduction in p_o in equation (5.7). One can think of this price reduction as either a reduction in the price of a year of schooling for a fixed quality (movement from A to B) or an increase in school quality for the same price per year of schooling (movement from A to C).

The implication of the above discussion is that models that examine the impact of the price of school quantity on fertility can also be used to assess the impact of changes in the price of school quality on fertility. This is possible because there is really only one price, changes in which can be interpreted as either changes in the price of quantity or changes in the price of quality. The

[17]See also equation (5.8) in Becker (1981), which concerns prices of child quantity and of child quality, but the same idea applies. An increase in p_c in that expression can be interpreted as an increase in the price of child quantity (if quality is fixed) or an increase in the price of child quality (if quantity is fixed).

question then arises of what those models can tell us about the impact of the price of schooling on fertility. While Becker does not explicitly address this question, it is examined by Rosenzweig (1982), who shows that the impact of a decrease in the price of schooling on the fertility decisions of today's parents is ambiguous. The reason for this is simple: a decrease in the price of schooling is effectively a decrease in the price of child quality. Price effects suggest that parents will buy more child quality and less child quantity and fewer consumption goods. However, income effects suggest that parents will buy more of all three goods. Thus a decrease in the price of school will clearly raise the average schooling of children (since the price and income effects move in the same direction), but the effects on the number of children and consumption of other goods will be ambiguous.[18]

In summary, there has been no theoretical work examining the impact of changes in school quality, or more generally the price of school quality, on the current fertility decisions of today's parents. However, one can derive such results from economic models of fertility because there is really no difference between the price of school quantity and the price of school quality. The impact of a decrease in the price of schooling, which is essentially the same as a decrease in the price of school quality (or an exogenous increase in school quality), has an ambiguous effect on fertility because the income and substitution effects work in opposite directions: the former effect raises fertility (assuming child quantity is a normal good), while the latter effect reduces it. This theoretical ambiguity means one must examine the empirical evidence, which is done in the next section.

Impact of School Quality on Future Fertility Decisions of Today's Children

The previous subsection focuses on the impact of school quality on the fertility decisions made by today's parents, but it also explains that parents are likely to increase the average education levels of their children if school quality improves. When these children become adults, they will make their own fertility decisions, which will be influenced by the higher levels of human capital they have as a result of past improvements in school quality. There is now a fairly large literature on the determinants of fertility in developing countries, and one of the almost universal findings is that higher education leads to reduced fertility (Schultz, 1993; United Nations, 1995; Ainsworth et al., 1996; see also Chapter 2). Thus, improved school quality today will lead to reductions in future fertility when today's children become adults. Of course, the mechanisms by which this

[18]Rosenzweig also points out that even the price effect alone can be ambiguous, but this simply reinforces the general finding that the overall effect is ambiguous.

comes about are quite complicated; Figure 5-3 depicts the various mechanisms involved.

For simplicity, Figure 5-3 does not distinguish between school quality and years of schooling. Together with other household and child characteristics (recall Figure 5-1), school quality and years of schooling affect children's values (arrow a), fertility knowledge (arrow c), and cognitive skills (arrow d).[19] Fertility knowledge will be acquired directly in school only if it is part of the curriculum, such as a family-life course.[20] Such knowledge can also be acquired indirectly through cognitive skill attainment; literacy acquired in school gives women (and men) the means to acquire fertility knowledge by reading various forms of written information (arrow f). These three direct products of schooling—values, fertility knowledge, and cognitive skills—have implications for young women in two different markets: the marriage "market" (arrows i, j, and k, respectively) and the labor market (arrow o).[21] Cognitive skills also affect women's ability to promote child quality, that is child health and schooling (arrow p).

A woman's value in the marriage market can be thought of as her marriage prospects (see also Basu, this volume). In general, better-educated spouses are more valuable as wives, though some men may prefer less-educated wives because they are thought to be more subservient. A woman's value in the marriage market, as well as her own values, will determine her spouse's characteristics and her age at marriage (arrows h and q, respectively). In the labor market, the impact of cognitive skills, and possibly years of schooling (arrow e), on the value of a woman's time is almost always positive; that is, education raises the woman's productivity in the labor market. Similarly, cognitive skills increase her ability to raise high-quality children (arrow p). In a penultimate step, a woman's fertility knowledge, her cognitive skills, the value of her time, her ability to raise high-quality children, and her spouse's characteristics will determine the woman's bargaining power in marriage (arrows m, n, s, t, and v, respectively).[22] The last step in Figure 5-3 shows how a woman's values, her spouse's characteristics and her age at marriage, her fertility knowledge, the value of her time, her bargaining

[19]The term "values" denotes ways of thinking that can be changed in some way. Thus values are assumed to be endogenous in that they can be altered by public policies. In contrast, the term "tastes" indicates preferences that cannot, by definition, be changed by public policies or by anything else.

[20]Of course, some knowledge may be acquired informally from classmates in school even if there is no such curriculum.

[21]It is possible that values and fertility knowledge, particularly the former, could directly affect the value of a woman's time in the labor market; to reduce clutter, this possibility is not shown in the diagram.

[22]For a general discussion of intrahousehold bargaining, see Alderman et al. (1995a), Behrman (1997), and Strauss and Thomas (1995).

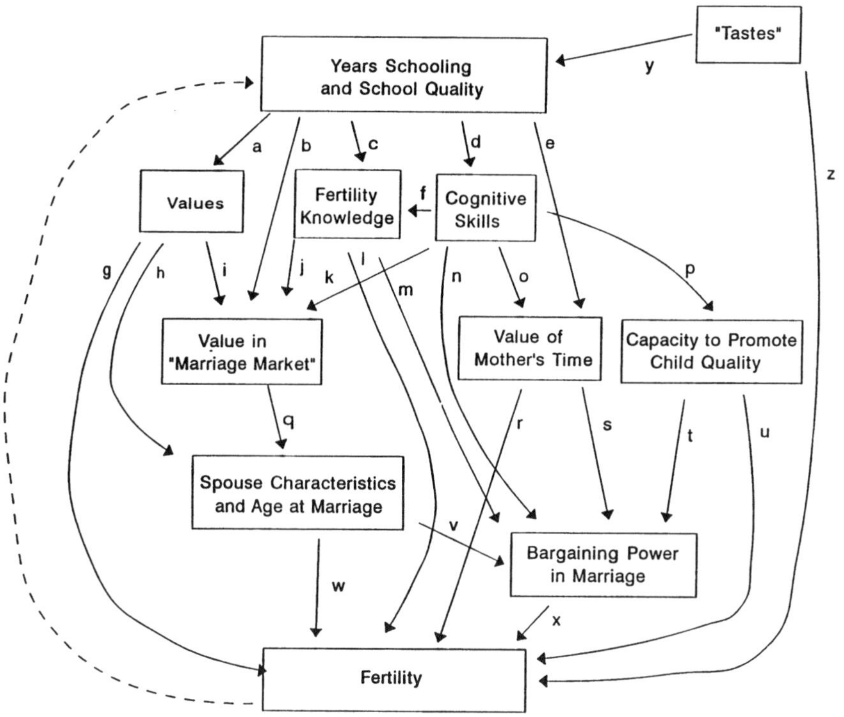

FIGURE 5-3 Relationship between schooling and fertility.

power within her marriage, and her ability to raise high-quality children (arrows g, w, l, r, x, and u, respectively) determine her fertility. A final point, noted earlier, is that it is also possible for fertility to affect schooling outcomes; a female student who has a child while in school may have to leave school. This arrow is dashed to indicate reverse causality.

The above discussion of Figure 5-3 is not intended to be an all-encompassing description of how education affects fertility. Indeed, the figure could be made even more complex.[23] However, the discussion does demonstrate the complexity of the impact of schooling, in terms of both years of schooling attained and school quality, on the future fertility of today's children. Yet there is one more aspect of the relationship between education and fertility that deserves mention because the connection is not causal at all. One can imagine that young women vary in their tastes for different choices to be made during their lives. These

[23]For example, see Chapters 2 and 3 for a discussion of other possible pathways by which education can affect fertility.

tastes can play a role in determining both schooling and fertility (arrows y and z).[24] In particular, women who are less family oriented and more career oriented will tend to have both higher levels of schooling and lower fertility, even in the absence of a causal link from the former to the latter; rather, the causality operates through a third factor, tastes. Because such tastes are not easily observed, this possibility further complicates attempts to understand the relationship between schooling and fertility in both developed and developing countries.

EMPIRICAL EVIDENCE ON THE IMPACT OF SCHOOL QUALITY AND FERTILITY

Impact on Current Decisions of Today's Parents

The present review revealed no empirical work that explicitly addresses the impact of school quality on the current fertility decisions of today's parents in developing countries. However, one can get at this issue by examining empirical work on the impact of school prices on fertility. While no studies were found that explicitly examine the impact of school prices, two studies examine the impact of availability of local schools, which can be interpreted as a price effect. The first is that of Rosenzweig (1982), which uses household survey data from India. It finds no significant impact of the availability of a local primary school on fertility rates. The second is that of Pitt et al. (1993), which uses district-level data from Indonesia. It finds that the presence of middle and high schools has no significant effect on fertility, while the presence of primary schools does have a small but significantly positive effect.

Of course, both of these studies can be criticized. Rosenzweig does nothing to control for the possible endogeneity of the presence of schools in a village; although the problem is noted, the conclusion is that nothing can be done to address it. In addition, variation in tastes for child quality and quantity are ignored. If some households or villages favor quantity while others favor quality, the results will be biased in favor of showing a negative effect of school availability on fertility. The implication is that an ambiguous result may mask a genuine positive relationship. Measurement error may also be a problem because the availability of a local school is a very crude indicator of school prices. The Pitt et al. (1993) study also has shortcomings. The data used include no information on household income or nonland assets, leading to possible omitted-variable bias (perhaps wealthier communities have more children, other things being equal, and also are able to lobby the government to build local schools). In addition, the fixed-effects estimates presented assume no interaction effects between observed variables and the fixed effects that are differenced out during estimation.

---

[24]The tastes involved may be those not only of the woman, but also of her parents.

In summary, there is a small amount of evidence on the impact of school quality on the fertility decisions of today's parents, which can be inferred by looking at the impact of school availability on fertility. One study finds an insignificant effect of primary schools, while another finds a small but significant effect of primary schools, but no significant effect of middle or high schools. While these studies constitute a sample size of two and can be criticized on methodological grounds, they are relatively careful as compared with the literature reviewed earlier. Thus the little evidence available suggests no sizeable effects of school quality on the fertility decisions of today's parents. Of course, school quality may affect fertility in the future. This possibility is examined in the next subsection.

Impact on Future Decisions of Today's Children

We turn now to the impact of improvements in school quality on the future fertility decisions of today's children. Figure 5-3 shows that the relationship between education and fertility, while complex, must work through one of the following four pathways: (1) changes in values brought about by schooling, (2) changes in fertility knowledge, (3) cognitive skills learned in school, and (4) a noncausal relationship whereby an individual's tastes determine both schooling outcomes and fertility. Knowledge of the relative importance of these pathways and of the distinct contributions (if any) of specific types of cognitive skills would provide a much clearer picture of the role played by school quality in affecting future fertility, and might even demonstrate how changes in school curriculum could lead to reductions in fertility.

There appear to be only three studies that attempt to disentangle the various pathways through which schooling leads to reduced fertility. The first, Lam and Duryea (1999), uses Brazilian data to look at the impact of years of schooling on both fertility and labor force participation. At low levels of schooling, the authors find strong effects of years of schooling on fertility, but only weak effects on labor supply. They also find strong effects of low levels of schooling on child health. While many studies have examined the impact of schooling on both fertility and labor force participation, the Lam and Duryea study is distinctive in that it uses the results to say something about the pathways by which schooling affects fertility. In particular, the authors interpret the evidence, especially the effects of low levels of schooling, as indicating that the effects of schooling on fertility work, at least in part, through pathways other than those based on the value of a mother's time in the labor market.

Although the analysis of Lam and Duryea is intriguing, some of the findings can be criticized. First, their regressions on the determinants of fertility assume that a mother's schooling and that of her spouse are exogenous, which can be questioned. In particular, the positive relationship between higher schooling and lower fertility may reflect, at least in part, the impact of tastes as depicted in

Figure 5-2. Second, part of the impact of mother's schooling may work through spouse's schooling, in that a better-educated woman will choose a better-educated spouse (see also Basu, this volume). Third, many other variables that may determine fertility, such as local family planning or health services, are not included in the regression. Fourth, the authors ignore the possibility that part of the causality underlying the relationship between schooling and fertility may run from the latter to the former as a result of pregnancy forcing young women to drop out of school.

A second study addressing the pathways by which schooling leads to reduced fertility is by Oliver (1997). It uses data on women's cognitive skills to understand the relationship between education and fertility. In particular, it uses the 1988-1989 Ghana Living Standards Survey to show that a woman's level of literacy, but not her level of mathematical ability, leads to reduced fertility.[25] In addition, it finds that years of schooling has a strong negative effect over and above the effect due to literacy. This finding suggests that either values, fertility knowledge, or perhaps cognitive skills other than literacy and numeracy can play a role in reducing fertility beyond the role played by the acquisition of basic cognitive skills.

Oliver's findings can be interpreted in terms of Figure 5-3. She shows that improvements in school quality reduce fertility by raising cognitive skills (arrow d in Figure 5-3). In addition, she shows that more years of schooling reduces fertility even after controlling for the effect that works through cognitive skills. This could occur because schooling changes students' values, their value in the marriage market, or their fertility knowledge (arrows a, b and c, respectively). Unfortunately, the data used by Oliver cannot distinguish among these alternative pathways.

Another intriguing aspect of Oliver's study is that it relates the impact of literacy and years of education on fertility to specific components of school quality. In particular, the study presents estimates of the impact of six middle school quality improvements on the number of children ever born, and for three of those a cost-effectiveness ratio is given. These results are shown in Table 5-2. The total impact of the different school improvements varies from a fertility reduction (measured in terms of children ever born) of 0.04 due to providing textbooks to a reduction of 0.64 due to providing blackboards. Note that much of this effect comes about because these schooling improvements also raise years of schooling (see column 2 of Table 5-2). Of the three schooling improvements for which cost-effectiveness figures are calculated, provision of blackboards is by far the least expensive avenue to reduce fertility. Repair of leaking classroom roofs is more expensive, and the costliest of the three is provision of textbooks. It would be interesting to compare these cost figures with the cost of reducing

---

[25]Both literacy and numeracy are measured in terms of scores on cognitive skills tests.

TABLE 5-2 Impact of Middle School Improvements on Children Ever Born in Ghana

Middle School Improvement	Impact on Children Ever Born: Reading Scores	Years of School	Total	Cost-Effectiveness[a]
Reducing travel time from 2 to zero hours	0.121	0.171	0.292	—
Raising average teacher experience from 2 to 10 years	0.112	0.158	0.270	—
Providing a school library	0.066	0.094	0.160	—
Repairing classrooms that cannot be used when it rains	0.288	0.153	0.441	1,273-2,545 cedis
Providing blackboards in schools where none exist	0.440	0.200	0.640	100-200 cedis
Providing 50 textbooks per room in schools that now have 25 per room	0.044	—	0.044	36,364-60,605 cedis

[a]These figures indicate the cost of reducing total predicted (future) children ever born to students in the improved classroom by 1. Note that the data presented here were collected in 1988-1989, at which time the exchange-rate value of the Ghanaian cedi was about 200 cedis per U.S. dollar.

SOURCE: Oliver (1997).

fertility through typical family planning programs; unfortunately, Oliver does not do this in her study.

Oliver's study does suffer from some methodological shortcomings. The schooling of the mother is assumed to be exogenous, which ignores the possible role of tastes in determining the relationship between schooling and fertility. It is also likely that omitted-variable bias is present because several variables that may determine fertility are not included, such as the availability of family planning and health services. Third, the possibility that fertility could reduce schooling because pregnant girls quit school is not considered. Finally, although the attempt to relate fertility reduction to specific changes in school quality is particularly valuable, the study does not address aspects of school quality that are likely to change a child's values. This is an admittedly difficult task, and it is questionable whether any existing data could be used to investigate this aspect of schooling and fertility.

A final study that sheds light on the impact of school quality on fertility is that of Thomas (see Chapter 6), who uses recent household survey data from South Africa to examine how schooling affects fertility. In particular, Thomas examines the effect of years of schooling and of scores on mathematics and reading comprehension tests on children ever born. His findings are similar to those of Oliver. Reading comprehension has an important effect, but mathematics skills have no significant effect, and even when both of these variables are included in the regression, years of schooling still has a strong independent effect. Unfortunately, Thomas' South African data cannot be used to examine how specific aspects of school quality determine the acquisition of cognitive skills.

As with the other two studies, Thomas' work suffers from several shortcomings, most of which cannot be corrected with the available data. The role of tastes in determining both schooling and fertility may seriously bias the estimates, or at least reduce what can be inferred from them. The possibility of reverse causality, that is, of women dropping out of school because of pregnancy, is not considered. Finally, the general problems of omitted-variable bias and measurement error are not addressed.

In summary, these three studies support the common finding that schooling is associated with reduced fertility. The studies of Oliver and Thomas show that reading comprehension skills, but not mathematics skills, directly affect fertility, and Oliver's paper shows the association between specific changes in school quality and reduced fertility. Finally, the results of all three studies imply that the impact of schooling on fertility is not just a matter of attaining mathematics and reading skills. However, much more remains to be learned. What can be done about this need is briefly discussed in the following subsection.

Recommendations for Future Research

The most obvious recommendation for future research on the impact of school quality on fertility is that much more of such research should be done. First, more research is needed on the impact of school quality on the current fertility decisions of today's parents. This work should examine the impact of school quality directly, as opposed to relying on the price of schooling or the availability of a local school. Second, much more can be done to examine the impact of current changes in school quality on the future fertility decisions of today's children. As in the study by Oliver (1997), this work can be divided into two parts: the impact of a variety of cognitive skills, knowledge, and even attitudes on fertility, and the impact of improvements in school quality on all of those determining factors. While some initial work has been done on the most basic cognitive skills, almost nothing has been done on other cognitive skills or on knowledge and attitudes.

As with the literature on the determinants of school quality, another obvious recommendation is that more useful data should be collected. Data are needed on school quality, fertility, and cognitive skills, plus attitudes and fertility knowledge (and other knowledge as well, such as health knowledge), from the *same* households. If data that follow young women over several years can be collected, a link can be made between specific schooling outcomes and subsequent fertility outcomes. Alternatively, if only cross-sectional data can be collected, the data should include the skills of adult women (determined by administering achievement tests) to see how those skills are related to fertility. Both types of data go well beyond what is usually collected in developing countries, which explains the paucity of research on the pathways by which school quality affects fertility.

Finally, the call for more randomized evaluations of education policies made earlier also applies here. Although this section has not gone into detail on the statistical problems that complicate attempts to estimate the impact of school quality on fertility (see Strauss and Thomas, 1995, for a discussion of this issue), many such problems do arise that are difficult to solve. Randomized evaluations can, in principle, get around almost all of these problems.[26] There have apparently been no randomized trials relating schooling to fertility in developing countries, perhaps because the time lag between a schooling intervention and the future fertility outcomes of today's children may be many years. Again, bilateral and multilateral aid agencies need to take the lead on this matter by building randomized evaluations into their development projects.

CONCLUSION

The main message of this chapter is that very little is known about what determines school quality in developing countries, and even less is known on how school quality affects fertility. This state of affairs exists even though a large number of studies have been done on the first topic—the relationship between school quality and learning. There are two main reasons that little is known about this relationship: (1) statistical tools have not been used very carefully, and (2) the data available are usually inadequate for the task. Both of these problems need to be addressed in future work. In addition, randomized evaluations of schooling interventions hold promise for addressing some of the more intractable statistical problems. Given the apparent inefficiencies in the way schools operate in developing countries, improving the general state of knowledge on which interventions are most cost-effective has the potential to bring about sizeable increases in learning, and eventually in the standard of living, in those countries.

While the relationship between the quantity of schooling and fertility has

---

[26]However, recall that poor design and/or implementation can compromise results based on randomized evaluations.

been documented numerous times, the effect of school quality on fertility has rarely been examined. Better knowledge of the various pathways involved in the latter could lead to policy recommendations that would ultimately help bring about further reductions in fertility. For example, the little evidence produced thus far suggests that spending more class time on reading skills and less on mathematics may reduce fertility. However, much more must be learned before such broad policy recommendations can be made, and one must bear in mind that fertility reduction is only one of many different schooling outcomes to be considered when contemplating such changes.

Finally, since this chapter was written from an economist's perspective, there is one more difficult question to raise: Why should the government concern itself with trying to alter households' fertility decisions? There is a tendency among many demographers to assume at the outset that fertility levels in developing countries are too high. This may be so, but it should be demonstrated instead of merely assumed. If demographers want to win the support of economists on this issue, more theoretical and empirical work may be needed.

ACKNOWLEDGMENTS

The findings, interpretations, and conclusions expressed in this paper are entirely those of the author. They do not necessarily represent the views of the World Bank, its executive directors, or the countries they represent. I would like to thank Andrew Foster, Bruce Fuller, Hanan Jacoby, Emmanuel Jimenez, the editors of this volume, and two anonymous referees for very useful comments on and/or discussion of previous drafts.

REFERENCES

Ainsworth, M., K. Beegle, and A. Nyamete
1996 The impact of women's schooling on fertility and contraceptive use: A study of fourteen sub-Saharan African countries. *World Bank Economic Review* 10(1):85-122.

Alderman, H., J. Behrman, S. Khan, D. Rose, and R. Scott
1995a Public schooling expenditures in rural Pakistan: Efficiently targeting girls and a lagging region. In D. van de Walle and K. Nead, eds., *Public Spending and the Poor: Theory and Evidence*. Baltimore, Md.: The Johns Hopkins University Press.

Alderman, H., P.A. Chiappori, L. Haddad, J. Hoddinott, and R. Kanbuv
1995b Unitary versus collective models of the household: Is it time to shift the burden of proof? *World Bank Research Observer* 10(1):1-19.

American Psychological Association
1995 *Intelligence: Knowns and Unknowns*. Report of a task force established by the Board of Scientific Affairs of the American Psychological Association. Washington, D.C.: American Psychological Association.

Becker, G.
1981 *A Treatise on the Family*. Cambridge, Mass.: Harvard University Press.

1995 *Human Capital and Poverty Alleviation.* HRO Working Paper No, 52. Human Resources Development and Operations Policy Vice Presidency. Washington, D.C.: The World Bank.

Behrman, J.

1997 Intrahousehold Distribution and the Family. In M. Rosenzweig and O. Stark, eds., *Handbook of Population and Family Economics.* Amsterdam: North Holland.

Behrman, J., M. Rosenzweig, and P. Taubman

1994 Endowments and the allocation of schooling in the family and in the marriage market: The twins experiment. *Journal of Political Economy* 102(6)1131-1174.

Cox, D., and E. Jimenez

1991 The relative effectiveness of private and public schools: Evidence from two developing countries. *Journal of Development Economics* 34:99-121.

Fuller, B., and P. Clarke

1994 Raising school effects while ignoring culture?: Local conditions and the influence of classroom tools, rules and pedagogy. *Review of Educational Research* 64(1)119-157.

Gertler, P., and P.Glewwe

1990 The willingness to pay for education in developing countries: Evidence from rural Peru. *Journal of Public Economics* 42:251-275.

Glewwe, P.

1998 *The Economics of School Quality Investments in Developing Countries: An Empirical Study of Ghana.* London: Macmillan.

Glewwe, P., M. Grosh, H. Jacoby, and M. Lockheed

1995 An eclectic approach to estimating the determinants of achievement in Jamaican primary school. *World Bank Economic Review* 9(2):231-258.

Glewwe, P., and H. Jacoby

1994 Student achievement and schooling choice in low income countries. *Journal of Human Resources* 29(3):843-864.

Glewwe, P., M. Kremer, and S. Moulin

1998 Textbooks and Test Scores: Evidence from a Propsective Evaluation in Kenya. Draft paper. Washington, D.C.: The World Bank.

Godfrey, L.G.

1988 *Misspecification Tests in Econometrics.* Cambridge: Cambridge University Press.

Hanushek, E.

1986 The economics of schooling: Production and efficiency in public schools. *Journal of Economic Literature* 25:1141-1177.

1995 Interpreting recent research on schooling in developing countries. *World Bank Research Observer* 10(August):227-246.

Hanushek, E., C. Benson, R. Freeman, D. Jamison, H. Levin, R. Maynard, R. Murnane, S. Rivkin, R. Sabot, L. Solomon, A. Summers, F. Welch, and B. Wolfe

1994 *Making Schools Work: Improving Performance and Controlling Costs.* Washington, D.C.: Brookings Institution.

Harbison, R., and E. Hanushek

1992 *Educational performance of the poor: Lessons from rural northeast Brazil.* New York: Oxford University Press.

Haveman, R., and B. Wolfe

1984 Education and economic well-being: The role of non- market effects. *Journal of Human Resources* 19:377-407.

Heckman, J., and J.A. Smith

1995 Assessing the case for social experiments. *Journal of Economic Perspectives* 9(2):85-110.

Hedges, L., R. Laine, and R. Greenwald
1994 Does money matter? A meta-analysis of studies of the effects of differential school inputs on student outcomes. *Educational Researcher* 23:5-14.
Heyneman, S.P., D.T. Jamison, and X. Montenegro
1984 Textbooks in the Philippines: Evaluation of the pedagogical impact of nationwide investment. *Educational Evaluation and Policy Analysis* 6(2):139-150.
Jamison, D., B. Searle, K. Galda, and S. Heyneman
1981 Improving elementary mathematics education in Nicaragua: An experimental study of the impact of textbooks and radio on achievement. *Journal of Educational Psychology* 73(4):556-567.
Jimenez, E., M. Lockheed, E. Luna, and V. Paqueo
1991 School effects and costs for private and public schools in the Dominican Republic. *International Journal of Education Research* 15:393-410.
Jimenez, E., M. Lockheed, and N. Wattanawaha
1988 The relative efficiency of public and private schools: The case of Thailand. *World Bank Economic Review* 2:139-164.
Kagitcibasi, C., D. Sunar, and S. Bekman
1993 *Long-Term Effects of Early Intervention.* Department of Education, Bogadzdi University, Istanbul, Turkey.
Kremer, M.
1995 Research on schooling: What we know and what we don't, a comment on Hanushek. *World Bank Researcher Observer* 10:247-254.
Kremer, M., S. Moulin, D. Myatt, and R. Namunyu
1997 *Textbooks, Class Size and Test Scores: Evidence from a Prospective Evaluation in Kenya.* Cambridge, Mass.: Department of Economics, Massachusetts Institute of Technology.
Lam, D., and S. Duryea
1999 Effects of Schooling on Fertility, Labor Supply, and Investments in Children, with Evidence from Brazil. *Journal of Human Resources.*
Lockheed, M.
1995 Educational assessment in developing countries: The role of the World Bank. In T. Oakland, ed., *International Perspectives on Academic Assessment.* Norwell, Mass.: Kluwer Academic Publishers.
Lockheed, M., and A. Verspoor
1991 *Improving Primary Education in Developing Countries.* New York: Oxford University Press.
Oliver, R.
1997 Fertility and women's schooling in Ghana. In P. Glewwe, ed., *The Economics of School Quality Investments, in Developing Countries: An Empirical Study of Ghana.* London: Macmillan.
Pitt, M., M. Rosenzweig, and D. Gibbons
1993 The determinants and consequences of the placement of government programs in Indonesia. *World Bank Economic Review* 7(3):319-348.
Rosenzweig, M.
1982 Educational subsidy, agricultural development and fertility change. *Quarterly Journal of Economics* 97(1):67-88.
Schultz, T.P.
1993 Returns to women's education. In E. King and A. Hill, eds., *Women's Education in Developing Countries: Barriers, Benefits, and Policies.* Baltimore, Md.: The Johns Hopkins University Press.

Strauss, J., and D. Thomas
1995 Human resources: Empirical modeling of household and family decisions. In J. Behrman and T.N. Srinivasan, eds. *Handbook of Development Economics, Volume IIIA*. Amsterdam: North Holland.

United Nations
1995 *Women's Education and Fertility Behavior: Recent Evidence from the Demographic and Health Surveys.* New York: Department for Economic and Social Information and Policy Analysis, United Nations.

United Nations Development Programme
1990 *Human Development Report.* New York: Oxford University Press.

Velez, E., E. Schiefelbein, and J. Valenzuela
1993 *Factors Affecting Achievement in Primary Education.* HRO Working Paper No. 2. Washington, D.C.: The World Bank.

World Bank
1990 *World Development Report.* New York: Oxford University Press.
1995 *Improving Basic Education in Pakistan: Community Participation, System Accountability and Efficiency.* Washington, D.C.: The World Bank, South Asia Region.

APPENDIX A
SIMPLE TWO-PERIOD MODEL OF SCHOOL CHOICE

To determine how the optimal (utility-maximizing) value of years of schooling is affected by changes in the parameters of the model given in the main text, assume first that school quality is given exogenously. As given in equation (5.6) in the text, the expression to be maximized with respect to S is:

$$U = Y_1 - pS + \delta Y_2 + [(1 - S + \delta)k\pi + \sigma]\alpha f(Q)g(S) \quad \text{(A-1)}$$

The first and second derivatives of U with respect to S are:

$$\partial U/\partial S = -p + \alpha f(Q)g'(S)[(1 - S + \delta)k\pi + \sigma] - k\pi\alpha f(Q)g(S) \quad \text{(A-2)}$$

$$\partial U/\partial S^2 = \alpha f(Q)g''(S)[(1 - S + \delta)k\pi + \sigma] - 2k\pi\alpha f(Q)g'(S) \quad \text{(A-3)}$$

Totally differentiating the first-order condition (the condition that equation (A-2) = 0) yields:

$$\begin{aligned}
&[2\alpha f(Q)g'(S)k\pi - \alpha f(Q)g''(S)((1 - S + \delta)k\pi + \sigma)]dS \\
&= [\alpha f(Q)g'(S)(1 - S + \delta) - \alpha f(Q)g(S)]dk\pi \\
&+ [f(Q)g'(S)((1 - S + \delta)k\pi + \sigma) - k\pi f(Q)g(S)]d\alpha - dp + [\alpha f(Q)g'(S)]d\sigma \\
&+ [af'(Q)g'(S)((1 - S + \delta)k\pi + \sigma) - k\pi\alpha f'(Q)g(S)]dQ \\
&+ [\alpha f(Q)g'(S)k\pi]d\delta \qquad \text{(A-4)}
\end{aligned}$$

It is immediately clear that the coefficient associated with dp (i.e., –1) is negative and that the terms associated with $d\sigma$ and $d\delta$ are positive. The fact that the second-order condition, (A-3), must be negative implies that the term associated with dS is positive. The fact that the first-order condition, (A-2), equals zero implies that the terms associated with $d\alpha$ and dQ are positive. Since k and π always appear together, their product can be treated as a single variable, denoted by $k\pi$. The term associated with $dk\pi$ cannot be signed unambiguously, but it will be positive if σ is relatively small.

Now turn to the case where school quality, Q, is a choice, and higher school quality implies a higher tuition fee. As given in equation (5.8) in the text, under the assumption that $f(Q) = Q^\beta$ and $g(S) = S^\gamma$, the expression to be maximized with respect to S and Q is:

$$U = Y_1 - p_o QS + \delta Y_2 + \alpha Q^\beta S^\gamma((1 - S + \delta)k\pi + \sigma) \quad \text{(A-5)}$$

The first and second derivatives of (A-5) with respect to S are:

$$\partial U/\partial S = -p_o Q + \alpha Q^\beta \gamma S^{\gamma-1}((1 - S + \delta)k\pi + \sigma) - k\pi\alpha Q^\beta S^\gamma \quad \text{(A-6)}$$

$$\partial^2U/SU^2 = \alpha Q^\beta\gamma(\gamma - 1)S^{\gamma-2}((1 - S + \delta)k\pi + \sigma) - 2k\pi\alpha Q^\beta\gamma S^{\gamma-1} \quad \text{(A-7)}$$

The first and second derivatives of (A-5) with respect to Q are:

$$\partial U/\partial Q = -p_o S + \alpha\beta Q^{\beta-1}S^\gamma((1 - S + \delta)k\pi + \sigma) \quad \text{(A-8)}$$

$$\partial^2U/\partial Q^2 = \alpha\beta(\beta-1)Q^{\beta-2}S^\gamma((1 - S + \delta)k\pi + \sigma) \quad \text{(A-9)}$$

Note that the requirement that both second derivatives equal zero implies, by (A-9), that $\beta < 1$, so that Q^β is a concave function of Q. Setting (A-6) and (A-8) equal to zero, dividing (A-6) by Q and (A-8) by S, and substituting (A-6) into (A-8) (i.e., substituting out p_o) yields:

$$\alpha Q^{\beta-1}\gamma S^{\gamma-1}((1 - S + \delta)k\pi + \sigma) - k\pi\alpha Q^{\beta-1}S^\gamma$$
$$= \alpha\beta Q^{\beta-1}S^{\gamma-1}((1 - S + \delta)k\pi + \sigma) \quad \text{(A-10)}$$

Dropping $Q^{\beta-1}$ from both sides of (A-10) and multiplying both sides by $S^{1-\gamma}$ yields the following optimizing solution for S:

$$S = (\gamma - \beta)(1 + \delta + \sigma/k\pi)/(1 + \gamma - \beta) \quad \text{(A-11)}$$

Clearly, this solution is only plausible if $\gamma > \beta$. Substituting (A-11) into (A-7) and noting that $\gamma > \beta$ implies that (A-7) is negative, which means that the second-order condition for maximization is satisfied. Setting (A-8) equal to zero, solving for Q, and replacing S with (A-11) yields the optimizing solution for Q:

$$Q = (\alpha\beta k\pi/p_o)(\gamma - \beta)^{\gamma-1}((1 + \delta + \sigma/k\pi)/(1 + \gamma - \beta))^\gamma \quad \text{(A-12)}$$

The impact of most of the parameters in (A-12) is clear. The exceptions are k and π, which again can be treated as a single variable $k\pi$. Differentiating Q with respect to $k\pi$ yields:

$$\partial Q/\partial k\pi = ((\gamma - \beta)^{\gamma-1}\alpha\beta/p_0(1 + \gamma - \beta)^\gamma)(1 + \delta + \sigma/k\pi)^{\gamma-1}$$
$$(1 + \delta + (1 - \gamma)\sigma/k\pi) \quad \text{(A-13)}$$

The expression in (A-13) will be positive if $(1 + \delta) + (1 - \gamma)\sigma/k\pi > 0$, and negative otherwise. Thus the impact of k and π on Q will depend on the values of δ, γ, σ, k, and π. Note that if σ is sufficiently small, this term will be positive even if $\alpha\gamma > 1$, which is a similar condition for the case when Q is exogenous.

6

Fertility, Education, and Resources in South Africa

Duncan Thomas

INTRODUCTION

South Africa has emerged from three-quarters of a century of apartheid, which placed comprehensive restrictions on the geographic and economic mobility of its population. As those restrictions are relaxed and the society moves toward integration, one of the greatest challenges facing the people of South Africa will be the absorption of a young and rapidly growing labor force into an economy undergoing dramatic restructuring. While South Africa appears to be ahead of other African countries in its demographic transition, there is tremendous diversity within the country. It seems safe to conjecture, therefore, that population policy will play a key role in influencing the success of social and economic development in the country (Chimere-Dan, 1993; African National Congress, 1994, 1995).

Using recently collected household survey data, this chapter examines an important consideration in the design of that policy: the relationship between fertility and resources, with a focus on the role played by maternal education. A vast number of studies have demonstrated that education and fertility tend to be negatively correlated in a wide array of contexts. In South Africa, education is a key correlate of fertility among all black women, but the association is less clear among women of other races, except, perhaps, those who are better educated. Over and above simply documenting these findings, this chapter examines three potential mechanisms in an attempt to provide insight into what underlies the observed association between education and fertility among South African blacks.

First, education is not randomly assigned within a population; rather, people choose how much they invest in schooling given the constraints and opportunities they face. In the extreme, it might be argued that schooling provides no value-added, but is simply a sorting mechanism: those who are more able spend more time at school in order to signal their ability to their future employers (or spouses). Placing the spotlight on educational attainment around natural exit points in the South African education system, the evidence suggests that self-selection in education does play some role in explaining the effect of education on fertility in a regression context. Thus, a naive interpretation of the effect as being entirely causal would be misleading.

Second, education and household resources tend to be correlated, so a woman's education may simply be a proxy for her, or her family's, income. To the extent that it can be tested with the available data, this interpretation does not appear to tell the entire story in South Africa. While household resources do affect fertility outcomes, even after controlling for spousal characteristics, household income, labor market choices, and community characteristics, female education continues to have a powerful negative association with fertility. Thus one can conclude that a substantial part of the effect of female education on fertility operates independently of resources. Spousal education is also negatively correlated with fertility (see Basu, this volume), and the impacts of male and female education are, in most cases, close in magnitude. In South Africa, men appear to have an important influence on demographic outcomes.

Third, one can attempt to isolate the relationship between skills likely to be learned in school and demographic outcomes. Drawing on a subsample of women who completed a short comprehension and quantitative test, one finds that, after controlling for income and education, performance on these tests has an independent impact on fertility. The impact of comprehension skills is particularly large in magnitude, suggesting that the acquisition and assimilation of information may be important in affecting family decision making.

The next section sets the stage for the main analysis of the chapter by placing fertility and educational attainment in South Africa in historical context. This is followed by three sections that use recently collected household survey data to examine in turn the three mechanisms discussed above. The final section presents conclusions.

FERTILITY AND EDUCATION IN HISTORICAL PERSPECTIVE

Given the central role played by population policy in the apartheid system of South Africa, it is remarkable how little solid evidence exists on the demography of the country. Even today, few of the data sources predating 1993 that contain information on fertility have been placed in the public domain. As a result, one must rely on reports that have not been subjected to the sort of scientific scrutiny they warrant (see Caldwell and Caldwell, 1993, for an excellent discussion). Fortunately, as the government has embraced the concept of openness and access to information, this situation has been remedied. Data collected by the Central Statistical Service and, in many cases, by units that are independent of the government are now routinely placed in the public domain; the Project for Statistics on Living Standards and Development (PSLSD) and the annual October Household Surveys are good examples.

The 1994 October Household Survey estimates South Africa's population at about 40 million, of whom over three-quarters are black; half the rest are white, nearly 9 percent are mixed-race coloreds, and fewer than 3 percent are Asians, mostly of Indian descent. That survey estimates the total fertility rate (TFR) to be 4.1, although the Central Statistical Service views this as a substantial underestimate, particularly among blacks.

Much of the historical data on fertility and family planning in South Africa is described by van Zyl (1994), who also documents the methodologies used for the main surveys conducted by the Human Sciences Research Council that form the basis of these estimates. There are good reasons to be skeptical about the quality of some of those surveys, not least of which is the fact that population policy was an important political issue in South Africa, and it is far from clear that, at least at that time, the Human Sciences Research Council played a role that was entirely divorced from the political system. It is also prudent to treat comparisons across time with considerable caution since the surveys are not always comparable, and several focused on specific subpopulations. For example, in many surveys, the so-called homelands (where many of the poorest South Africans lived) were excluded from the samples, and in some surveys, fertility questions were asked only of married women. Setting aside the fact that the definition of marriage is complex in this society, many women who would not declare themselves as married have borne children, and teenage pregnancy rates are very high. According to the 1994 October Household Survey, about 33 of every 100 women have given birth out of wedlock. (See, for example, Preston-Whyte, 1990, for an insightful discussion.)

While remaining mindful of these caveats about data quality, it is useful to attempt to place South Africa's fertility rate in historical context. TFR estimates for 1950 through 1990 for each of the four main racial groups in South Africa are presented in the upper panel of Figure 6-1.[1] According to these estimates, in 1950, the TFRs of blacks, coloreds, and Indians were all high (above 6) and reasonably close to one another, whereas that of whites was much lower (slightly above 3). By 1990, the picture was dramatically different: TFRs among coloreds and Indians had been reduced by more than half and were very close to that of whites. The TFR of blacks, however, remained much higher, around 5.0. While fertility among blacks had declined sharply during the 1970s and early 1980s, it had remained virtually constant during the earlier two decades. It appears that

---

[1]The data are drawn from Lucas (1992) and van Zyl (1994).

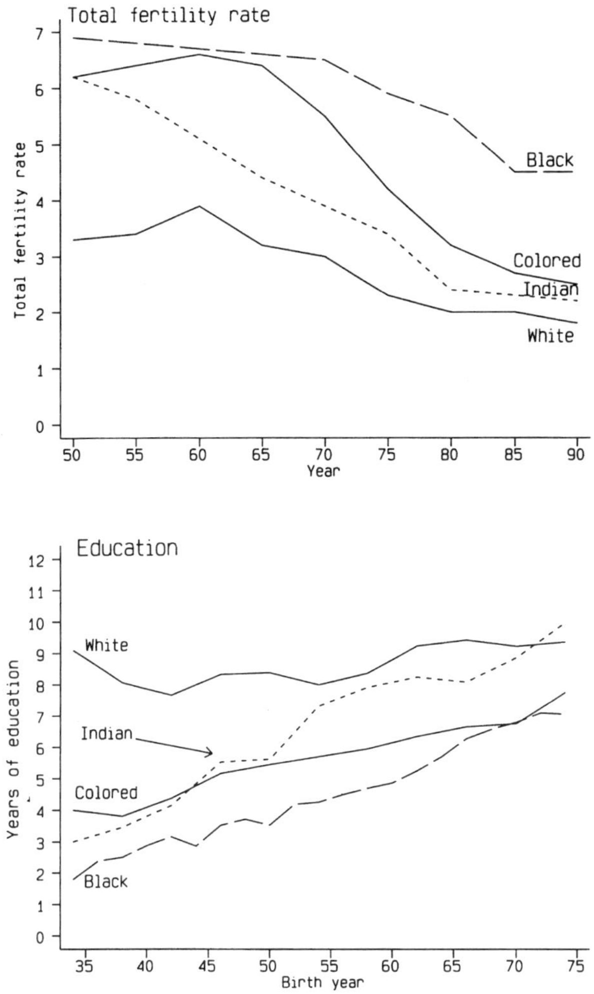

FIGURE 6-1 Total fertility rates and education of females, South Africa, 1950-1990.

among blacks, the demographic transition began to accelerate only around a quarter-century ago. In sharp contrast, there were rapid declines in fertility among Indians dating back to the 1950s, and their fertility stabilized around 1980. Coloreds fall between these two groups: their fertility actually rose in the 1950s, so that in the early 1960s, the TFRs of blacks and coloreds were almost identical (around 7), but the TFR of coloreds declined during the following quarter-century to a level that is now very close to that of Indians. The fertility of whites changed very little during the period, having risen slightly during the 1950s and declined slowly since then to below replacement levels.

If these estimates reflect reality, several questions arise. First, what underlies the differences in the timing of fertility decline among Indians, coloreds, and blacks? Second, why has the fertility of coloreds and Indians fallen so dramatically, while that of blacks has remained at levels comparable with those of neighboring Botswana and Zimbabwe, whose populations are substantially poorer and less well educated?

A plausible hypothesis centers around differences in community resources, specifically access to family planning services. There is, however, little direct evidence on the relationship between the fertility of individual women in South Africa and their access to services, and the evidence in both Botswana and Zimbabwe suggests that access to services alone cannot explain fertility decline there. Nevertheless, casual inspection of the evidence in South Africa does suggest that service availability may have played a role.

Prior to the mid-1960s, government had little involvement in family planning, and it seems likely that only whites, and possibly Indians, would have had good access to services. Public investments in family planning began in the mid-1960s and were targeted largely toward urban dwellers: this coincides with the decline in fertility among colored women, the majority of whom live in urban areas. In the mid-1970s, the National Family Planning Programme was established, and access to services was massively expanded, with special attempts being made to serve rural women. In 1972, for example, there were fewer than 250 family planning clinics in the country, but by the early 1980s, that number had risen to more than 36,000 (Lucas, 1992). It was also during this period that the decline in black fertility took hold.

Yet even today, access to family planning services is probably not universal in South Africa. Evidence for this conclusion is provided by data from the PSLSD indicating that there is a family planning clinic in the community for over three-quarters of Indian women aged 15 to 49, about half of colored women, but only one-third of black women.[2]

---

[2]These discrepancies are likely to be underestimates of differences in service availability for at least two reasons. First, many women in South Africa obtain family planning services from places other than family planning clinics, and blacks are the least likely to use alternative sources. Second, the estimates are based on data collected at the community level, and it is well known that those data are difficult to collect in a survey setting and are therefore prone to serious measurement error. (See Frankenberg and Sudharto, 1995, for a general discussion, and Thomas and Maluccio, 1996, for a specific description of the nature and extent of problems that are evident in a community survey conducted in Zimbabwe in 1990.) Two issues are of special importance. First, it is not entirely clear how to define "community," particularly in urban and metropolitan areas, and the definition may not mean the same thing to all respondents. Second, the so-called "community informants" who are "prominent members of the community such as school principals, priests and chiefs" (Project for Statistics on Living Standards and Development, 1994:v) may themselves not be very well informed. For example, the PSLSD reports a family planning clinic in two-thirds of urban communities, one-third of rural communities, but only one-quarter of metropolitan communities. Yet it is the metropolitan communities that are likely to be best served of all.

Racial differences in fertility rates may also be explained by differences in household resources. The benefits of growth and development in South Africa have not been distributed evenly across races, and the society is marked by very high levels of inequality. This inequality is reflected, for example, in differences in education as depicted in the lower panel of Figure 6-1, which displays mean educational attainment for women, by birth cohort, as reported in the 1993 PSLSD.[3] Among women born in 1935, whites are much better educated than coloreds, Indians, and blacks: the average white woman had completed 9 years of schooling, whereas the average black had completed less than 2. The educational attainment of all groups except whites—especially Indians and, to a lesser extent, blacks—has increased substantially since then. Thus among women born in 1975, Indians are at least as well educated as whites, and blacks are nearly as well educated as coloreds. While the convergence of average educational attainment across races is striking, it is well known that there are substantial differences in the quality of schooling between racial groups, so it is unlikely that a year of education means the same thing to a black and a white.

A comparison of the upper and lower panels of Figure 6-1 does suggest that educational attainment and fertility are negatively correlated. However, it remains difficult to explain the timing of declines in TFRs for each race using an argument based on the average education of women. Digging a little more deeply and examining changes in other parts of the education distribution, a more complex picture emerges.

Thomas (1996) exploits the large sample sizes of the 1991 South African Census to explore rates of growth in educational attainment at each quartile of the education distribution. He reports that among those born between 1920 and 1970, an Indian woman would have spent 1.5 more years in school if she had been born a decade later, and the growth was most rapid among the least educated; for example, growth rates were 1.8 years at the bottom quartile and 1.2 years at the top quartile of the distribution. A similar pattern emerges for coloreds, although their average growth rate was only 0.7 years per decade. In sharp contrast, however, the least-educated blacks were largely excluded from the increase in education, which was, instead, concentrated among the better educated

[3]Completed years of education is defined as 1 if the woman completed sub-A, sub-B, or Standard 1, with another year being added for each grade completed until Standard 10, when most students take the matriculation (matric) examination. In the survey, postsecondary schooling is not reported in years, but in terms of qualifications. Diplomas, technical degrees, teacher training, nursing training, and completion of some university education are assigned 12 years of schooling. Completion of a university degree is assigned 14 years of schooling. Since only 5 percent of women report attending school beyond Standard 10, the impact of making different reasonable assumptions about years of schooling for these women is likely to be small. Moreover, the specifications for the regressions discussed in detail below are sufficiently flexible to ensure that coefficient estimates are not biased by this assumption.

of that group. There is a positive note in this dismal picture for the poorest black South Africans since, among those born in the latter part of the period, increases in education have occurred across all black women. This more recent extension of the fruits of development to the poorest may well be related to the tardiness of the fertility decline among blacks.

While they are suggestive, these aggregate data can give only a very incomplete picture of the relationship between fertility and education at the micro level. Therefore, in the following sections, survey data from the PSLSD are used to examine not only the correlation between fertility and education, but also some of the mechanisms that underlie that correlation. Before doing that, however, it is useful to take a slight detour and examine the determinants of educational attainment in South Africa. Ideally, one would like to be able to say something about how much of the increase in educational attainment in South Africa over the last half-century can be attributed to public policies such as investments in school infrastructure, teachers, and teacher training. It is not possible to answer that question directly with the available data, but it is possible to turn the question around and assess the extent to which resources in the home and in the community have affected the educational outcomes of adults and children.

We begin with completed schooling of adults. Respondents in the South African Social Stratification Survey (1991-1994)[4] report their own education; a migration history, including information on the type of house and community they lived in at birth; and characteristics, including education and occupation, of the people they viewed as their father- and mother-figure at age 14. Regressions in the upper panel of Table 6-1 report the impact of maternal and paternal years of schooling on the completed years of education of adult children aged 20 to 70 at the time of the survey. Parental education is a powerful predictor of own education: fully 26 percent of the variation in educational attainment among blacks is explained by parental education alone. Intergenerational mobility has risen over time, as indicated by the larger coefficients on education for older than younger blacks; this change is particularly striking for the impact of maternal education. While mobility remains lower among blacks relative to whites, even for whites an additional year of parental schooling is associated with one-fifth of a year more schooling for the respondent.

How much of the impact of parental education can be attributed to the role of household and community resources? It is difficult to imagine any household survey measuring resources in the home 50, 40, or even 20 years prior to the interview with any degree of accuracy. Fortunately, the South African Social

[4]The survey was conducted by Don Treiman in collaboration with the Human Sciences Research Council. One (randomly chosen) adult respondent was interviewed from each of 9,000 households in South Africa. See Treiman (1996).

Stratification Survey does provide proxies for resources in the home and community when the respondent was a child. Drawing on this information, the regressions were reestimated to include controls for the occupation of the parents when the respondent was age 14, location of birth, type of residence at birth, and language spoken at home. In addition, to capture variation in access to schools and possibly quality of schools, as well as other infrastructure at the community level, the reestimated regressions include fixed effects for town of birth. Results are reported in Panel B of Table 6-1.

Among blacks, over half the variation in educational attainment is explained by the controls, and the effects of parental education, particularly that of fathers, are significantly reduced. This suggests that household and community resources do matter and that paternal education is, in part, proxying for those resources. Further support for this interpretation is provided by the fact that among the covariates, paternal occupation is key. If a respondent's father had a job working in the wage sector or for the government or if the father was self-employed, the respondent is likely to have completed half a year of additional schooling, but a third of a year less if the father was a farm laborer; the excluded category includes informal-sector workers, communal farmers, and those not working at all.[5]

The additional controls do little to diminish the impact of maternal education, especially among older blacks, suggesting that a woman's education has an independent effect on the human capital of her children over and above the role of resources. Among whites, the additional controls do reduce the impact of parental education, but the differences are relatively small and not significant. This may be because variation in household and community resources is less important among whites or because the measures of these resources are too crude to be informative.

To provide some evidence on that question, one can examine the effects of parental education and resources on the educational attainment of children still resident at home using data from the PSLSD.[6] An advantage of these data is that they contain information on household per capita expenditures, a longer-run measure of resources available to the family; the disadvantage is that one is forced to restrict attention to only those children who are still resident in the

---

[5]The regressions include controls for whether the respondent was born in an urban, peri-urban, or squatter area, along with town-of-birth fixed effects. Paternal occupation is not, therefore, simply proxying for rural-urban differences. The negative effect of occupation if the father was a farm laborer is greater (and significant) among the younger cohort, suggesting that it may partly capture the effect of the Verwoerdian policy of "putting a school on every farm." The quality of those schools has been roundly criticized (see, for example, Department of Education, 1996).

[6]The PSLSD is a nationally representative survey of some 9,000 households conducted in South Africa during October through December 1993, a few months before the first democratic elections in April 1994.

TABLE 6-1 Intergenerational Transmission of Education

ADULTS	BLACKS (by age in years)			WHITES (by age in years)		
	ALL	20-39	41-70	ALL	20-39	41-70
A. Education only						
Maternal education	0.296*	0.258*	0.419*	0.201*	0.224*	0.185*
	[0.02]	[0.02]	[0.04]	[0.02]	[0.03]	[0.04]
Paternal education	0.264*	0.235*	0.337*	0.178*	0.164*	0.194*
	[0.02]	[0.02]	[0.05]	[0.02]	[0.03]	[0.03]
B. Full set of controls						
Maternal education	0.258*	0.211*	0.397*	0.176*	0.156*	0.194*
	[0.02]	[0.03]	[0.05]	[0.03]	[0.04]	[0.05]
Paternal education	0.178*	0.155*	0.215*	0.177*	0.160*	0.187*
	[0.03]	[0.03]	[0.08]	[0.03]	[0.04]	[0.04]
R^2	0.52	0.46	0.57	0.42	0.43	0.50
Sample size	4,533	2,964	1,569	2,161	1,133	1,028

C. CHILDREN	BLACKS (by age in years)					WHITES
	ALL	10-11	12-13	14-15	16-17	ALL
Maternal education	0.073*	0.038*	0.076*	0.102*	0.115*	0.003
	[0.01]	[0.01]	[0.01]	[0.02]	[0.02]	[0.01]
Paternal education	0.056*	0.021+	0.046*	0.063*	0.073*	0.015
	[0.01]	[0.01]	[0.02]	[0.02]	[0.02]	[0.01]
ln(per capita expenditure)	0.373*	0.200*	0.289*	0.415*	0.529*	0.066
	[0.05]	[0.05]	[0.06]	[0.09]	[0.10]	[0.12]
R^2	0.56	0.26	0.32	0.35	0.34	0.85
Sample size	6,609	1,706	1,729	1,658	1,516	577

NOTE: Dependent variable is years of completed education. Adult regressions based on respondents aged 20-70 in South African Social Stratification Survey, 1991/94. Adult "education only" regression includes controls for gender and (linear spline in) age of respondent, whether education of parent is missing, and whether father-figure and mother-figure are biological parents. "Full set of controls" adds controls for occupation of father and mother (at respondent's age 14), language spoken in home at respondent's age 14, type of place lived in at birth, type of house lived in at birth, and fixed effect for town of birth. Child regressions based on children aged 10-17 in PSLSD, 1994. Regressions include dummies for gender of child, each year of age of child, and whether urban or rural dweller.

home. The focus here is on children aged 10 through 17, but recognizing that a substantial fraction of older children are likely to have left the nest, the analyses are stratified into 2-year age bands. Panel C of Table 6-1 presents the regression results.

Educational attainment of black children is significantly correlated with parental education and household per capita expenditures, and all the effects increase with the age of the child. Among whites, there is no evidence that parental education or household resources are correlated with child educational attainment. One can conclude, therefore, that while there has been substantial intergenerational transmission in educational attainment among whites, resource constraints and limited access to schools are unlikely to have had a large impact on this group's educational attainment. Among blacks, however, resources do seem to matter, indicating that there is substantial scope for public interventions designed to raise schooling levels. Corroborating evidence is reported by Case and Deaton (1995), who show that even crude measures of teacher-pupil ratios are correlated with educational attainment among blacks, but not whites. The interpretation has considerable intuitive appeal in view of the history of South Africa, where racially segregated education was a central pillar of the apartheid system, state policies sought to restrict blacks' access to schooling, and a very well-funded system for whites coexisted with a substantially poorer system for blacks. In 1975, for example, the year before the Soweto school riots, public expenditures on education of the average white school-age child were more than 15 times greater than expenditures on the average black child.

RELATIONSHIP BETWEEN FERTILITY AND EDUCATION

Having shown that parental education and, for blacks, family and community resources play an important role in determining the educational attainment of the next generation, the discussion now turns to the correlation between education and fertility. The following analyses are based on the PSLSD, in which female respondents aged 15 to 49 reported the number of children ever born (CEB), how many survived to age 1 and how many to age 5, and how many were alive at the time of the survey. Unfortunately, fertility in the last year (or last 5 years) was not recorded. We must therefore focus on CEB as our sole measure of fertility.[7]

Summary statistics for the 10,500 female respondents are reported in Table 6-2. Three-quarters of the women in the survey were black and, as indicated in Figure 6-1, they had borne more children than coloreds, Indians, or whites. But

[7]It is also unfortunate that the limited set of information reduces the scope for undertaking internal consistency checks in these data—an issue of considerable import given the concerns raised about data quality above.

TABLE 6-2 Means and [Standard Errors]

Characteristic	Black	Black Lit. sample[a]	Colored	Indian	White
No. children ever born	2.106	1.785	2.002	1.604	1.535
	[0.026]	[0.079]	[0.068]	[0.088]	0.044]
(among those aged 40-49)	5.000	4.781	4.250	2.949	2.503
	[0.117]	[0.230]	[0.273]	[0.277]	0.107]
Woman's characteristics					
Years of education	5.654	6.139	6.489	8.023	9.140
	[0.036]	[0.107]	[0.094]	[0.160]	0.113]
Fraction completed					
Standard 0	0.109	0.066	0.041	0.041	0.074
Standard 1	0.041	0.032	0.022	0.006	0.003
Standard 2	0.048	0.039	0.025	0.006	0.004
Standard 3	0.061	0.058	0.047	0.021	0.006
Standard 4	0.075	0.067	0.074	0.032	0.026
Standard 5	0.114	0.096	0.115	0.035	0.014
Standard 6	0.127	0.150	0.162	0.120	0.042
Standard 7	0.099	0.140	0.134	0.091	0.041
Standard 8	0.118	0.145	0.165	0.170	0.161
Standard 9	0.088	0.091	0.071	0.123	0.055
Standard 10	0.091	0.091	0.108	0.276	0.324
Diploma/> Standard 10	0.029	0.025	0.028	0.044	0.135
University degree	—	—	0.008	0.035	0.118
Age	28.472	25.887	30.150	30.704	32.544
	[0.105]	[0.338]	[0.318]	[0.535]	[0.290]
Fraction worked in last year	0.176	0.126	0.335	0.290	0.433
ln (wage)	6.140	6.158	6.562	7.000	7.508
	[0.026]	[0.098]	[0.049]	[0.059]	[0.025]
Monthly Wage (Rs)	705.730	790.271	929.008	1327.217	2102.629
	[17.226]	[64.935]	[36.406]	[98.809]	[55.561]
Fraction in urban sector	0.173	0.213	0.357	0.531	0.248
Fraction in rural sector	0.651	0.591	0.069	0.003	0.077
Fraction ever married	0.546	0.365	0.567	0.660	0.750
Spouse's characteristics					
Fraction dead	0.058	0.000	0.053	0.040	0.016
Fraction absent	0.292	0.327	0.122	0.053	0.049
Fraction present	0.650	0.673	0.825	0.907	0.935

Table continued on next page

TABLE 6-2 Continued

Characteristic	Black	Black Lit. sample[a]	Colored	Indian	White
Years of education	2.975	3.194	5.589	8.049	9.778
	[0.053]	[0.206]	[0.160]	[0.264]	[0.146]
Fraction completed					
Standard 1	0.051	0.065	0.018	0.004	0.005
Standard 2	0.040	0.049	0.022	0.013	0.001
Standard 3	0.038	0.019	0.045	0.004	0.000
Standard 4	0.059	0.061	0.049	0.004	0.012
Standard 5	0.074	0.107	0.079	0.027	0.004
Standard 6	0.078	0.071	0.152	0.080	0.028
Standard 7	0.034	0.049	0.079	0.049	0.016
Standard 8	0.057	0.049	0.165	0.147	0.118
Standard 9	0.027	0.039	0.067	0.120	0.025
Standard 10	0.047	0.039	0.087	0.298	0.264
Diploma	0.015	0.013	0.033	0.044	0.257
University degree	0.005	0.010	0.010	0.084	0.164
Household income	1143.240	1135.677	2382.135	4483.229	6936.798
	[17.251]	[42.084]	[65.842]	[492.055]	[312.383]
ln (household income)	6.577	6.611	7.469	7.994	8.545
	[0.012]	[0.037]	[0.031]	[0.049]	[0.024]
Sample size	8,142	788	896	341	1,084

[a]Literacy assessment sub-sample.

in contrast with the TFRs in Figure 6-1, the gap between blacks and coloreds is very small: blacks reported 2.1 children on average, whereas coloreds reported 2.0. Indians and whites reported about .5 child less—1.6 and 1.5, respectively. This clustering of coloreds with blacks and Indians with whites matches the education levels presented in the lower panel of Figure 6-1 and is also reflected in the fertility of women aged 40 to 49. (Because the sample sizes of coloreds and Indians are small, the present analysis uses the fertility of this relatively broad age group as the measure of completed fertility, although it is important to recognize that many women in this age group will continue to have more children.) The 1994 October Household Survey reports a birth history for each female respondent; among those aged 40 to 49, the fertility rates of whites and Indians are remarkably close to those reported in the PSLSD. (For whites, completed fertility is 2.39 in the October Household Survey and 2.50 in the PSLSD. For Indians, it is 2.89 and 2.95, respectively.) However, for coloreds and blacks, reported fertility is much lower in the October Household Survey than in the PSLSD (3.31 versus 4.25 for coloreds and 2.49 versus 5.00 for blacks in the October Household Survey and PSLSD, respectively). The Central Statistical Service argues that the fertility estimates for blacks in the October Household Survey are almost certainly underestimates; the same is probably true for coloreds.

Precisely what underlies the discrepancy between the October Household Survey and PSLSD estimates is not clear, although an important factor may be that the former survey was conducted by the government, whose agencies during apartheid had a history of discouraging fertility among blacks, while the PSLSD was conducted by a consortium of private and quasi-government survey teams.[8] Whatever the reasons, the PSLSD estimates cast a shadow of doubt on the reliability of the time series of TFR estimates presented in Figure 6-1 and raise serious questions about what is thought to be known about fertility in South Africa.

Returning to the PSLSD, the correlation between fertility and education is reported in the first line of Table 6-3, which presents the coefficient (and standard error) from a linear regression of CEB on completed years of education, controlling for age (splines), and indicator or dummy variables for urban or rural residence (with metropolitan areas excluded). There is a powerful association between fertility and education among black women: an additional year of education is associated with 0.12 fewer children. The correlation is almost as large for coloreds, half as large for Indians, and relatively small for whites.

While the above is a simple summary of the data, it is not obvious that the relationship between fertility and education should be linear. Figure 6-2, which presents the mean CEB for each year of completed education, indicates that the relationship is, in fact, not linear. Those estimates confound the role of age and education, which we know from Figure 6-1 are negatively correlated because of the tremendous growth in education across cohorts. Thus, Panel C of Table 6-3 reports the analogous regression estimates, controlling for age and location (which are also reported).

Before discussing those results, it is useful to examine the distribution of education reported in Panel B of Table 6-2. Primary school ends at Standard 5; many women exit secondary school at Standard 8 (after completing their Junior Certificate); and Standard 10 is the terminal year of secondary school, at which time women write matric examinations (which are used for entry into universities, tecnicons, and training programs). Looking first at black women, there is clear evidence of stacking of the distribution at the natural exit points, but there are many women who left school at other times. Note in particular that a substantial fraction of women left in the year immediately prior to completing primary school (Standard 4) and in the first year of secondary school (Standard 6). Moreover, fully one-third of black women did not complete primary school, and among those who attended secondary school, only 12 percent completed matric (Stan-

---

[8]There is, for example, anecdotal evidence of enumerators in the 1980s lecturing respondents about the virtues of small family sizes.

TABLE 6-3 Children Ever Born and Female Education, Women Aged 15-49

Explanatory Variable	Black	Black Rural	Colored	Indian	White
A. Linear					
Years of education	–0.117	–0.119	–0.094	–0.056	–0.037
	[0.006]	[0.007]	[0.018]	[0.023]	[0.009]
B. Spline					
0-5 years	–0.106	–0.103	0.051	0.172	0.185
	[0.013]	[0.015]	[0.044]	[0.067]	[0.034]
6-10 years	–0.134	–0.134	–0.168	–0.175	–0.160
	[0.012]	[0.016]	[0.033]	[0.045]	[0.027]
> 10 years	–0.059	–0.119	–0.175	–0.046	–0.070
	[0.041]	[0.053]	[0.092]	[0.066]	[0.022]
C. Semiparametric					
Standard 1	–0.128	–0.156	0.874	0.388	–0.566
	[0.102]	[0.119]	[0.398]	[0.882]	[0.638]
Standard 2	–0.079	–0.208	0.236	1.432	0.117
	[0.097]	[0.111]	[0.385]	[0.875]	[0.556]
Standard 3	–0.338	–0.383	0.529	0.679	–0.045
	[0.090]	[0.107]	[0.322]	[0.538]	[0.460]
Standard 4	–0.423	–0.371	0.731	1.681	0.151
	[0.085]	[0.102]	[0.294]	[0.472]	[0.239]
Standard 5	–0.592	–0.650	0.578	1.021	0.429
	[0.076]	[0.092]	[0.275]	[0.456]	[0.307]
Standard 6	–0.623	–0.589	0.163	0.849	0.726
	[0.075]	[0.093]	[0.266]	[0.360]	[0.203]
Standard 7	–0.699	–0.660	0.252	0.285	0.862
	[0.081]	[0.102]	[0.271]	[0.383]	[0.210]
Standard 8	–0.921	–0.933	0.015	0.460	0.515
	[0.077]	[0.100]	[0.265]	[0.350]	[0.147]
Standard 9	–0.961	–0.969	–0.047	0.329	0.447
	[0.083]	[0.106]	[0.299]	[0.365]	[0.188]
Standard 10	–1.274	–1.331	–0.283	0.179	0.009
	[0.083]	[0.108]	[0.282]	[0.341]	[0.135]
Diploma	–1.401	–1.577	–0.785	–0.009	–0.303
	[0.117]	[0.153]	[0.371]	[0.435]	[0.152]
University degree	—	—	–0.990	–0.078	–0.223
			[0.592]	[0.460]	[0.156]

dard 10). The shape of the distribution of education for coloreds is very similar (although it is shifted to the right relative to blacks). Indians and whites, however, display different patterns: only about 15 percent had not completed primary school, while more than one-third of Indians and more than half of white women had completed matric. Whereas most whites left school at either Standard 8 or Standard 10, the distribution is much smoother for Indians. The stark differences

TABLE 6-3 Continued

Explanatory Variable	Black	Black Rural	Colored	Indian	White
Age spline					
< 30	0.185	0.193	0.161	0.164	0.158
	[0.005]	[0.006]	[0.014]	[0.020]	[0.012]
30-39	0.161	0.180	0.162	0.079	0.091
	[0.007]	[0.010]	[0.019]	[0.026]	[0.013]
40-49	0.109	0.123	0.068	0.006	0.004
	[0.011]	[0.014]	[0.027]	[0.037]	[0.015]
(1) if urban	0.195	—	–0.159	0.012	0.142
	[0.060]		[0.105]	[0.130]	[0.078]
(1) if rural	0.498	—	0.203	–0.456	0.270
	[0.049]		[0.201]	[1.170]	[0.126]
Intercept	–2.763	–2.511	–2.889	–3.329	–3.242
	[0.140]	[0.161]	[0.419]	[0.562]	[0.313]
F(all covariates)	579.87	480.27	57.17	20.59	49.21
R^2	0.533	0.560	0.525	0.520	0.440
Sample size	8,142	5,303	896	341	1,084

NOTE: Standard errors below coefficients; p-values below F statistics.

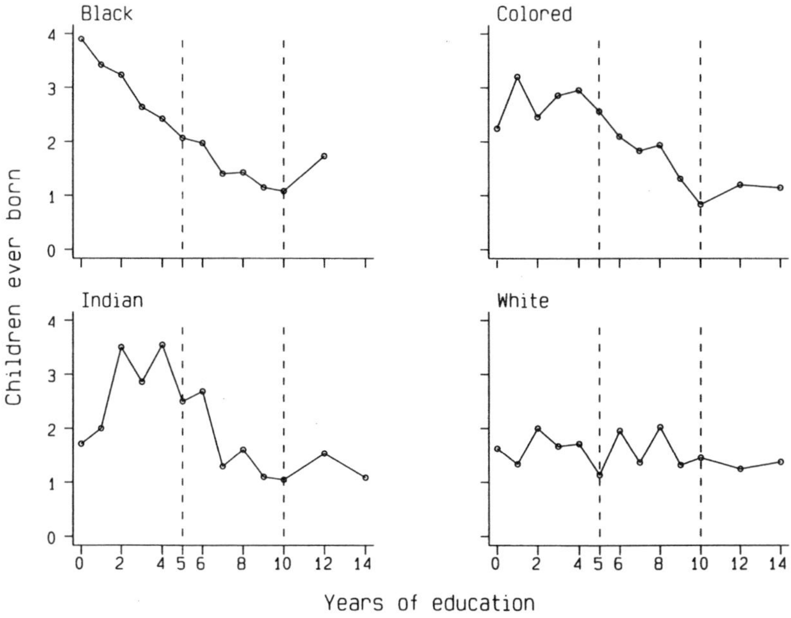

FIGURE 6-2 Children ever born and female education.

in the shapes of these distributions are, in large part, a reflection of state policies during apartheid.

The semiparametric estimates of the association between education and fertility in Panel C of Table 6-3 impose no restrictions on the shape of the fertility-education function since each year of completed education is represented by an indicator variable. Because the excluded education category is zero years, the coefficients should be interpreted as the impact of that level of schooling relative to not having attended school. For example, black women who completed Standard 5 had 0.59 children fewer than those who reported no schooling; those who had completed Standard 10 had 1.27 fewer children. Because so few blacks had a university degree (less than 0.5 percent), postmatric schooling is combined into a single category.

The semiparametric estimates provide several important new insights beyond those revealed by the linear regressions in Panel A. First, the relationship between fertility and education is not linear for any of the racial groups. Second, focusing on blacks, the negative association between fertility and education is relatively weak at the bottom of the education distribution and is significant only among women with at least 3 years of schooling. Third, the marginal effect of an additional year of schooling is largest at schooling levels that are natural exit points in the schooling system. For example, women who had completed matric (Standard 10) had 0.39 fewer children than those who had completed only Standard 9. This is three times larger than the average effect for each year of schooling, which, from Panel A, is 0.12 fewer children. Similarly, the marginal effect of completing Standard 8 relative to Standard 7 is 0.22 fewer children. If this reflects an increasing marginal impact of education with more years of schooling, women who had completed Standard 9 should have had many fewer children than those who had graduated Standard 8. They did not: the marginal difference is a mere 0.04 child.

A similar pattern emerges around completion of primary school. The difference between women who fell just short of completing primary school (Standard 4) and those who completed Standard 5 is 0.17 child, but another year of schooling is associated with only 0.03 fewer children. Among rural blacks, women who had started secondary school but completed only 1 year (Standard 6) actually had more children than those who had exited at the end of primary school (the effects being –0.59 and –0.65, respectively). While this upward turn in the fertility-education function is not significantly different from a flat, it is striking that the first 2 years of secondary schooling are associated with virtually no decline in fertility among rural women, whereas there is a huge impact associated with completing the third year, Standard 8, when the Junior Certificate examination is taken.

There may be important age and education interactions since younger women are better educated in South Africa, and fertility rises with age. To further isolate the relationship between fertility and education, Table 6-4 repeats the same re-

TABLE 6-4 Children Ever Born and Female Education, Women Aged 40-49

Explanatory Variable	Black	Black Rural	Colored	Indian	White
A. Linear					
Years of education	–0.136*	–0.152*	–0.124*	0.010	–0.054*
	[0.023]	[0.031]	[0.062]	[0.053]	[0.020]
B. Spline					
0-5 years	–0.150*	–0.175*	0.146	0.172	0.233*
	[0.040]	[0.052]	[0.130]	[0.134]	[0.071]
6-10 years	–0.140*	–0.085	–0.362*	–0.145	–0.249*
	[0.066]	[0.114]	[0.129]	[0.117]	[0.061]
> 10 years	0.016	–0.265	–0.026	0.154	–0.069
	[0.193]	[0.338]	[0.292]	[0.196]	[0.051]
C. Semiparametric					
Standard 1	–0.053	–0.010	1.249	—	–1.381
	[0.290]	[0.351]	[1.094]		[1.281]
Standard 2	–0.058	–0.106	1.572	-0.546	0.258
	[0.300]	[0.347]	[1.226]	[1.706]	[0.921]
Standard 3	–0.505+	–0.668+	1.343	0.731	0.497
	[0.280]	[0.350]	[0.886]	[0.880]	[0.772]
Standard 4	–0.659*	–0.680+	2.595*	1.710*	0.397
	[0.270]	[0.344]	[0.804]	[0.827]	[0.511]
Standard 5	–0.930*	–1.069*	1.424+	1.188	1.710
	[0.260]	[0.345]	[0.782]	[0.850]	[1.285]
Standard 6	–0.677*	–0.716*	0.459	0.565	0.995*
	[0.235]	[0.323]	[0.775]	[0.700]	[0.406]
Standard 7	–0.753*	–0.391	0.991	0.017	0.847
	[0.361]	[0.662]	[0.834]	[0.959]	[0.567]
Standard 8	–1.140*	–1.222*	0.345	0.089	0.315
	[0.306]	[0.604]	[0.788]	[0.781]	[0.289]
Standard 9	–1.367*	–1.703+	0.542	0.945	0.212
	[0.465]	[0.925]	[1.038]	[0.830]	[0.415]
Standard 10	–1.649*	–1.592+	0.953	0.318	–0.075
	[0.472]	[0.805]	[2.154]	[0.882]	[0.275]
Diploma	–1.424*	–1.782*	0.743	0.829	–0.965*
	[0.446]	[0.621]	[1.366]	[1.013]	[0.338]
University degree	—	—	–1.047	0.809	–0.263
			[1.604]	[1.125]	[0.334]

Table continued on next page

gressions for women aged 40 to 49. Among black women, reported in the first two columns, the same pattern emerges. Only 5 percent of women reported more than Standard 8 schooling, so we focus on completion of primary school. There is a very large decline in fertility for women who had completed Standard 4 as compared with those who had completed Standard 5. In terms of completed fertility, those who had stayed at school for 1 more year (until Standard 6) look

TABLE 6-4 Continued

Explanatory Variable	Black	Black Rural	Colored	Indian	White
Age in years	0.104*	0.133*	0.056	0.045	0.063*
	[0.024]	[0.032]	[0.056]	[0.075]	[0.025]
(1) if urban	0.660*	—	–0.202	–0.297	–0.029
	[0.227]		[0.335]	[0.371]	[0.172]
(1) if rural	1.192*	—	1.063	—	0.241
	[0.192]		[0.686]		[0.276]
Intercept	–0.204	-0.266	0.509	0.424	–0.434
	[1.072]	[1.435]	[2.614]	[3.417]	[1.141]
F(all covariates)	11.190	4.200	2.290	0.880	3.080
	[0.000]	[0.000]	[0.006]	[0.579]	[0.000]
R^2	0.103	0.057	0.164	0.139	0.140
Sample size	1,377	852	191	85	300

much more like the Standard 4 women than do those who had exited at Standard 5, and it is only those who had completed Standard 8 who reported fewer children than the Standard 5 women.

In sum, the fertility-education profile for black women in South Africa is characterized by a generally downward slope that is punctuated by steeper steps at natural exit points and flats (or upward shifts) immediately afterward. A traditional human capital interpretation of this evidence would conclude that particular years of schooling are especially productive (at least in terms of their impact on reproduction), while others are, frankly, of little value. Or put another way, if more women were only to pass their examinations, such as the Junior Certificate in Standard 8 or matric in Standard 10, fertility would decline even more rapidly. This seems a very unlikely scenario.

A more plausible interpretation of the evidence recognizes the fact that education is not randomly distributed across women, but is the outcome of a set of choices made by each woman and her family when she was an adolescent. Those women who did not quite complete an important school hurdle, such as passing the Standard 8 examinations, are likely to be different in both observable and unobservable ways from women who did pass those exams. To attribute all the differences in the observed relationship between education and fertility to productivity effects associated with schooling itself and ignore the role of the unobserved attributes of the women is likely to be very misleading. Following the same logic, women who started secondary school but completed only the first year (Standard 6) before dropping out may be even less able than those who exited at the end of primary school. Thus, the small impact of education for those women does not mean that Standard 6 is unproductive, but that the women who exit at that point are selected from a different part of the distribution of tastes and, possibly, abilities than those who exit at Standard 5.

It is worth emphasizing that schooling decisions are not made in a vacuum, but reflect the choices of individuals and families given the opportunities and constraints they face. The fact that under apartheid South Africa, many government policies seriously curtailed the opportunities open to blacks does nothing to diminish the import of the argument that education is not randomly assigned in the population. On the contrary, it seems reasonable to suppose that self-selection may be particularly germane in this context, where state policies actively sought to limit the education opportunities of blacks (Samuel, 1990).

An alternative explanation for the nonlinearities in the effects of education has been proposed in the labor economics literature. In estimates of wage functions, evidence of steps and flats around completion of particular levels of education (or particular examinations) has been interpreted as "certification" effects. However, that interpretation has little appeal in a fertility context. Rather, interpreting the steps and flats as reflecting self-selection in educational attainment is a plausible explanation for both the wage- and fertility-education relationships.[9] (See Weiss, 1995, for a review and discussion in the context of wage functions.)

To be sure, the evidence in Tables 6-3 and 6-4 cannot say anything conclusive about the productivity of education in terms of its impact on fertility. The powerful negative correlation certainly suggests there may be a causal link, but without taking account of the potential endogeneity of education, one cannot be certain. However, the evidence does indicate that a naive causal interpretation of the magnitude of the association is probably flawed, and that failure to take account of the selection process underlying educational achievement is likely to lead to substantially incorrect inferences.

The same pattern of steps and flats is apparent in the association between contraceptive use and education in neighboring Zimbabwe, as demonstrated by Thomas and Maluccio (1996). They show that Zimbabwean women who have completed primary school are twice as likely to use modern contraceptives as those who have dropped out in the year before completion (a step) and that primary school graduates are more likely to use contraceptives than those who

[9]Evaluating these interpretations of education in the context of fertility rather than wages has an important additional advantage: wages are earned only by those who are working in the labor market, and that choice needs to be taken into account in the estimation. Unfortunately, there are no good instruments for measuring labor market participation in the PSLSD. However, there is some evidence that self-selection in education is important for black women since the probability a woman works is nearly twice as high if she completed Standard 5 (9 percent) than if she completed Standard 4 or Standard 6 (5 percent). Conditional on working, women who complete Standard 8 have wages only 6 percent lower than those who leave school at Standard 9, but their wages are fully 75 percent higher than those of women who exit school at Standard 7. Both female labor force participation and wage functions in South Africa are, therefore, also characterized by steps and flats.

have attended 1 year of secondary school (a flat). Using data from Brazil, Lam and Duryea (1995) demonstrate a similar pattern for the fertility of women aged 30 to 34. The pattern of steps and flats is, therefore, not unique to South Africa.

Turning to the remaining three columns in Tables 6-3 and 6-4, the fertility of coloreds appears to rise with education until around Standard 4, whereupon it declines rapidly, following the inverted-U shape that has been observed in many other countries and is discussed, for example, by Cochrane (1983). As a simplified summary of the evidence, Panel B of the two tables reports a spline specification with knots at 5 and 10 years of schooling. Among women with more than 5 years of schooling, there is a powerful negative association between education and fertility: each year of education is associated with around 0.17 fewer children, which is larger in magnitude than the decline among similar black women. The fertility of Indian women also increases until around the completion of primary school and then falls dramatically (at about the same rate as that among coloreds) until completion of Standard 10, at which point it seems to stabilize. Thus, Indian women with no schooling have, on average, the same number of children as women with more than 10 years of education. A roughly similar pattern emerges for white women, with the exception that the peak in fertility is observed among women with Standard 7 education, although fewer than 15 percent of white women had not completed at least Standard 8.

INFLUENCE OF HOUSEHOLD RESOURCES ON DEMOGRAPHIC OUTCOMES

It has been argued above that the education effects reported in Tables 6-3 and 6-4 are likely to reflect in part the impact of observable and unobservable characteristics of the woman. It is very difficult to take account of unobservable differences among women in a survey unless the survey incorporates a special experimental design that permits comparisons among otherwise identical women with different levels of education. See, for example, Ashenfelter and Krueger (1994), who compare the wages and educational attainment of monozygotic twins; even that design is not without potential flaws, since identical twin pairs with different levels of education may also be different in unobserved ways. However, it is possible to take into account observable differences among women, and this is the approach taken in this and the next section, which exploit some of the breadth and richness of the PSLSD. In this section, the focus is on a set of proxies for income, wages, and community characteristics; in the following section, attention is turned to alternative measures of human capital accumulation.

By controlling for observed characteristics, one cannot uncover "pure" estimates of the effect of education. In some sense, the reduced-form estimates discussed above are "pure" or "full" estimates of those effects. Rather, by adding controls to the regression, one can better understand the mechanisms through which education affects fertility choices. In so doing, one is trading off the (possible) purity of reduced-form estimates with estimates that include outcomes of choices as regressors that are potentially endogenous. However, in view of the argument above that education itself is a choice, converting to purism now would appear to be somewhat inconsistent.

The first column of Table 6-5A repeats the CEB regression in the first column of Table 6-3 for black women. Additional covariates are included, and their effects are reported in Table 6-5B for the flexible regression with a semi-parametric specification for women's education. For reference, the associated linear and spline estimates with the same sets of additional controls are reported in Panels A and B of Table 6-5A. Results for the other three races are discussed below but not shown.

A natural starting point is the inclusion of spousal characteristics. While most women in South Africa do get married, slightly over half of the black women in the survey had ever been married by the time of the survey.[10] Among those who were married, only two-thirds were living with their husbands; this finding reflects, in part, massive migration by black South African men, typically to urban areas for employment reasons, leaving their wives and families behind. Fertility was higher among married women and highest among those whose husbands were present, who had 1.5 children more than unmarried women. In contrast, relative to not being married, a woman whose husband was absent had only .25 child more on average. It is unfortunate that the PSLSD provides so little information about these absent husbands and does not even report their education or location. Knowing more about the welfare of these families, including the noncoresident members, as well as understanding the strategies they adopt in times of crisis, would likely yield important behavioral insights that would, in turn, be important for policy design.

Among those black women who were married and whose spouses were in the household at the time of the survey, the correlation between their educational levels is 0.58 (which is considerably higher than among any of the other racial groups).[11] Thus the inclusion of spousal characteristics in the fertility regression is associated with a decline of about one-third in the estimated effects of female education, and this decline is essentially constant across the entire education distribution. The estimated spousal education effects in Table 6-5B indicate that around the time of completion of primary school, husband's education has a larger depressing effect on fertility than does wife's education. However, as husband's education increases, the impact on fertility does not increase much, so

[10]This is because the PSLSD is a random sample of women, and many in the survey were too young to have been married by the survey date. The age of the average black female respondent is 28.

[11]The correlations are 0.5, 0.4, and 0.3 for coloreds, Indians, and whites, respectively.

TABLE 6–5A Children Ever Born, Female Education, and Household and Community Resources, Black Women Aged 15–49

	Baseline (1)	Add Spouse Characteristics (2)	Add Household Income OLS (3)	Add Household Income IV (4)	Add Wages and LFP (5)	Include Community Fixed Effects (6)
A. Linear						
Years	–0.117*	–0.080*	–0.073*	–0.065*	–0.072*	–0.068*
	[0.006]	[0.006]	[0.006]	[0.007]	[0.006]	[0.007]
B. Spline						
0-5 years	–0.106*	–0.071*	–0.069*	–0.067*	–0.069*	–0.071*
	[0.013]	[0.013]	[0.013]	[0.013]	[0.013]	[0.013]
6-10 years	–0.134*	–0.089*	–0.079*	–0.067*	–0.080*	–0.070*
	[0.012]	[0.012]	[0.012]	[0.013]	[0.012]	[0.013]
> 10 years	–0.059	–0.067+	–0.051	–0.027	–0.004	–0.014
	[0.041]	[0.040]	[0.041]	[0.042]	[0.041]	[0.042]
C. Semiparametric						
Standard 1	–0.128	–0.016	0.001	0.001	–0.013	–0.050
	[0.102]	[0.099]	[0.100]	[0.100]	[0.099]	[0.100]
Standard 2	–0.079	0.075	0.120	0.142	0.094	0.044
	[0.097]	[0.094]	[0.096]	[0.097]	[0.094]	[0.096]
Standard 3	–0.338*	–0.179*	–0.184*	–0.174*	–0.176*	–0.187*
	[0.090]	[0.088]	[0.089]	[0.090]	[0.088]	[0.090]
Standard 4	–0.423*	–0.235*	–0.217*	–0.207*	–0.216*	–0.245*
	[0.085]	[0.083]	[0.085]	[0.086]	[0.083]	[0.085]
Standard 5	–0.592*	–0.385*	–0.368*	–0.353*	–0.368*	–0.371*
	[0.076]	[0.076]	[0.077]	[0.078]	[0.076]	[0.079]
Standard 6	–0.623*	–0.390*	–0.372*	–0.350*	-0.373*	–0.402*
	[0.075]	[0.075]	[0.076]	[0.077]	[0.075]	[0.078]
Standard 7	–0.699*	–0.437*	–0.402*	–0.375*	–0.415*	–0.421*
	[0.081]	[0.081]	[0.082]	[0.083]	[0.081]	[0.083]
Standard 8	–0.921*	–0.561*	–0.512*	–0.462*	–0.525*	–0.497*
	[0.077]	[0.078]	[0.079]	[0.081]	[0.078]	[0.081]
Standard 9	–0.961*	–0.572*	–0.527*	–0.475*	–0.548*	–0.547*
	[0.083]	[0.083]	[0.085]	[0.087]	[0.083]	[0.087]
Standard 10	–1.274*	–0.829*	–0.764*	–0.693*	–0.768*	–0.746*
	[0.083]	[0.083]	[0.085]	[0.089]	[0.084]	[0.087]
> Standard 10	–1.401*	–0.992*	–0.874*	–0.739*	–0.739*	–0.747*
	[0.117]	[0.118]	[0.121]	[0.130]	[0.125]	[0.129]

TABLE 6–5A Continued

	Baseline (1)	Add Spouse Characteristics (2)	Add Household Income OLS (3)	Add Household Income IV (4)	Add Wages and LFP (5)	Include Community Fixed Effects (6)
D. Test statistics						
F(all covariates)	579.87	359.03	336.15	334.40	311.16	35.70
	[0.00]	[0.00]	[0.00]	[0.00]	[0.00]	[0.00]
Overidentification test	—	—	—	1.09	—	—
				[0.37]		
R^2	0.533	0.570	0.571	0.569	0.573	0.599

NOTE: OLS = ordinary least squares; IV = instrumental variables; LFP = labor force participation. In all regressions, 8,142 observations used. Standard errors below coefficients; p–values below F statistics. See Table 6–5B for additional controls. Specifications A, B, and C all include those controls, along with maternal education specification as denoted. Results reported in Table 6–5B correspond to the semiparametric specification, C, as do test statistics, D. Instruments for income used in column 4 are seven indicator variables for ownership of a bicycle, radio, television, telephone, refrigerator, electric stove, and primus (gas) stove. Overidentification test is generalized method of moments (GMM) test for validity of instruments; it is distributed as an F statistic with 7 degrees of freedom.

at the top of the education distribution, it is the wife's education that plays a dominant role. The evidence is succinctly summarized in a linear spline specification: husband's education is associated with 0.087 fewer children for each year of schooling between 1 and 5, whereas wife's education is associated with only 0.071 fewer children. The relative importance of male and female education reverses for those who attended secondary school, with the effect of husband's education being smaller (0.061 per year) and that of wife's education being larger (0.089 per year).[12]

In many studies conducted in a wide range of contexts, it has been shown that relative to the education of a mother, her husband's schooling has a smaller effect on both the quantity of children and their quality, as indicated by, for

[12]Since the effect of husband's education is relatively constant across the education distribution, the effect of wife's education increases with education, and there is a constant proportionate decline in her education effect. When spouse's education is added to the regression, the correlation between the education of spouses must rise with education. It does: for women who did not complete primary school, the correlation is 0.25; for those who did, the correlation is 0.54.

TABLE 6–5B Children Ever Born, Female Education, Household and Community Resources, Black Women Aged 15–49

	Baseline (1)	Add Spouse Characteristics (2)	Add Household Income OLS (3)	IV (4)	Add Wages and LFP (5)	Include Community Fixed Effects (6)
Spouse's characteristics						
Standard 1	—	–0.112	–0.099	–0.096	–0.103	–0.159
		[0.121]	[0.123]	[0.124]	[0.121]	[0.122]
Standard 2	—	–0.073	–0.113	–0.110	–0.080	–0.112
		[0.134]	[0.138]	[0.138]	[0.133]	[0.135]
Standard 3	—	–0.212	–0.202	–0.194	–0.222	–0.254+
		[0.136]	[0.137]	[0.138]	[0.135]	[0.137]
Standard 4	—	–0.280*	–0.202+	–0.174	–0.286*	–0.253*
		[0.117]	[0.118]	[0.120]	[0.117]	[0.118]
Standard 5	—	–0.448*	–0.467*	–0.440*	–0.451*	–0.405*
		[0.110]	[0.112]	[0.112]	[0.110]	[0.111]
Standard 6	—	–0.604*	–0.628*	–0.589*	–0.608*	–0.557*
		[0.108]	[0.110]	[0.111]	[0.108]	[0.110]
Standard 7	—	–0.231	–0.191	–0.170	–0.258+	–0.260+
		[0.144]	[0.147]	[0.147]	[0.145]	[0.146]
Standard 8	—	–0.681*	–0.644*	–0.584*	–0.656*	–0.620*
		[0.120]	[0.122]	[0.124]	[0.122]	[0.123]
Standard 9	—	–0.554*	–0.537*	–0.491*	–0.566*	–0.571*
		[0.158]	[0.161]	[0.163]	[0.160]	[0.161]
Standard 10	—	–0.785*	–0.732*	–0.647*	–0.765*	–0.719*
		[0.129]	[0.131]	[0.135]	[0.133]	[0.134]
> Standard 10	—	–0.532*	–0.461*	–0.316	–0.481*	–0.343+
		[0.185]	[0.187]	[0.194]	[0.194]	[0.198]
(1) if dead	—	1.023*	1.014*	0.965*	1.026*	1.002*
		[0.107]	[0.110]	[0.112]	[0.107]	[0.108]
(1) if absent	—	0.251*	0.243*	0.237*	0.266*	0.371*
		[0.053]	[0.054]	[0.054]	[0.053]	[0.058]
(1) if present	—	1.524*	1.511*	1.480*	1.599*	1.569*
		[0.081]	[0.083]	[0.083]	[0.086]	[0.088]

example, survival rates and health status. This finding is often attributed to the fact that men tend to bear less of the time burden associated with childrearing. If men spend no time on child care and if women's leisure time is weakly separable from that of their husbands, then male education will have only an income effect on fertility. These are strong assumptions and unlikely to be true, although they are often made in empirical studies of household choices. We can make some progress in testing these assumptions by including income in the fertility regression.

The primary focus here is on the extent to which the association between

TABLE 6–5B Continued

	Baseline (1)	Add Spouse Charac-teristics (2)	Add Household Income OLS (3)	IV (4)	Add Wages and LFP (5)	Include Community Fixed Effects (6)
Income and wages						
ln(HH income)	—	—	–0.069*	–0.186*	—	—
			[0.018]	[0.044]		
ln(female wage)	—	—	—	—	–0.223*	–0.217*
					[0.047]	[0.051]
(1) if employed	—	—	—	—	–0.216*	–0.155*
					[0.049]	[0.052]
ln(spouse's wage)	—	—	—	—	0.129*	0.076
					[0.053]	[0.059]
(1) if spouse employed	—	—	—	—	–0.191*	–0.041
					[0.059]	[0.063]
Woman's age (spline)						
< 30	0.185*	0.136*	0.136*	0.136*	0.139*	0.139*
	[0.005]	[0.005]	[0.005]	[0.005]	[0.005]	[0.006]
30–39	0.161*	0.144*	0.144*	0.145*	0.148*	0.149*
	[0.007]	[0.007]	[0.007]	[0.007]	[0.007]	[0.007]
40–49	0.109*	0.102*	0.107*	0.109*	0.101*	0.102*
	[0.011]	[0.010]	[0.011]	[0.011]	[0.010]	[0.010]
Location						
(1) if urban	0.195*	0.085	0.136*	0.110*	0.121*	—
	[0.060]	[0.076]	[0.059]	[0.059]	[0.058]	
(1) if rural	0.498*	0.189	0.367*	0.305*	0.352*	—
	[0.049]	[0.122]	[0.049]	[0.054]	[0.048]	
Intercept	-2.763*	–2.160*	–1.709*	–0.935*	–1.662*	–1.143*
	[0.140]	[0.140]	[0.185]	[0.326]	[0.415]	[0.481]

NOTES: See Table 6–5A.

maternal education and fertility is simply capturing the role of household resources. Thus, in column 3 of Tables 6-5A and 6-5B, (the logarithm of) household income is added to the regression. The male and female education effects are only slightly reduced (by less than 10 percent). Among parents with little education, the reduction is trivial, but for those who are better educated, especially men and women with some secondary schooling, the declines are larger, suggesting that part, but only part, of the effect of education does reflect the role of household resources.

The regressions also indicate that current income does have a significant, albeit small, effect on fertility. For example, a threefold increase in income would be associated with a 20 percent decline in fertility. There are, however, at least two problems with the analysis of income effects. First, one can expect income to be measured with error in any household survey. Second, current income is not the appropriate concept in a regression of cumulative fertility. Ideally, one would like to examine the effect of income—and changes in income—on fertility decisions over the life course. This is not possible with a single cross-section in which respondents report only CEB and current income. Under the assumption that there is a good deal of serial correlation in income, one might interpret current income as a proxy for long-run household resources, but since it is at best an error-ridden proxy for resource availability over the life course, the estimated income effect is likely to be downward biased. This raises a question regarding the interpretation of education effects as being net of income since education is likely to be correlated with long-run income.

One strategy for reducing the impact of measurement error is to use predicted income, based on longer-run measures of resources. We use household ownership of seven assets that are likely to be related to wealth and present instrumental variables estimates in the fourth column of Tables 6-5A and 6-5B.[13] Consistent with the measurement error hypothesis, the estimated income effect is much larger: if income were to double, fertility would be predicted to fall by about 20 percent. The key point for present purposes is that the estimated maternal education effects remain large and significant. For example, the impact on fertility of doubling income is about the same as the difference between a woman who completed Standard 9 and one who completed Standard 10.

We have examined nonlinearities in the effect of income in some detail. The results of including quadratic and cubic terms in log (income) indicate that a linear effect cannot be rejected. This inference was checked using nonparametric methods to estimate the fertility-income function (both unconditionally and conditional on the woman's age, education, and location, as well as her spouse's education). The relationship is linear in logs for all women except those whose household income is in the top decile, for whom income and fertility are positively associated. There are two reasons for concluding that this result is due to measurement error in household income that is correlated with income. First, nonlinear instrumental variables estimates indicate that the income effects are negative throughout the income distribution, and most negative at the top of the

[13]The instruments are ownership of a bicycle, radio, television, telephone, refrigerator, electric stove, and primus (gas) stove. The first-stage regression explains 30 percent of the variation in (log) household income, and the instruments are significant predictors of income ($F_{35,8106} = 269.55$) after controlling for other observables in the regression in column 4. In addition to being good predictors of income, the assets should not be correlated with residuals from the second-stage regression. They are not: the Generalized Method of Moments (GMM) overidentification test reported at the bottom of Table 6-5A is not significant.

distribution. Second, nonparametric estimates of the relationship between fertility and household expenditures, which may be a better indicator of longer-run household resources than income, suggest a negative correlation at the top of the expenditure distribution. The estimated education effects are essentially unchanged by including nonlinearities in income or replacing income in the regressions with expenditure, so we conclude that the education effects do not reflect purely the role of household resources in fertility.

The estimated effects of income on fertility reflect a combination of two mechanisms. First, better-educated people tend to earn higher wages, which implies a higher market value of their time and, assuming that rearing children is time-intensive, a reduction in the number of children a woman will want to have. Second, higher income implies more resources for the family to spend, which, assuming children are valued, raises the demand for children. The fact that the impact of income is negative suggests that the first of these mechanisms, the substitution effect, dominates.

Following the same argument, increases in the value of time as education rises are likely to contribute to the negative correlation between fertility and education. To investigate this issue, the regression in the fifth column of Tables 6-5A and 6-5B includes the woman's (log) wages, her spouse's (log) wages, and controls for whether they had worked during the year prior to the survey. Not only is working associated with fewer children, but women who earn higher wages tend to have smaller families. Working spouses also tend to be associated with fewer children, but conditional on the spouse's working and his education, higher wages are associated with more children. This association might be interpreted as a pure income effect.[14]

The coefficients on maternal education are very close to those in the third column of Tables 6-5A and 6-5B. Dropping the woman's education from the regression yields a female wage effect of -0.38 (and a standard error of 0.04), suggesting that changes in the value of the woman's time and in her tastes for children are mutually reinforcing as education increases. Thus, we conclude that a higher value of time does not fully explain the negative correlation between education and fertility. The positive wage effect for males indicates that men whose wages are higher than would be expected, given their education, desire larger families. Dropping the spouse's education from the regression yields a wage effect that is zero (0.02, with a standard error of 0.05), suggesting that, in contrast to females, a higher value of time among better-educated men is offset by a desire for a larger family.

[14]As with income, one must assume there is sufficient serial correlation in wages so that current wages (conditional on age) are informative about wages over the life course.

Causality in this model is not unidirectional. On the one hand, if childrearing costs rise with the number of children, the shadow price of time for women who have borne more children will be higher, and, ceteris paribus, they will be less likely to participate in the labor market. On the other hand, women with higher wages, holding age and education constant, are more productive in the labor market and so are less likely to leave the labor market to bear children. Part of this higher productivity may be a result of more labor market experience, in which case it is the fact the woman has had fewer children that underlies her higher wages and its impact on fertility.

In principle, if there is a set of instruments that predicts labor market choices but has no direct bearing on fertility, an instrumental variables approach will make it possible to disentangle the influences in each direction. At least two classes of instruments have been suggested in the literature: nonlabor or asset income, and indicators of local labor market demand. In the context of a static model, it may be argued that both are valid instruments. By their nature, however, fertility and labor supply choices demand a dynamic modeling framework: current fertility is the cumulation of choices from adolescence, and there is evidence of substantial state dependence and serial correlation in labor market choices. Given the South African data, estimation of a dynamic model of labor supply and fertility is well beyond the scope of the present analysis, but see Hyslop (1996), who demonstrates the empirical importance of taking seriously unobserved heterogeneity and state dependence in a dynamic model of labor supply and fertility choices. In the context of a dynamic model, treating nonlabor income or ownership of assets as predetermined is not very appealing since it is, to a large extent, the culmination of prior savings, and thus reflects previous labor supply and consumption choices.[15] Note that this is a substantially different motivation for using instrumental variables than that which applied earlier in the discussion of concerns about measurement error in income.

The second class of instruments is indicators of local labor demand. They are not exogenous if women are mobile, and employment opportunities affect their choice of residential location. In South Africa, where pass laws have restricted family and, particularly, female mobility in response to earning opportunities, treating local labor demand as exogenous appears to be the lesser of two evils. For example, only 6 percent of women in the sample reported having moved during the 5 years prior to the survey.

Implementation of the instrumental variables approach using local labor demand as the instruments involves empirically characterizing the local labor market (which is not straightforward), along with indicators of other local infrastructure (which is virtually impossible with these data; see note 2 above). As an

[15]In addition, that approach does a poor job of predicting each of the labor market factors in the first stage, so that estimates in the second stage are very imprecise, and none is significant.

alternative approach, in the direction of accounting for unobserved heterogeneity, the regressions were reestimated controlling for community fixed effects, with the communities being defined as sampling cluster units, or Census Enumerator Subdistricts.[16] These controls absorb all observable and unobservable local market and community characteristics that are fixed across households. They therefore absorb all possible measures of local labor demand and thus any instruments that might be constructed at the local market level. If the only source of unobserved heterogeneity that affects the choice to work is fixed at the community level, the fixed effects estimates in column 5 of Tables 6-5A and 6-5B will be unbiased. The community fixed effects estimates also remove the influence of all formal and informal local information and infrastructure, which may include, for example, local family planning programs and messages, as well as the role of community-level social networks.

While the impact of female labor force participation on fertility decreases with the inclusion of community fixed effects, the association with female wages is little changed. Both female employment characteristics remain important and significant correlates of fertility choices. Male labor market choices, however, are all but eliminated: the effect of spouse's employment is trivial, and the impact of his wage is almost halved (and is not significant). These results suggest that much of what would be attributed to a male employment effect in column 4 of Tables 6-5A and 6-5B is in fact associated with community resources and infrastructure. Further evidence along these lines is provided by reestimating the regression in column 3, which includes (log) household income, with community fixed effects: the estimated income effect is reduced from -0.069 to -0.019 (with a standard error of 0.019). This result suggests that community services may play a role in affecting fertility outcomes, although identification of the critical services involved is not possible with the available data.

In contrast with income and male employment, the estimated roles of male and female education in the fertility function are remarkably robust to the inclusion of community fixed effects. Both sets of covariates remain significant and, in terms of magnitude, remain very close to one another, as well as the instrumental variables estimates in column 4. Caldwell (1977, 1979) has suggested that the nature of information in the community, as measured by community-level educational attainment, is a more important determinant of demographic outcomes than an individual woman's education. To the extent that the sampling clusters proxy the local community, the fixed effects estimates remove community-level education; thus the results suggest that in South Africa, individual education does remain an important correlate of demographic choices.

To directly investigate the relative importance of community education, the

---

[16]There are 295 clusters in this sample, and the median cluster contains 28 women aged 15 to 49.

regressions in columns 3 and 4 of Tables 6-5A and 6-5B were reestimated with the race-specific mean and standard deviation of education of women aged 15 to 49 in the community being included. The male and female education effects in this specification are very close in magnitude and significance to those in the fixed effects specification in column 6. Moreover, the mean educational level in the community has a significant negative association with fertility, while the standard deviation of education in the community is not significant. These results suggest that mean education in the community is a good proxy for all community characteristics, and it may be a sufficient statistic for heterogeneity in the community.

However, that inference is not supported by the evidence on the impact of household income. Recall that when community fixed effects are included in the model, the impact of household income is reduced to zero. When community characteristics are proxied by average education, the impact of income remains virtually unchanged (and significant) in both the ordinary least squares and instrumental variables estimates.

In contrast with community-level education, the first two moments of (log) household income in the community are good at capturing unobserved community-level heterogeneity. Reestimating the model while replacing community-level education with community-level income yields two results. First, the community mean of (log) income has a significant negative impact on fertility that is at least as large as that of the household's own income, suggesting that community resources are important. Second, greater inequality in a community, as measured by the standard deviation of (log) household income, is associated with higher fertility, indicating that community resources do not benefit everyone equally. After controlling for community-level income, household income has no effect on fertility, the estimated education effects are very similar to those in column 6 of Tables 6-5A and 6-5B, and both the mean and standard deviation of education in the community are unrelated to fertility.[17]

These results raise an important question regarding the ability to separate out the impacts of community characteristics and local income on demographic outcomes. Intuitively, one assumes that communities served by good infrastructure tend to be wealthier, so it is difficult to interpret the effects of community services in models of fertility or child health that fail to control fully for household or at least local income levels. Since income is, at best, sketchy in surveys such as the Demographic and Health Surveys, this is a serious concern for studies based on such data.

[17]The coefficient (and standard error) on the community mean of (log) income is –0.20 (0.04) and –0.15 (0.06) in the ordinary least squares and instrumental variables regressions, respectively. The corresponding coefficients (and standard errors) on the standard deviation of (log) income are 0.23 (0.07) and 0.21 (0.07).

Restricting attention to black women aged 40 to 49 yields essentially the same results. To summarize the differences, female education effects are slightly larger, and the magnitude of household income effects is also slightly larger (but significant only in the instrumental variables regression). The largest differences emerge in the relationship between fertility and current labor market behavior: while the woman's wages are negatively associated with fertility, neither her labor market participation nor her husband's wage or participation is correlated with family size. These results warrant an especially cautious interpretation since a dynamic framework that simultaneously models labor market and fertility choices over the life course would seem particularly germane among women at the end of their childbearing.

Differences among the four main South African racial groups in the relationships between fertility and education, income, and community resources are striking. First, among colored women with at least 5 years of schooling, the effect of her education is negative and large, and persists even after controlling for income, wages, and community fixed effects. Spousal education effects are smaller, and among labor market choices, only female wages are associated with fertility. Second, the effect of own education on the fertility of Indian women follows an inverse-U shape (peaking toward the end of primary school). The effect is dramatically reduced when spouse's education is controlled, and his education plays a more important role in determining family size than does female education. Among Indians, moreover, income effects and labor market factors are relatively unimportant, suggesting that education, particularly male education, captures differences in tastes rather than the value of time. Third, the education of white women also follows an inverted U-shape, but spousal education, income, and even labor market characteristics do not seem to affect the shape of the relation. Working women and women with higher wages have substantially smaller families, and the results are little affected by the inclusion of community fixed effects. Labor market factors appear to be important correlates of fertility among whites.

In sum, education of both men and women has a powerful association with fertility outcomes in South Africa. Among blacks, household resources, labor market factors, and community characteristics are significant determinants of fertility, but only a relatively small portion of the association between female education and family size can be attributed to those factors. The evidence suggests that the estimated education effects can be attributed in part to the role of unobserved characteristics of women who self-select into particular school grades. However, the magnitude of the education coefficients—and their persistence across the education distribution—suggests there may be some productivity gains associated with education itself. To explore that idea in more depth, the next section examines the relationship between fertility and performance on a set of cognitive tests conducted as part of the PSLSD.

ROLE OF OTHER MEASURES OF HUMAN CAPITAL

As noted above, there were vast differences in public investments in education across racial groups under apartheid in South Africa, and according to data in the PSLSD, these gaps were reinforced by private expenditures on schooling. There are therefore dramatic differences in school quality across races, regions, and socioeconomic groups. Eight years of schooling probably does not mean the same thing to every South African woman. Even the standard examinations, such as matric, had their own race- and region-specific boards, and standards were not uniform across those boards. The Indian board, for example, has a reputation of setting the highest standard.

In an effort to capture some of these differences in the meaning of schooling, a Literacy Assessment Module (LAM) was fielded in conjunction with the PSLSD. The LAM sought to measure three sets of basic skills: reading comprehension (6 questions), listening comprehension and practical mathematics (2 questions), and computational skill (6 questions). The specific questions appear in Appendix A. Fuller et al. (1995) provide an extensive description of the data.

The LAM was intended to be given to a random subsample of 25 percent of all households. Within each household, the enumerator was instructed to choose randomly two household members for the test; one was to be aged 13 to 18 and the other aged 18 to 50. Unfortunately, the sampling scheme that was implemented in the field was not random. The LAM was completed in only 15 percent of households, and because the sample sizes are small, the present analysis focuses on black women. The characteristics of the LAM subsample are reported in the second column of Table 6-2. A regression of the probability that a woman is in the LAM subsample provides a simple way of summarizing the differences between the subsample and the women in the full sample. That regression indicates that enumerators tended to select younger, never-married, urban women. In large part, this presumably reflects the fact that these women were more likely to be at home and that younger (and therefore better-educated) respondents would complete the module more quickly. However, conditional on age, there is no evidence of differences between women in the LAM subsample and the full sample in terms of their education and household income.

The effect of the selection is reflected in the first column of Table 6-6, which reports the results of regressing fertility on education, controlling for age and location, based on data from the 778 black women who completed the LAM. The comparable regression, based on the entire sample of black women, is reported in the first column of Table 6-5A. The correlation between education and fertility is stronger among women in the LAM subsample and, as is apparent from column 2 of Table 6-6, so are income effects.

Within this subsample, the inclusion of raw test scores has a substantial

TABLE 6-6 Children Ever Born and Cognitive Test Scores, Black Women Aged 15-49

	Baseline	HH Income	Test: Total	Test: Separate	Income & Tests	Access Information	All
Years of education							
Woman	–0.147*	–0.102*	–0.089*	–0.087*	–0.082*	–0.096*	–0.079*
	[0.016]	[0.016]	[0.018]	[0.018]	[0.018]	[0.017]	[0.018]
Spouse		–0.057*	–0.066*	–0.066*	–0.056*	–0.057*	–0.056*
		[0.025]	[0.025]	[0.025]	[0.025]	[0.025]	[0.025]
ln(HH income)	—	–0.147*	—	—	–0.133*	–0.142*	–0.130*
		[0.045]			[0.045]	[0.045]	[0.045]
Test scores							
Total	—	—	–-0.052*	—	—	—	—
			[0.017]				
Comprehension	—	—	—	–0.076*	–0.068*	—	–0.067*
				[0.033]	[0.033]	—	[0.033]
Quantitative	—	—	—	–0.033	–0.030	—	–0.028
				[0.028]	[0.028]		[0.028]
(1) if read paper in last 2 weeks	—	—	—	—	—	–0.099	–0.061
						[0.096]	[0.097]
F(all human capital)	—	—	28.27	19.09	15.87	20.12	11.99
			[0.00]	[0.00]	[0.00]	[0.00]	[0.00]
F(test scores)				5.04	4.06		3.72
				[0.01]	[0.02]		[0.02]
F(all covs.)	279.14	179.93	179.49	164.54	154.09	165.04	143.00
R^2	0.69	0.72	0.72	0.72	0.72	0.72	0.72

NOTES: In each regression, 778 women were included. Sample characteristics are reported in column 2 of Table 6-2. Standard errors in parentheses below coefficients; p-values below F test statistics. Regressions include controls for age (spline); spouse present, absent, or dead; and location of residence.

impact on the effect of education: the effect is reduced by more than one-third.[18] Moreover, the tests themselves are negatively correlated with fertility. Specifically, it is the reading comprehension test that is of particular relevance. A woman with better-developed comprehension skills (who answered all six questions correctly) would, on average, have nearly half a child less than a woman who failed to answer any of the questions correctly.

Since women who score well on such tests are likely to earn more and live in higher-income households, the impact of the test scores may simply reflect the role of household resources. Controlling for income, however, has very little impact on the estimates. More directly, in a regression of (log) wages on age, education, and test scores among black women, it is computational skills that appear to be rewarded in the labor market: an additional correct answer to the computational questions is associated with a 15 percent higher wage (t statistic is 2.5), whereas a correct comprehension answer is associated with only a 7 percent higher wage (t statistic is 1.3). Thus if test scores are simply a proxy for income, computational skills should have a larger impact on fertility than do comprehension skills. In fact, the reverse is true.

Why do comprehension skills affect demographic outcomes, but not wages? Women with better comprehension skills may be better able to access and assimilate information in the community. They may thus be likely to be better informed than their peers and therefore better able to use community services effectively.

In one attempt to examine this hypothesis, test scores were replaced with a control for whether the woman reported that she had read a newspaper in the previous 2 weeks. Slightly fewer than half of the women in the sample had done so. Clearly, reading a newspaper is a choice, so the interpretation of the regression is not ambiguous; however, the covariate is not significantly correlated with fertility, and its inclusion in a regression with the test scores does not affect the estimated impact of comprehension skills.

An alternative strategy for examining the information hypothesis is to include community fixed effects that capture all community-level information and services available to women. If women who score well on the tests live in communities with services that affect fertility, these effects will be absorbed by the fixed effects. While the impact of the total test score is robust to their inclusion (its impact is –0.047 with a standard error of 0.022), the impact of the comprehension score is halved, and it is not significant. (In contrast, the impact of the quantitative score rises.) This result suggests that access to information may play an important role in explaining the link between fertility and test scores, and therefore education.

---

[18] Put another way, test scores and education are highly correlated in these data. For example, among black women, controlling for age and location, an additional year of schooling is associated with a 0.21 higher score on the quantitative tests and a 0.22 higher score on the comprehension test. Standard errors are 0.02 in both cases.

CONCLUSIONS

Female education is a powerful predictor of fertility outcomes among women in South Africa, particularly those who are black or colored. Drawing primarily on survey data from the PSLSD, this chapter has investigated some of the mechanisms that underlie this relationship. The discussion has focused on black women, among whom an additional year of schooling is associated with about 0.12 fewer children ever born.

Part of this effect reflects assortative mating in the marriage market (see Basu, this volume). The education of husbands and wives is positively correlated, and controlling for the education of the spouse, the effect of maternal education on children ever born is reduced by about a third. This reduction is greatest among the least-educated women. The results indicate that with regard to fertility choices, men matter in South Africa, particularly among the poorest groups, suggesting that family planning outreach should be directed toward both men and women.

It is difficult with the available data to determine the precise magnitude of the effect of household resources on fertility with much confidence. There can be no doubt, however, that income significantly depresses childbearing. Higher rates of female labor force participation and higher wages are also associated with lower fertility. Thus, policies designed to increase growth in income, particularly female income, are likely to lead to slower population growth.

There is suggestive evidence from aggregate data on the timing of fertility declines in South Africa that greater access to family planning services may have been associated with lower fertility. Evidence from the PSLSD demonstrates that community characteristics do indeed affect fertility outcomes, although the impact apparently varies within communities. It is, however, not possible, using the PSLSD, to identify the specific factors that are important or who benefits most. This is unfortunate since investments in community infrastructure and services can play a central role in public policy interventions, particularly in the social sector, and in policies that are targeted toward particular subpopulations, such as the poorest.

While household and community resources are important determinants of fertility outcomes, the key finding for this analysis is that they can explain at most half of the correlation between maternal education and fertility, and most of the difference can be attributed to the role of husband's education. Parental education, particularly schooling of the mother, is also a powerful predictor of the educational outcomes of children, after controlling for family and community resources. Thus as maternal education increases, there is both a decline in the quantity of children desired and an increase in their quality. One can conclude, therefore, that maternal education has an important independent association with fertility and investments in the human capital of the next generation.

Part of the influence of maternal education is related to skills that are likely to be learned in school; in particular, comprehension skills appear to play a special role in affecting demographic outcomes (see also Diamond et al., this volume). Thus raising cognitive functioning by improving the quality of schooling of today's students and also, perhaps, by providing adult education programs may yield returns beyond the direct economic benefits through the additional impact on demographic and social outcomes.

However, part of the association between education and fertility appears to have nothing to do with the education production function per se, but is a reflection of the fact that education is not randomly distributed across the population. Specifically, women and their families choose their educational attainment given the opportunities and constraints they face, so the better educated are a self-selected sample of the underlying population. This is an important insight as it suggests that a naive interpretation of the correlation between education and fertility as entirely causal is likely to be misleading and to lead to an overstatement of the potential impact of increased levels of female schooling on population growth.

In sum, this chapter has identified several mechanisms through which the correlation between fertility and maternal education operates. A small part of the correlation can be attributed to the role of family and community resources, a larger part to the role of husband's schooling, and part to the acquisition of cognitive skills. An indeterminate fraction of the correlation is associated with unobserved heterogeneity, reflecting the fact that educational attainment is ultimately a choice made by individuals.

ACKNOWLEDGMENTS

I am grateful to SALDRU and The World Bank for providing access to the survey data used here. The comments of Caroline Bledsoe, John Bongaarts, John Casterline, Barney Cohen, Elizabeth Frankenberg, Simon Mpele, Ingrid Woollard, and three anonymous referees have been very helpful.

REFERENCES

African National Congress

1994 *The Reconstruction and Development Programme.* Johannesburg, South Africa: Umanyano Publications.

1995 *Population Policy for South Africa*? Green Paper. Pretoria, South Africa: Ministry of Welfare and Population Development.

Ashenfelter, O., and A. Krueger

1994 Estimates of the economic return to schooling from a new sample of twins. *American Economic Review* 84(5):1157-1173.

Caldwell, J.

1977 The economic rationality of high fertility: An investigation illustrated with Nigerian survey data. *Population Studies* 31(1):5-27.

1979 Education as a factor in mortality decline: An examination of Nigerian data. *Population Studies* 33(3):395-413.

Caldwell, J., and P. Caldwell
1993 The South African fertility decline. *Population and Development Review* 19(2):225-261.

Case, A., and A. Deaton
1995 School quality and educational outcomes in South Africa. Princeton, N.J.: Princeton University. (mimeographed)

Chimere-Dan, O.
1993 Population policy in South Africa. *Studies in Family Planning* 24(1):31-39.

Cochrane, S.
1983 Effects of education and urbanization on fertility. In R. Bulatao and R.D. Lee, eds., *Determinants of Fertility in Developing Countries*. New York: Academic Press.

Department of Education
1996 *The Organisation, Governance and Funding of Schools*. Education White Paper 2. Pretoria: Department of Education.

Frankenberg, E., and P. Sudharto
1995 *Community-Facility Data Collection in the Indonesian Family Life Survey*. Santa Monica, Calif.: RAND. (mimeographed)

Fuller, B., P. Pillay, and N. Sirur
1995 *Literacy Trends in South Africa: Expanding Education While Reinforcing Unequal Achievement?* Cambridge, Mass.: Harvard University. (mimeographed)

Hyslop, D.
1996 *Estimation of a Dynamic Model of Female Labor Force Participation*. Industrial Relations Working Paper. Princeton, N.J.: Princeton University.

Lam, D., and S. Duryea
1995 *Effects of Schooling on Fertility, Labor Supply and Investments in Children, with Evidence from Brazil*. Ann Arbor, Mich.: University of Michigan Population Studies Center. (mimeographed)

Lucas, D.
1992 Fertility and family planning in Southern and Central Africa. *Studies in Family Planning* 23(3):145-158.

Preston-Whyte, E.
1990 Qualitative perspectives on fertility trends among African teenagers. In W.P. Mostert and J.M. Lotter, eds., *South Africa's Demographic Future*: Pretoria: Human Sciences Research Council.

Project for Statistics on Living Standards and Development
1994 *South Africans Rich and Poor: Baseline Household Statistics*. Cape Town: Southern African Labor and Development Research Unit.

Samuel, J.
1990 The state of education in South Africa. In B. Nasson and J. Samuel, eds., *Education: From Poverty to Liberty*. Cape Town: David Philip.

Thomas, D.
1996 Education across generations in South Africa. *American Economic Review* 86(2):330-334.

Thomas, D., and J. Maluccio
1996 Fertility, contraceptive choice and public policy in Zimbabwe. *World Bank Economic Review* 10(1):189-222.

Treiman, D.
1996 On the backs of the blacks: Apartheid and Afrikaner upward mobility. Unpublished manuscript. Los Angeles, Calif.: Department of Sociology, University of California, Los Angeles.

van Zyl, J.
1994 History, scope and methodology of fertility and family planning surveys in South Africa. Pretoria: Human Sciences Research Council. (mimeographed)

Weiss, A.
1995 Human capital vs. signalling explanations of wages. *Journal of Economic Perspectives* 9(4):133-155.

APPENDIX A
SALDRU, UNIVERSITY OF CAPE TOWN

Project for Living Standards and Development

LITERACY ASSESSMENT MODULE [LAM]

Section A: Listening, Comprehension, and Practical Math (about 5 minutes)

Question 1: "Imagine that you are taking a trip on the bus to a township that is located 280 kilometres away. The bus driver says that he will drive at a speed of 80 kilometres per hour. How many hours will the trip take to complete?"

Question 2 : [in Mother Tongue] "Meshack would like to set up a fruit stand in the town market. The manager of the market says that Meshack must pay him R 100 to set up his stand. He must also pay R 25 per month to the market manager. Over the first year, how much in total must Meshack pay to the manager?"

Section B: Reading Comprehension (15 minutes)

Question 3: "When Mbaya was a child, he got very excited when his mother, Corfu, asked if he would like to go to the meat market with her. As they walked into the centre of town, the wonderful odours of meat—both fresh and spoiled—could be smelled up to one kilometre away. The hundreds of market stalls formed a row of almost 1 and 1/2 kilometres long. It took almost one hour to walk slowly from one end of the meat market to the other.

"Sometimes Corfu would let Mbaya choose what meat they would buy that morning. The smell of fresh beef was Mbaya's favorite. But sometimes Mbaya would accidentally choose the beef that was not fresh. Corfu would go up close to the big piece of meat hanging from the rack and smell it. Once she was close to it, Corfu could tell immediately that the beef was not fresh. Then she would laugh at Mbaya and tease him for picking spoiled meat. The meat seller would be angry, as Corfu let on to other shoppers that his beef was not fresh. Mbaya would then start looking around for beef that seemed more fresh, no longer trusting that his nose is the best instrument for finding fresh meat."

Q3a. How long was the row of meat stalls, from one end to the other end?
- a. 1 and 1/2 kilometres long.
- b. 1 kilometre long.
- c. It was very close from one end to the other end.
- d. Hundreds of stalls were lined up.

Q3b. What did Mbaya most like to do inside the meat market?
- a. Try to find spoiled meat.
- b. Walk from one end to the other end of the market.
- c. Have his mother tease him when he found spoiled meat.
- d. Find fresh beef for his mother to buy.

Q3c. What did not happen when Mbaya would choose a spoiled piece of meat?
- a. The meat seller would get angry.
- b. Mbaya and his mother would leave the market.
- c. Corfu would tease Mbaya.
- d. They would keep shopping for fresh meat.

Question 4: "Zenariah was riding to work in her usual combi. The driver and the woman sitting next to him, named Roseline, were arguing over whether it was any use for the woman's son to stay in school. The son, named Philemon, was 16. His secondary school had been closed for many days over the past 6 months. Teachers often did not show up for work. But the woman felt that if he could pass matric, Philemon could eventually find a good job, perhaps as a clerk or office worker. The driver, however, claimed that even university graduates were having difficulty finding jobs as clerks. Zenariah had graduated from the University of the Western Cape, and it had taken her 3 months to find her job as an assistant accountant. She was sympathetic to the woman's position, but also had to agree that until the economy improved, education would not guarantee a good job."

Q4a. When Zenariah goes to work in the morning . . .
- a. She usually takes the combi.
- b. She always sits next to Roseline.
- c. She tries to find different drivers and combis.
- d. She usually talks about her son, Philemon, in the combi.

Q4b. What kind of job did Philemon's mother hope he would find?

a. Assistant accountant.
b. Combi driver.
c. Office worker.
d. Teacher.

Q4c. What was the combi driver's position?

a. Schools are of high quality.
b. Philemon should go to the University of the Western Cape.
c. Completing school will lead to a good job.
d. Schooling does not guarantee a good job.

Section C: Computational Problems (15 minutes)

Question 5: 103 kg – 37 kg = _____ kg

Question 6: R 35.50 × 7 = R _____

Question 7: 25% of R 228 = R _____

Question 8: R 22.25 – R 7.88 = R _____

Question 9: "According to the doctor, the mother must buy 0.30 litres of cough mixture for her two sick children. She can either buy three bottles, each containing 0.10 litres, for R 9.50 per bottle *or* she can buy four bottles, each containing 0.08 litres, for R 7.00 per bottle. What is the *least amount of Rand* she needs to spend to get the 0.30 litres required by the doctor?

Question 10: "Namane was trying to figure out her transport costs from the township to the city to get to her job. The combi cost R 2.00 each day. If she took a combi, then a taxi for part of the trip, she would have to spend R 3.50 each day. How much more would the taxi plus the combi cost for the week, than just taking a taxi, if she went to work five days during the week?"

Section E: Spoken Languages and General Reading

Question 11: What language do you speak?

a. At home or when talking with friends?
b. At work (if currently working, otherwise go to Q12).

Question 12: During the past two weeks, did you read any parts of the following items?

a. A newspaper?
If yes, in what language?

b. A magazine?
If yes, in what language?

c. A book of any kind?
If yes, in what language?

7
Which Girls Stay in School? The Influence of Family Economy, Social Demands, and Ethnicity in South Africa

Bruce Fuller and Xiaoyan Liang

INTRODUCTION

Considerable evidence demonstrates the influence of formal schooling on women's fertility and child health practices, as reviewed in earlier chapters. Notwithstanding important exceptions observed in Africa, longer schooling for girls and young women appears to alter an important range of fertility and child health behaviors (Cochrane, 1979; Hill and King, 1993). Accumulating evidence also shows that spending more of one's childhood in school usually results in higher levels of learning—despite uneven levels of school quality and a still hazy understanding of how classroom processes alter girls' knowledge or beliefs in ways that affect fertility and maternal health practices (Lockheed and Verspoor, 1991).

We are operating largely in the empirical dark, however, on a parallel issue, which is the focus of this chapter: What local forces—operating from both within the family and the surrounding economic and institutional environment—lead some girls to stay in school longer while many others drop out?

International agencies are moving ahead rapidly with ambitious programs aimed at increasing female school enrollment. But when we focus on impoverished communities and low-income families, we find very little empirical evidence on the factors that explain why some daughters stay in school while others exit. Western models of school attainment, relying on mobility traditions within industrialized societies, are partially useful in illuminating the economic and cultural forces that may explain girls' educational attainment in developing-country settings (Fuller et al., 1995a; Haveman and Wolfe, 1995). The purpose of this chapter is to advance theoretical understanding of the role of the family's character and practices, especially variability in the work and social demands parents place on daughters, in determining when girls leave school.

First, we review how sociologists and economists have represented the school attainment process within developing-country settings. Second, we report on our household-level study of female school attainment among young black South Africans. After reviewing the economic and social factors that explain local variation in girls' school attainment, we examine how those factors help explain whether and when girls leave school. The final section presents a summary and conclusions. We find that the propensity of daughters to remain in school is associated with the family's economic consumption levels, the family's social structure, and labor and social demands placed on young females. We also find significant variability among black ethnic groups in when daughters typically leave school, variation that corresponds in part to regional histories and school supply. Our analysis suggests that unless policy and program designers take local institutions and particular conditions into account, their well-meaning interventions may be costly and ineffective.

HOUSEHOLD AND INSTITUTIONAL DETERMINANTS OF GIRLS' SCHOOL ATTAINMENT

We often confound how parents make decisions about fertility behavior with whether, or how, parents press their children to stay in school. Working from a rational-choice framework, household economists and demographers argue that (1) parents come to see that more individualized ("higher-quality") childrearing holds greater economic utility, and (2) this realization leads to more determined family planning, lower birth rates, and stronger motivation to keep daughters in school for longer periods of time (Easterlin and Crimmins, 1985). Beyond the household are macroeconomic and institutional forces: evolving labor demand for female workers, shifts in family income, modern forms of social status, and women's variable commitment to reproductive independence (Caldwell and Caldwell, 1990).

A major ingredient of this shifting institutional context is the expansion of mass schooling. Through mass education, the state attempts to define the legitimate social roles that girls should normatively fill. Yet only recently has a family-level literature emerged from sociology that attempts to link the household's immediate economic situation to the broader institutional and cultural context by examining how forces at these two levels of social organization shape girls' school attainment (e.g., Walters and James, 1992). The first conceptual step is to separate household-level processes from both the economic context and social institutions, such as the state and school, that may variably condition family-level action.

Neoclassical Household Decision Making

Recent work by Haveman and Wolfe (1995:1832) reiterates the neoclassical claims by which variation in children's educational attainment is often explained:

> Economists have viewed the process of children's school attainment to be an aspect of the theory of family behavior. The family is viewed as a production unit which employs real inputs in order to generate utility for its members. Adults ...make decisions regarding the generation of family economic resources [and] determine the uses of these resources. Parents make a variety of other choices such as fertility, location, and family stability that influence the returns to productive efforts. The amount of family resources allocated to children, the nature of these resources, and the timing of their distribution influence the school attainment of children.

This model is cross-generational with regard to school attainment: it argues that parents' decisions about their fertility behavior and family structure occur concurrently with choices about their children's school attainment. These decisions, although bundled by the rational parent, aim to advance the individual child's human capital, thereby advancing the family's long-term welfare (Becker, 1976).

Caldwell's earlier work (1976) borrows heavily from this framework, arguing that the "emotional and economic nucleation" of the family occurs as parents come to see, within modernizing contexts, that bearing more children will not necessarily lead to greater long-term wealth or security in old age. As firms and institutions, especially the state and modern schools, exogenously come to associate social status with greater human capital investment, parents factor this into their calculus for allocating household-level resources and labor demands in ways that boost their children's school attainment. Becker and Tomes (1976:S148) note that as parents become upwardly mobile, they invest more heavily in the quality rather than the quantity of children, and they often move to communities where "public contributions to their children's schooling would be greater."

Here the argument shifts to the contextual or institutional level: the commercializing and modernizing context, highly variable across local regions, is changing the structure of wage labor and economic opportunity. In addition, the formal school gains the authority to allocate youths to status and social-class positions. Even household economists are now struggling to incorporate context, rather than simply postulating that preferences are exogenous to the intrafamily utility-maximization process. Haveman and Wolfe (1995:1837), for example, move beyond the family unit by arguing that governments make choices to improve poor families' economic and social context. Parents are viewed as "choosing" various family practices from their environment: "the sort of monitoring, disciplinary, nurturing, and expectational environment in which their children are raised." Drawing on the notion of "social capital" advanced by Loury (1977) and Coleman (1988), Haveman and Wolfe argue that the state can act in ways that strengthen family and kin support and guide both the character and intensity of parents' investments in their children. The family thus mediates information and resources emanating from institutions to improve intrahousehold socialization practices and advance school attainment.[1] The households and surrounding institutional arrangements are therefore acting in tandem.

Institutional Resources and Constraints That Bound Family Choices

We must delineate more crisply those institution-level forces which condition intrafamily decision making. Indeed, many of the quandaries over the education-fertility link expressed by demographers and others interested in population issues may stem from an inadequate understanding of how household-level processes and institutional arrangements operate simultaneously. In demographic circles, for instance, the grand theory of demographic transition has proven to be of limited utility in some African contexts: in countries such as Botswana or Kenya, economic commercialization unfolds, modern rules emerge, female enrollment rises, but fertility behavior changes only slightly (Isiugo-Abanihe, 1994). Similarly, school attainment levels have been highly uneven among societies and within particular regions, despite steady modernization and huge investments in mass education since the 1960s. Females comprise about 25 percent of all secondary school pupils in Chad, versus 56 percent in Namibia. Fewer than half of all children in sub-Saharan Africa reach grade 5, and girls complete 1.5 fewer school years on average relative to boys (World Bank, 1995).

Such variability in the way local parents make decisions about their children's schooling, and over time their own fertility behavior, might be explained by three institution-level forces.

First, the organization of job opportunities varies in ways that establish long-term or immediate returns to staying in school. Labor demands operate differently on girls versus boys. In many parts of Botswana and South Africa, for example, we observe that daughters actually stay in school longer than sons, a phenomenon that can be explained in part by centuries of male labor migration to either commercial centers or cattle fields. In addition, subsistence crop yields are often quite low in arid regions of Southern Africa, so that there is ample discretionary time for daughters to pursue schooling without cutting into time required for domestic chores (Kossoudji and Mueller, 1983).

---

[1]These arguments also depart from the earliest mobility or status-school attainment studies of sociologists from the 1960s forward. This work has focused on how parents, with variable education levels and occupational status, attempt to reproduce the family's position through human capital investment. The question of mobility has been central to this line of work: Can offspring move up the status hierarchy independently of their parents' class position? This work has not, however, been able to incorporate changes in context, other than to see context as a residual set of exogenous factors that cannot be captured by within-family variables (e.g., Campbell, 1983).

Second, the state's educational policies, formulated over time, can induce family demand for female schooling. African countries have expanded their secondary school systems at widely varying rates since the 1960s. The Demographic and Health Surveys of the late 1980s, for instance, showed that just over half of all women aged 20-24 in Zimbabwe had completed some secondary schooling, versus just 2 percent in Mali and 10 percent in Ghana (Bledsoe and Cohen, 1993). The state also can influence norms about the legitimate location and role of young females. When the Botswana government reduced the terminal year of junior-secondary school from grade 10 to grade 9, female enrollment rates quickly began to decline after grade 9 (Fuller et al., 1995a). In addition, the state can influence parents' expressed demand for schooling by lowering the direct costs of enrollment, relieving labor demand for young girls (by investing in water wells or child-care centers), offering free lunches, and encouraging female enrollment through all-girls schools or targeted scholarship programs (Hill and King, 1993; Glewwe, 1994; Bradshaw and Fuller, 1996). School quality and student assessment processes can influence enrollment demand, as well as the extent to which girls are encouraged to achieve at high levels. In one study from Kenya, more than a third of all girls achieving in the bottom quartile dropped out of secondary school because of pregnancy, compared with just one-seventh of the top students (Division of Family Health, 1988, cited in Bledsoe and Cohen, 1993). Distance to school and the presence of female teachers also may encourage higher school attainment among young females (DiStefano, 1993; Fuller and Clarke, 1994).

Third, parents' cultural commitments and social practices, extracted from a modernizing institutional environment, may further explain variability in female school attainment. A variety of cultural practices have received empirical attention in Africa: the argument that sexual and marriage practices are culturally determined, occasionally altered by modernizing values (Whiting and Whiting, 1991); the role of polygyny and resulting demands placed on young women (Lesthaeghe, 1989); bride price and the extent to which schooling is factored in; initiation rites and role conflicts for young females who are now culturally ordained as "adults"; and the role of kin, not only the husband and wife, in making reproductive decisions (see Bledsoe and Cohen, 1993; Hyde, 1993).

Locally Situating the Household Model

How can we situate the family within variable local contexts to better explain girls' school attainment? A family-economy model has emerged recently in sociology. This model situates the household's actions within (1) local economic demands and (2) more localized social or cultural commitments that stem from a shared set of evolving institutions, at times situated within a common ethnic history. The household is still seen partly in neoclassical terms as a social collective that actively seeks to optimize its members' welfare, not dissimilar to a neoclassical model similar to Becker's (1976). But the family's "rationality" and opportunities are set by both local labor demands and institutional norms, and the family is seen as mediating these macro forces in allocating children's time between work and schooling.

How has this model—attempting to balance economic and social forces—been applied to the question of school attainment at the child level? As an example, the new family-economy model has helped explain an early contradiction in the school attainment literature: as societies industrialized from an agricultural or commercial base, enrollment rates often grew most rapidly in rural areas, not within industrializing centers where neoclassical theory accurately predicted higher economic returns to more schooling (Fishlow, 1966). In the United States, the historical evidence on household decision making shows that parents took into account immediate labor demands and income opportunities, not longer-term optimization or human capital strategies. Urban parents could move their children into factory or early service jobs, pulling them out of school to advance the household's immediate welfare. In rural areas, children experienced more discretionary time between planting and harvest seasons. This economic dynamic interacted with rural parents' Calvinist commitment to formal education, boosting secondary school attainment levels for girls and boys above those observed in urban centers (Walters and O'Connell, 1988). These family-economy theorists emphasize the state's contextual role in expanding the supply of schooling, reducing private costs, and regulating child labor—factors that boosted school attainment (Walters and James, 1992).

We recently extended the family-economy framework to explain rising female school attainment observed in Botswana villages since independence (Fuller et al., 1995a). Two major findings emerged from this study.

First, economic dynamics mediated by the household must be culturally situated and seen in gender-specific terms. Daughters were more likely to persist further through secondary school, for instance, when the number of household chores they were assigned was closer to the number assigned to sons. The presence of younger children and additional child-care obligations contributed to adolescent daughters' greater propensity to leave school. We also found a tendency to stay in school longer among daughters in father-absent households in the two southernmost villages, those located closest to the South African job market. While not always statistically significant, this finding is consistent with Schultz's (1990) report that when mothers serve as the household head, resources for schooling are allocated more equally to daughters. Studying several African societies, Lloyd and Blanc (1996) found that school attainment for both sons and daughters was higher in female-headed households, after taking into account economic factors (including generally lower income levels).[2]

[2]The presence and authority of the father also have implications for the mother's relative power over fertility decision making, as discussed by LeVine et al. (1994a) and Mburugu (1994).

Our second major finding was that mothers' attributes and social demands helped explain how far their daughters went in secondary school, again after taking into account the household's economic characteristics (within a survival analysis framework). In these Botswana villages, variability in the mother's schooling, assessed literacy level, perceived utility of formal education, family planning practices, and childrearing objectives all contributed to her daughter's school attainment. As posited by the new family-economy model, the discretionary time afforded by the economic context and parents' allocation of children's time between work and school contributed to daughters' school attainment.

Next, we clarify how the family-economy model can be applied to variable regions and ethnic groups within South Africa. We then assess empirically how household-level factors help explain why girls' school attainment varies among poor black families. This family-level analysis reveals cross-ethnic and regional differences in female school attainment, leading us back to the institution-level force of school supply and action by local states. We turn first to a consideration of how economic and social forces, observed within the household, can be more clearly conceptualized.

SOUTH AFRICA: EXPLAINING LOCAL VARIATION IN GIRLS' SCHOOL ATTAINMENT

Poor Families Mediating Economic and Social Linkages

The family-economy model posits that as parents consider the utility of keeping their children in school, they operate from preferences and anticipated streams of monetary benefits. Yet these "preferences" are viewed as stemming from variable economic demands and institutional norms, observable within the household, that pertain to childrearing aims and commitments to schooling. Parents attend to these (variable) local economic and social demands on the basis of the material and human resources they can draw from the environment. The family's linkages to the economic and social context vary in character across local regions. For example, in historically diverse and balkanized societies, such as South Africa, ethnic membership frequently corresponds to the family's regional location or designated "homeland," a point to which we will return.

Economic Linkages

Borrowing from the neoclassical household model, sociologists have emphasized the importance of economic resources and labor demands as parents allocate their children's time between work and school. Families are situated within specific labor structures that provide variable levels of income and job opportunities. These labor demands may compete for youths' time that otherwise would be available for schooling. Under the family-economy model, the resources and demands inherent in the organization of work are augmented by state action, especially government's ability to legitimate school attendance, rather than full-time work, as the norm for youths (Horan and Hargis, 1991; Walters and James, 1992). In our empirical model of daughters' school attainment, we include the household's variable economic resources and indicators of labor demand.

Social Linkages

The desire to go beyond macrostructural explanations of family decision making has renewed interest in situating children within a local social or cultural network. Anthropologists, of course, have long been focused on the situational norms and cultural models that guide childrearing and early socialization (Ogbu, 1978; Whiting and Whiting, 1991; LeVine et al., 1994). Rather than focusing on the content of socialization, however, Coleman (1988) examines the basic architecture of social relations, especially levels of obligation and trust within the family, and how these normative obligations may influence children's propensity to stay in school and achieve at higher levels. Under his construction of "social capital," he delineates structural features of the family that he and Schneider relate empirically to children's school attainment (Schneider and Coleman, 1993). The presence of parents or kin and their obligatory expectations are posited to constrain (or advance) children's school attainment levels through a number of mechanisms: the absence of one parent, a mother who works outside the home, a greater number of siblings, little talk at home about the child's life or schoolwork, and parents' low expectations and lack of pressure on the child to go on to college (Coleman, 1990:595). The presence of parents and the pressure they place on children to do well in school have in turn been linked to the household economy. Astone and McLanahan (1991), for instance, detail how working single parents spend less time supervising their children's homework or discussing their school lives.

This framework assumes that family-level linkages offer social resources to children: moral encouragement and specific strategies for doing well in school. Household economists are trying to incorporate the social capital construct, defining parental time as a resource or an investment made in children's development (Haveman and Wolfe, 1995:1836). As originally coined by Loury (1977), the term "social capital" referred to social linkages and obligations that enhance (or constrain) initial entry and advancement in the job market. Yet certain social linkages and obligations place social demands on children that pull them out of school. This is especially so in impoverished contexts where secondary schooling is not a fully legitimated institution, including developing-country settings where girls' school attendance is not taken for granted. The dampening effect of fathers' presence on their daughters' school attendance in Botswana, for example, may be due to domestic and marital obligations imposed by the father (see also Lloyd and Blanc, 1996).

A second element of the social capital construct—the content of social obligations and expectations between parent and daughter—has yet to be specified or related to female school attainment. While endorsement of the modern school is acquired from a modernizing institutional environment, it is manifest and observable within the household (Caldwell, 1986; United Nations, 1995). We take modest steps here to assess whether observable social resources and social demands placed on daughters, stemming from their parents' education and literacy levels, contribute to daughters' school attainment in South Africa. In the discussion, we return to what little is known about the content of these evolving social expectations.

Variability Among Poor Provinces and Households

The above intrafamily dynamics may be conditioned by the regional economic and institutional context in which the household is situated. Given its history of apartheid and racist migration controls, South Africa shows significant variation across regions and ethnic groups in the strength of regional economies, rates of father absence, and maternal schooling levels (see also Thomas, this volume). We focus on variability among regions populated by black ("African") families. Population growth rates, for instance, currently range from 2.6 to 3.9 percent in regions populated by Xhosa versus North Sotho and Venda communities (Erasmus, 1994). The separation of black ethnic groups into "homelands" also led to variability in the availability and quality of secondary schooling.

Outside white communities, South African families suffer from extreme levels of poverty. Fifty-three percent of all South Africans currently live below the poverty line, recently established as US$97 in monthly household expenditures per capita (1993 prices),[3] and blacks comprise 94 percent of this total. Indeed, two-thirds of all blacks, totaling 21 million adults and children, live in poverty. About two-thirds of all poor households are located in the three provinces on which our analysis focuses: the Eastern Cape (populated primarily by Xhosa speakers), KwaZulu/Natal (Zulu speakers), and the Northern Transvaal Province (North Sotho, Venda, and smaller groups). Figure 7-1 shows locations. Almost 70 percent of all female-headed households subsist below the poverty line, as compared with 44 percent of families with a resident father. Note that the old provincial boundaries were still in effect in 1993.

Secondary school enrollment rates are much lower among youths living in poverty. For households in the first and second poorest quintiles, just 46 and 57 percent, respectively, of children aged 13-17 are enrolled in school. In contrast,

---

[3]The poverty line is based on the 40th percentile of all households, using household income per adult equivalent, adjusting for family composition. Data and exchange rates are for 1993 (Reconstruction and Development Programme, 1995).

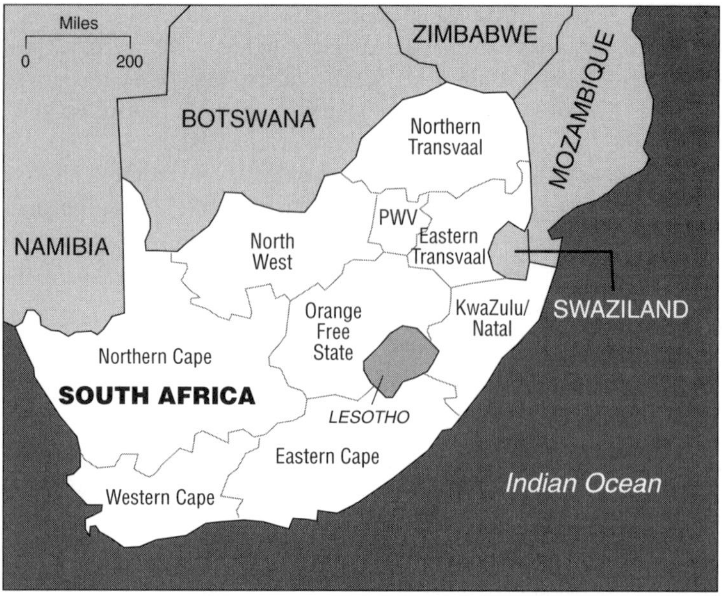

FIGURE 7-1 Map of South Africa.

this rate is 83 percent for families in the most affluent quintile.[4] Among the poor, just one-fifth have electricity, and almost half use wood as their main source of energy. South Africa's infant mortality rate remains at 53 per 1,000 live births; the total fertility rate stands at 4.1 (Erasmus, 1994; Reconstruction and Development Programme, 1995).[5]

Variability Across Regional Contexts

Our analysis focuses on girls' school attainment among the largest black ethnic groups. We begin by focusing on the context and attributes of the three

[4]The percentage of females enrolled in secondary schools exceeds that of males in most provinces. In the old black homeland areas in 1990, 58 percent of all grade 10 students who sat for the matriculation exam were females; females comprised just over half of all who passed the national exam. But relatively few black women enter a college or university. At the University of Cape Town and the Witwatersrand University, African females comprise just 9 and 7 percent of total enrollment, respectively (Truscott, 1994).

[5]White and colored populations are relatively affluent, compared with African families. But income inequality is stark: the richest 10 percent of all households, comprising just 6 percent of the population, accounts for 40 percent of all consumption. The lowest 40 percent, representing 53 percent of the population, accounts for less than 10 percent of total consumption (Reconstruction and Development Programme, 1995).

most populous communities: Zulu, Xhosa, and North Sotho speakers. Table 7-1 presents descriptive statistics for the three groups and for the respective province within which the majority of each resides. "Sample count" refers to the number of households for which data were reported for a mother and daughter pair, that is the eldest daughter still resident in the household, age 11-25. Our subsample, stemming from a 1993 national probability sample, equaled 1,503 households, including households belonging to one of the five largest black groups and reporting household consumption levels at or below two times the poverty line (which included over 90 percent of all sampled households from these ethnic groups).[6]

Mean per capita income for 1988 across the three provinces was uniformly low but variable. The Northern Transvaal province showed the lowest income level, equaling just US$319 (1988 exchange rate and prices), compared with $841 in KwaZulu/Natal. Per capita income averaged $1,116 nationally. An estimated 61 percent of all Zulus live below the poverty line, versus 92 percent of Xhosas and 83 percent of North Sothos.

Despite a more rural and weaker economy than the other two provinces, North Sotho adults display similar school attainment levels, which may historically have been specific to males. In 1993, the proportion of adults who had completed secondary school equaled 13.4 percent among North Sothos, versus 10.8 percent among Zulu households. Young adolescents in North Sotho communities currently display much higher rates of persistence through secondary school: in 1993, 54 percent of all children who began grade 1 had persisted to grade 11, whereas this figure equaled just 26 and 11 percent, respectively,[7] among Zulu and Xhosa youths. Our earlier analysis showed no literacy advantage among young North Sotho males or females, and the lower level of selectivity associated with lower dropout rates probably contributes to a lower matric pass rate among North Sotho secondary graduates (28 versus 43 percent for Zulu graduates; see Fuller et al., 1995b).

Household and Daughter Sample

The attributes of young females, shown in Table 7-1 for eldest daughters residing in sampled households differ across the three ethnic groups. The percentage of females enrolled in school ranged from about 60 percent and 57

---

[6]These data are from a national probability sample from 360 randomly selected clusters that yielded data on 8,848 households nationwide. The sampling plan is detailed in Project for Statistics on Living Standards and Development (1994). Gender-related analyses of school attainment and assessed literacy levels appear in Fuller et al. (1995b).

[7]For North Sotho communities, grade 12 enrollment counts are actually higher than those for grade 11, as youths reportedly stay in school to sit repeatedly for the matriculation exam. This rise in grade 12 enrollments is not observed in Zulu or Xhosa communities overall.

TABLE 7-1 Characteristics of Three Major Black Ethnic Groups by Principal Home Province, 1988-1993

Characteristic	Zulu Speakers	KwaZulu/Natal Province	Xhosa Speakers	Eastern Cape Province	No. Sotho Speakers	No. Transvaal Province
Population (1993)						
Total population (millions)	9.1	7.0	7.4	5.8	3.7	5.0
% in "home province"	74		76		78	
Sample count (households)	519	421	381	340	261	219
% in "home province"	81		85		82	
Contextual Conditions						
Per capita income in 1988 Rand (US$)		1,910 ($841)		1,358 ($598)		725 ($319)
Annual population growth rate (1985-1993)		2.8		2.6		3.9
% population in poverty[a]	61	53	92	78	83	77
Dependency ratio		2.3		3.7		4.8
% households with absent fathers		14		31		28
% labor force female		54		56		59
% adults who have completed secondary school	10.8		9.0		13.4	
% pupils who persist to grade 11[b]	26		11		54	
Matric exam pass rate[c]	43		44		28	
Literacy index, adults aged 19-34	5.3		5.2		—	
Sampled Eldest Daughters (n = 1,389)[d]						
Mean age (years)	19.6		18.9		19.7	
% in school aged 11-25[e]	45.9		57.0		59.8	
School attainment if out of school (years)[f]	5.6		5.9		6.7	

Sampled Households (n = 1,389)			
Monthly household expenditures (1993 Rand)[e]	1,331	780	920
Females fetch water (% of households)[e]	29	29	53
Children in household under age 18[e]	4.1	3.7	3.8
Males in household over age 18 e,g[e]	1.5	1.1	1.2
Mother's school attainment (years)[e,g]	3.6	3.8	2.8
Father's school attainment (years)	3.7	3.3	3.7
% mothers in clerical or laborer jobs[e]	22	16	15

NOTES:

[a]Poverty figures calculated from 1993 household survey for provinces and homelands within provinces. Figure for Xhosa-speaking households pertains to Transkei. Corresponding figure for Ciskei equals 73 percent. Poverty line is established at monthly expenditures of 301 Rand per adult equivalent. In 1993 prices, this equals US$97 per month.

[b]Figures are for homeland school departments. Percentage for Xhosas applies to the larger Transkei homeland. Percentage for the smaller Ciskei region equals 37 percent.

[c]Percentage pass rates for 1990 in the homeland areas of KwaZulu, Ciskei, and Transkei combined, and Lebowa.

[d]Includes daughters from the five principal ethnic groups—Zulu, Xhosa, North Sotho, South Sotho, and Tswana—with deletion of missing data by each individual variable.

[e]For sampled households and daughters, MANOVA tests were performed to assess differences among ethnic groups. $p < .01$ or stronger.

[f]For sampled households and daughters, MANOVA tests were performed to assess differences among ethnic groups. $p < .05$.

[g]Among sampled households, many North Sotho mothers (42 percent) reported they had completed no schooling. Median school attainment (in years) for Zulus, Xhosas, and North Sothos was 3, 3, and 1, respectively.

SOURCES: Education Foundation (1993), Erasmus (1994), Project for Statistics on Living Standards and Development (1994), Verwey and Munzhedzi (1994), Fuller et al. (1995b), Reconstruction and Development Programme (1995).

percent among North Sothos and Xhosas, respectively, to about 46 percent among Zulus. Labor demands also vary: 53 percent of all North Sotho households require female members to carry wood or water, versus just 29 percent of Zulu and Xhosa households. Zulus have larger families, with an average of 4.1 children under age 18 residing in the household, as compared with 3.8 for North Sotho and 3.7 for Xhosa families.

Importantly, mothers' school attainment for this sample is lowest in North Sotho households, just 2.8 years on average. Thus the school attainment advantage among young North Sotho females appears to be a relatively recent phenomenon, perhaps attributable to educational expansion in the old North Sotho homeland of Lebowa over the two decades following the 1976 Soweto uprising (Fuller et al., 1995b).

Ethnic Differences in Female Attainment

We now assess empirically how family economic and social factors influence daughters' school attainment across the five ethnic groups in our subsample (including Tswana and South Sotho households in addition to the three groups discussed above). We model a discrete-time hazard function that assesses whether and when young females leave school. First, however, we focus on descriptive differences in female school attainment across the five ethnic groups.

Figure 7-2 displays the percentage of females age 13-24 (n = 1,129) who were still enrolled in school at the time of the survey (1993-1994) for the three major black groups discussed previously. The North Sotho advantage relative to Zulu and Xhosa enrollment rates depends on the daughter's age. The 5-year secondary school cycle officially includes youths aged 13-17, but many enrolled students are over age 17. Among those aged 17-18, the enrollment rate of North Sotho females is 10 percent higher than that of Zulu females. Among those age 19-20, the North Sotho rate is 59 percent, versus 29 percent for Zulus and 48 percent for Xhosas.

Figure 7-3 focuses only on those girls who had left school by the time of the survey and reported their school attainment. Recognizing that right-censoring of cases is occurring, here too we see significant ethnic differences in school attainment levels for daughters: 5.6 and 5.9 years, respectively, for Zulu and Xhosa females, versus 6.7 years for North Sotho females ($p < .05$).[8]

For many young females, leaving school may coincide with becoming pregnant. Our hazard-rate models enable us to examine whether pregnancy substitutes for the effect of family-level factors in estimating the likelihood of leaving school. Figure 7-4 helps us understand descriptively the relationship between pregnancy and leaving school. Toward the end of the normal school-going age

[8]Note that the difference in the mean age of sampled daughters is not statistically significant, ranging between 18.9 and 19.7 years of age (Table 7-1).

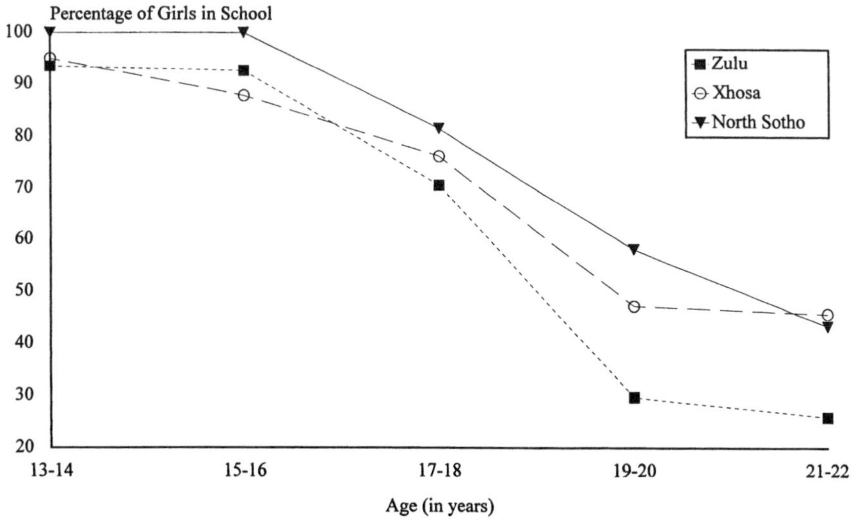

FIGURE 7-2 Percentage of girls in school by age and ethnic group. NOTE: For Zulu, n = 321; Xhosa, n = 331; North Sotho, n = 201.

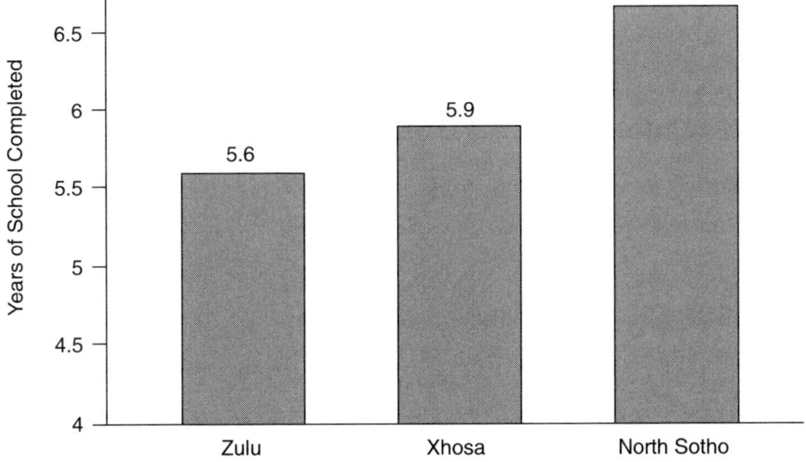

FIGURE 7-3 Average years of school completed for girls by ethnic group. (NOTE: Sample restricted to girls, aged 11-25, who have left school. For Zulu, n = 177; Xhosa, n = 138; North Sotho, n = 85.)

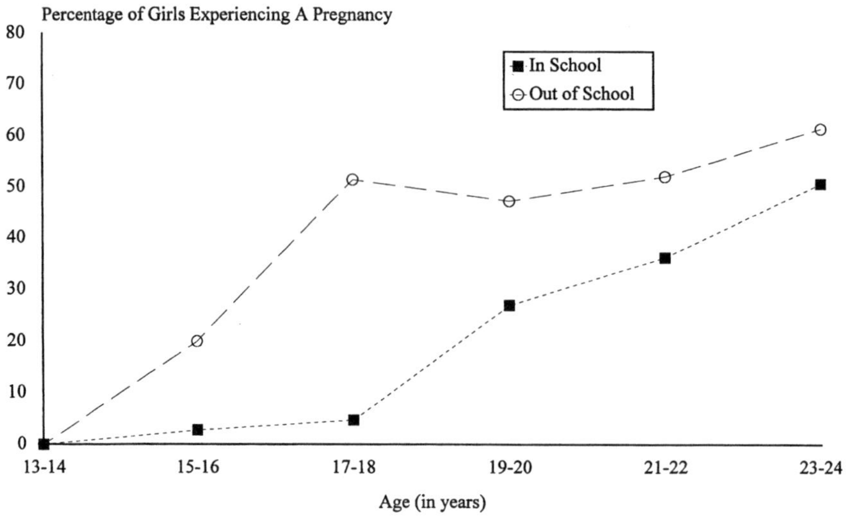

FIGURE 7-4 Percentage of girls experiencing a pregnancy by age and school enrollment. (NOTE: For girls who are still in school, n = 794; For girls who have left school, n = 709.)

(17-18), very few girls who were still enrolled had become pregnant; in contrast, just over half of all out-of-school females had experienced one pregnancy. Importantly, as the incidence of pregnancy becomes significant for young females, after age 19, many are still enrolled in school, having returned to or remaining in secondary school or postsecondary education.

HOW FAMILY-ECONOMY AND SOCIAL FACTORS INFLUENCE GIRLS' SCHOOL ATTAINMENT

We now examine how the household's economic and social attributes—particularly its resources and demands pertaining to daughters—help explain whether and when young females leave school. We rely on survey measures of the family economy and the household's social architecture. We also examine the strength of ethnic differences in explaining variations in school attainment, focusing on the three largest black groups. The discussion includes qualitative evidence to supplement the survey findings.

Household Attributes That May Influence Girls' School Attainment

Economic Resources

Within poor South African communities, families vary greatly in whether and how members are linked to the wage sector. To the extent that the family earns more cash income from wages or remittances from kin members, resources are available to cover school expenses (for books, uniforms, and combi fares in urban townships). Three survey measures were available to assess how basic resources are related to daughters' school attainment: monthly expenditures as reported by the household respondent; an index of durable goods owned by the family (refrigerator, bicycle, telephone, and electric kettle); and whether the family had credit and owed money for purchased items to a local shop. Monthly expenditures were moderately correlated with the durables index (r = .43). Earlier we found in Botswana that durables and housing quality measures, reflecting accumulated wealth or an investment attitude, were more consistently related to daughters' school attainment than were short-term consumption measures (Fuller et al., 1995a).[9]

Economic Demands

Labor demands faced by daughters can stem from adults' own involvement in the wage, informal cash, or agrarian sectors and from the family's demographic structure. It is often assumed that women's income from wages or informal-sector involvement will be related to household consumption levels. We found no correlation, however, between the mother's employment in a clerical or laborer job (including domestic work) and monthly household expenditures (r = .03 for both coefficients). This finding may be due to the low incidence of maternal employment (22 percent of Zulu and 15 percent of North Sotho mothers) or simply to sporadic and low wage income.[10]

Labor demands may be greater for eldest daughters whose mothers are employed outside the household: with mothers away at work, domestic duties may fall more heavily on the daughter's shoulders. This is one of our principal reasons for focusing our study on the eldest daughter. As discussed earlier, we included a direct measure of whether females are required to carry water or wood (Table 7-1). We also used measures to capture the fact that adolescent daughters

---

[9]The credit-linkage variable was modestly correlated with household expenditures (r = .21), but not with the durables index. Exploratory analyses also included remittance income, but this variable did not contribute to the explanatory power of the models.

[10]We have also restricted variation on all predictor and school attainment variables by deleting black households from the full national sample with incomes exceeding two times the poverty line (they represent just 6 percent of all black households sampled, 366 of 6,167 families).

often must care for younger siblings and cousins in the compound (Bozzoli, 1991) and that daughters likely feel greater labor demand in families with more and younger children. We originally used three such measures: the number of children under age 18 residing in the compound, the age of the youngest child, and the difference in age between the youngest child and the eldest daughter. The latter predictor proved to be highly collinear with the first, however, and was dropped. We also included the age of the second-eldest resident sibling who might relieve labor demands placed on the eldest daughter.

Social Resources

Coleman's (1988, 1990) delineation of how children may benefit from social linkages that raise school attainment represents one theoretical framework. Coleman stops short, however, of specifying the character and meaning of intra-household obligations, expectations, and forms of supervision over domestic chores and school work—social processes that undoubtedly vary across and within ethnic groups. As a first step, one can assess whether the presence of adult actors and social linkages helps predict daughters' school attainment levels (see also Schneider and Coleman, 1993). We included the number of women and men residing in the household as indicators of the intensity of adult supervision. We also examined whether the household received in-kind services from kin or friends living outside the household, including child-care support, repairs in the compound, meals, and other forms of nonmonetary support. Among Zulu and North Sotho families, 20 percent reported receiving such support, versus just 7 percent for all Xhosa households. Our final social-resource measure is whether the household contributed to a local church. Among Zulu households, 35 percent reported doing so, compared with 27 percent for both North Sotho and Xhosa families. Contributions were modestly related to overall household expenditures ($r = .21$).

Social Demands

The social-capital construct, derived from North American settings, assumes that a stronger presence of adults will increase children's school attendance. However, initial evidence from African settings, cited above, suggests that a father's absence may actually contribute to higher school attainment among daughters. Almost half (48 percent) of all black individuals live in female-headed households (Fuller et al., 1995b).[11] We also postulate that the mother's

[11]Among sampled Zulu households with a resident daughter age 11-25, 16 percent reported having an absent father. The incidence was 20 percent for North Sothos and 21 percent for Xhosas. The household study included a liberal definition of household "residency," including persons who have lived in the compound or homestead at least 15 days out of the past year, share meals from a common source, or contribute to a common resource pool.

and father's schooling levels lead to differing social demands for daughters, including the way their social roles are defined within the household and the relative time allocated to work versus school. Qualitative studies in Botswana, Kenya, and South Africa substantiate this assumption (Bozzoli, 1991; LeVine et al., 1994b). The importance of mothers' schooling levels for their daughters' school attainment has been established in several African countries; evidence on the importance of fathers' education in shaping pro-education social demands is less consistent (Hill and King, 1993). Among our sampled low-income households, maternal and paternal school attainment levels were moderately correlated (r = .43).

Our preliminary analyses revealed that the basic family-level model did not predict well whether the eldest daughter had experienced a pregnancy, with the exception of one explanatory variable—mother's level of schooling. Among eldest daughters, aged 11-25, who had left school, 53 percent reported having experienced at least one pregnancy; just 14 percent of these females were aged 19 or younger. Among daughters still attending school at the time of the survey, 15 percent had experienced at least one pregnancy.[12] Finally, we added pregnancy as an exogenous predictor of school attainment, assessing the extent to which pregnancy substitutes for the other predictors of female attainment.[13]

Surviving Secondary School: Explaining Which Girls Leave School and When

To assess the influence of the above family-economy and social factors on when young females leave school, we constructed discrete-time hazard models (Tuma and Hannan, 1984; Singer and Willett, 1993). Doing so involved estimating hazard functions for the 1,103 daughters aged 13-24 for whom complete data were available. This form of survival analysis assesses whether and when girls leave school, taking into account the fact that many observations are right-cen-

---

[12]Sampled mothers (of eldest daughters) reported four pregnancies on average (median). Of daughters who had been pregnant, 24 percent had experienced one infant death; the child of an additional 15 percent had died between the ages of 1 and 5. Maternal education was related to the number of pregnancies reported by the mother (r = –34), and the latter variable was related to the number of infant deaths (r = .41).

[13]Poor South African families are concentrated in rural areas. About 53 percent of the population resides in rural areas or outside of small towns; of these families, 74 percent live in poverty. In contrast, 41 percent of all urban families are impoverished. We found, however, that rural location made no consistent difference in explaining daughters' school attainment for our low-income sample. This finding may be due to overall poverty levels or to the fact that many rural households are linked to the wage sector through jobs in towns or remittances. Fewer than one-third of the sampled families had access to lands for crops or grazing. The representation of rural families in our sample approximated the national average; just over half the entire sample was living in traditional rural structures of mud, waddle, or daub.

sored: many girls will have left school after the survey was conducted, and a fair number of young females who dropped out of school because of pregnancy will have reentered later on.

Some selection bias may occur in choosing the eldest resident daughter on whom we have focused our analysis. We had three reasons for making this design decision. First, eldest daughters are at the age of greatest risk for leaving school: during the secondary-school years and (for a limited number of female matriculating graduates) the initial years of postsecondary education. Figure 7-5, panel A, shows that 88 percent of daughters (again from low-income families) complete primary school, corresponding to grade 4 (the old Standard 5). As girls progress through secondary school, survival rates begin to decline: the hazard or probability of leaving school increases for each successive year. Just half of all young females complete Form 4 and their matriculation exam (indicated by grade level 10). About 32 percent complete any postsecondary education, including teacher education (indicated as grade level 11). Panel B of Figure 7-5 reports the hazard rate (probability) of girls leaving school in any particular period given that they were in school during the prior period.

Our second reason for focusing on eldest daughters is that they are most likely to be subjected to labor demands by adult household members, especially if the mother is employed outside the home in the wage sector. In such cases, the social obligation of providing childcare and performing other domestic tasks linked to siblings is assumed to be significant.

The third reason is that the most complete data were available on resident children. The household interview contained no questions on children who had left the home or were fostered out. Countering possible concerns about selection bias, we found that children's outmigration rates were not significantly different across black ethnic groups.[14] In our initial analyses, we also included a control variable for the proportion of children who had migrated from the household, but this predictor was never significant.

Very little information is available on the differences between the school experiences of South African children who remain resident and those who are fostered out to other households. Without such data, it is difficult to estimate how selection bias may operate in the present analysis. Future work could focus on the school attainment and literacy levels of these two groups. Yet modeling of such educational events, based on the features of these two types of households, becomes very complex and could not be supported by this data set.

[14]A significantly greater number of daughters age 11-25 remained resident in Zulu households (1.8) relative to North Sotho daughters (1.6). But this finding is more strongly related to differences in family size than to outmigration rates, which were not statistically different.

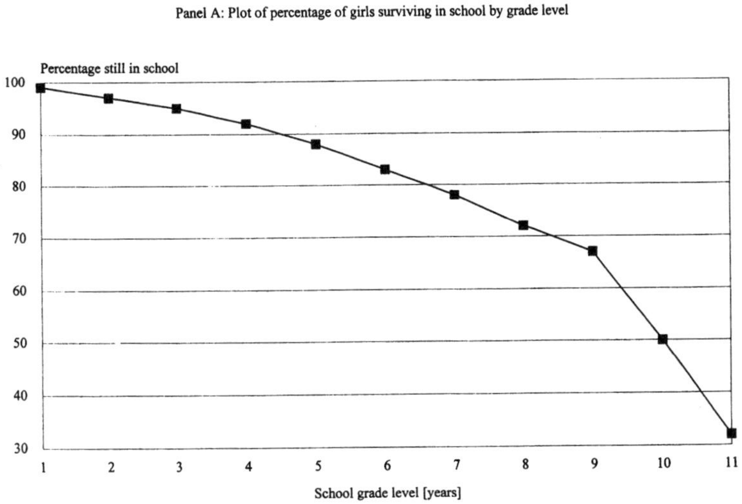

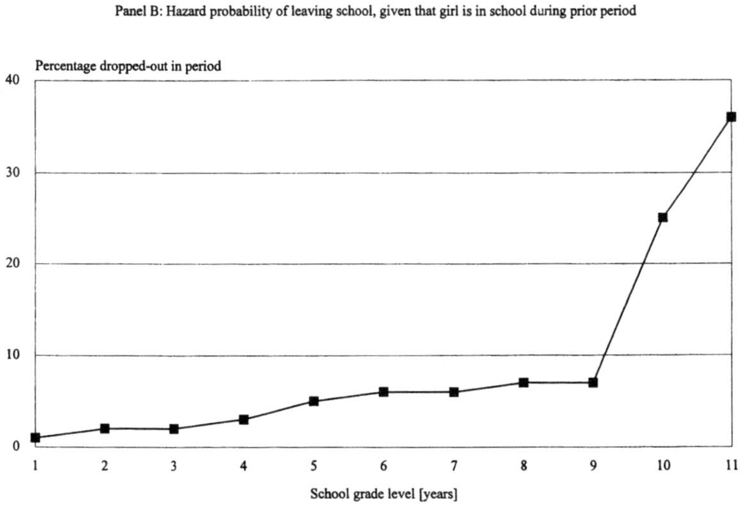

FIGURE 7-5 Survival and hazard plots of when girls leave school.

Influence of Family-Economy and Household-Level Social Factors

Results from our hazard-rate models appear in Table 7-2. We first report a baseline model that simply includes period dummies for each school attainment point. Model 2 then adds the family-economy predictors suggested by the theory, as specified above for the South African context. Note that we are estimating the

TABLE 7-2 Estimating the Hazard Function of When Daughters Leave School: The Influence of Family-Economy and Social Factors (n = 1,103 daughters, parameter estimates and standard errors reported)

Independent Variables	[1] Baseline model	[2] Adding economic factors	[3] Adding social factors	[4] Adding ethnic membership	[5] Adding pregnancy control
Baseline period dummies					
Year 1	–4.57[a]	–3.89[a]	–3.09[a]	–2.87[a]	–2.89[a]
	(0.30)	(0.31)	(0.35)	(0.36)	(0.37)
Year 2	–3.91[a]	–3.22[a]	–2.31[a]	–2.10[a]	–2.10[a]
	(0.22)	(0.23)	(0.29)	(0.30)	(0.31)
Year 3	–3.75[a]	–3.06[a]	–2.03[a]	–1.84[a]	–1.83[a]
	(0.21)	(0.22)	(0.30)	(0.30)	(0.31)
Year 4	–3.56[a]	–2.86[a]	–1.71[a]	–1.53[a]	–1.51[a]
	(0.20)	(0.21)	(0.29)	(0.31)	(0.32)
Year 5	–3.02[a]	–2.29[a]	–1.05[a]	–0.87[b]	–0.84[b]
	(0.16)	(0.18)	(0.28)	(0.30)	(0.30)
Year 6	–2.77[a]	–2.02[a]	–.67[c]	–.49	–.46
	(0.15)	(0.17)	(0.29)	(0.30)	(0.31)
Year 7	–2.78[a]	–2.00[a]	–.52	–.37	–.33
	(0.16)	(0.19)	(0.31)	(0.32)	(0.33)
Year 8	–2.53 [a]	–1.72[a]	–.12	.02	.07
	(0.17)	(0.19)	(0.32)	(0.33)	(0.34)
Year 9	–2.56 [a]	–1.73[a]	–.03	.11	.14
	(0.20)	(0.22)	(0.35)	(0.36)	(0.37)
Year 10	–1.08 [a]	--11	1.75[a]	1.94[a]	2.04[a]
	(0.13)	(0.18)	(0.34)	(0.35)	(0.36)
Year 11	--56	.64	2.55[a]	2.71[a]	2.81[a]
	(0.62)	(0.67)	(0.77)	(0.78)	(0.80)

Economic resources and demands				
Household expenditures	−.0007[a]	−.0004[a]	−.0006[a]	−.0005[a]
	(.0001)	(.0001)	(.0001)	(.0001)
Household durables index	−.08	−.008	.05	−.002
	(0.09)	(0.09)	(0.10)	(0.09)
Family has loan from shop	−.38[c]	−.52[b]	−.60[a]	−.55[b]
	(0.16)	(0.17)	(0.18)	(0.17)
Family receives in-kind services	−.12	−.06	.04	−.01
	(0.16)	(0.17)	(0.03)	(0.18)
Females collect wood and/or water	.08	.15	.24[b]	.16
	(0.08)	(0.08)	(0.08)	(0.09)
Mother holds a clerical job	.17	.63[a]	.54[b]	.50[b]
	(0.17)	(0.18)	(0.19)	(0.19)
Mother holds a laborer or domestic job	.08	.38[c]	.33	.34
	(0.18)	(0.18)	(0.19)	(0.19)
Social resources and demands				
Mother's school attainment		--.08[a]	−.09[a]	−.08[a]
		(0.02)	(0.02)	(0.02)
Father's school attainment	−.05[c]	−.04[c]	−.06[b]	
		(0.02)	(0.02)	(0.02)
Father absent from household	−.34[c]	−.30	−.31[d]	
		(0.17)	(0.17)	(0.17)
Age of target daughter	−.07[a]	−.06[b]	−.09[a]	
		(0.02)	(0.02)	(0.02)
Age of second-oldest daughter	−.01	−.01	−.005	
		(0.01)	(0.01)	(0.01)
Age of youngest daughter	−.11[a]	−.12[a]	−.07[a]	
		(0.02)	(0.02)	(0.02)
Number of resident females > age 18	.17 [b]	.16 [b]	.10	
		(0.05)	(0.05)	(0.05)
Number of resident males > age 18	.02	−.005	−.01	
		(0.06)	(0.06)	(0.06)

Table continued on next page

TABLE 7-2 Estimating the Hazard Function of When Daughters Leave School: The Influence of Family-Economy and Social Factors (n = 1,103 daughters, parameter estimates and standard errors reported)

Independent Variables	[1] Baseline model	[2] Adding economic factors	[3] Adding social factors	[4] Adding ethnic membership	[5] Adding pregnancy control
Ethnic membership					
North Sotho				-1.15^{a}	-1.09^{a}
				(0.19)	(0.19)
South Sotho				–.24	–.21
				(0.21)	(0.21)
Xhosa				$-.36^{c}$	$-.30^{d}$
				(0.16)	(0.16)
Tswana				–.09	–.07
				(0.20)	(0.20)
Ever pregnant [control]					1.08^{a}
					(0.14)
Full equation					
–2 log likelihood	2,730.49	2,601.84	2,423.81	2,382.00	2,319.00
Change in *df*	—	7	9	4	1
Decrement to χ^2	—	128.65	178.03	41.81	63.00
Critical value	—	14.07	16.92	9.49	3.84

NOTES: The –2 log likelihood without covariates = 10670.31. The base for ethnic membership predictors is the largest black group, Zulu.

$^{a}p < .001$
$^{b}p < .01$
$^{c}p < .05$
$^{d}p < .07$

risk of leaving school; therefore, negative coefficients indicate that the predictor lower the risk of dropping out. Household expenditures and access to credit (family has a loan from a neighborhood shop) significantly lower the daughter's risk of leaving school. Recall that all these families have quite low incomes. Yet consumption levels show variations that have implications for which daughters stay in school longer.

Model 3 adds the social factors that may influence female school attainment. Overall, these social factors exert a greater influence on reducing the model's chi-square statistic than do the family-economy factors (bottom of Table 7-2). Particularly influential in reducing the risk of leaving school are mother's and father's school attainment levels, father's absence from the home, target daughter's age, and age of the youngest daughter. As suggested earlier, the father-absent effect tends to confirm Schultz's (1990) finding that female-headed households, despite lower income levels, generally allocate resources more equitably to daughters relative to sons than do households headed by the father.

In Model 3 we also now observe significant effects from the mother's involvement in the wage sector: such involvement places daughters at greater risk of leaving school, perhaps because these daughters face greater labor demands within the household. Girls are also more likely to leave school if more adult females are resident in the household. This finding suggests either that adult females do not share the labor demands of the household, or that these families perpetuate more traditional social roles for young females, including less integration in the female labor market.

Model 4 adds another social factor: the daughter's ethnic membership. Girls in North Sotho communities are much less likely to leave school. Xhosa females display a lower risk of dropping out as well, although the difference is less than for North Sothos (Zulus form the base group). These patterns are consistent with descriptive results reported earlier (Figure 7-3). Thus the economic and social factors studied at the family level are not substituting for these striking ethnic differences.

In Model 5 we add the control predictor indicating whether the young female has ever experienced a pregnancy. This factor understandably raises the risk of leaving school. However, it substitutes for just two earlier observed effects: the number of resident adult females in the household and (partially) Xhosa ethnic membership. The former substitution effect supports the argument that households with more resident females either face more limited job opportunities or hold more traditional beliefs about gender roles.

Comparative Risks of Leaving School

Figure 7-6 presents comparative hazards of leaving school for eldest daughters situated in different kinds of households. Panel A shows a significantly higher likelihood of completing the matric (10 percent lower) or completing

Panel A: Hazard differences by maternal education level

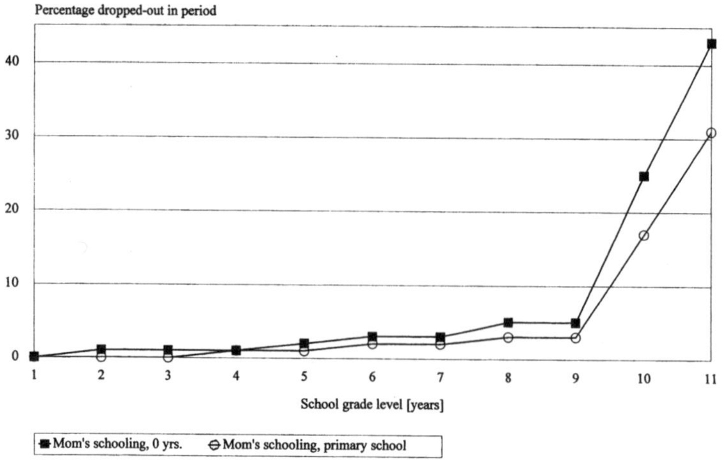

Panel B: Hazard differences for father present and father absent households

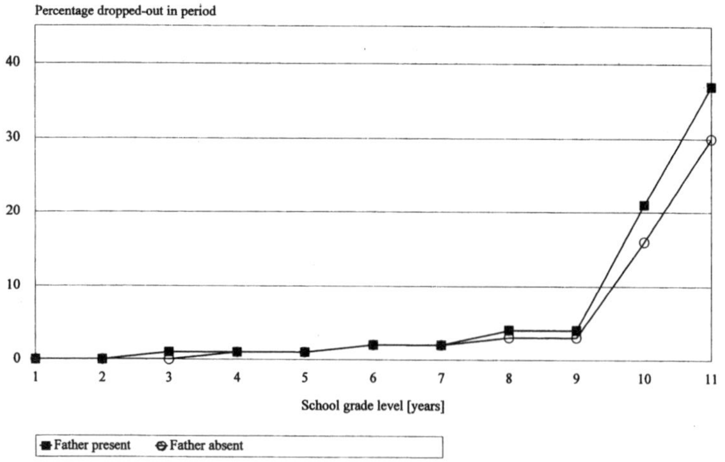

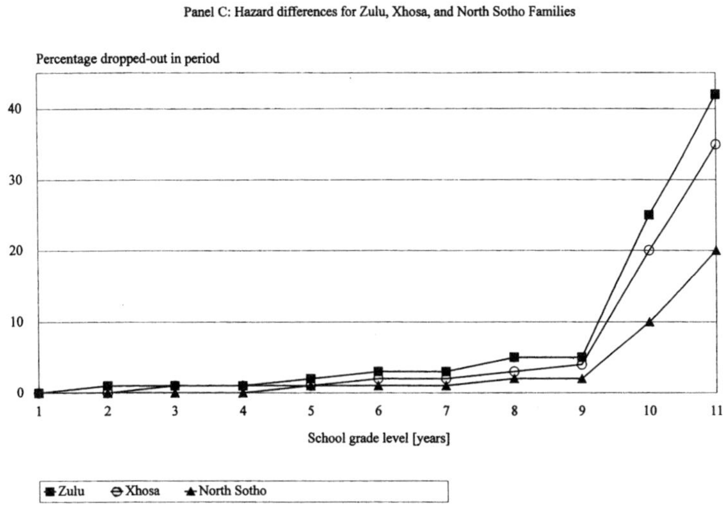

FIGURE 7-6 Comparative hazards of leaving school by social characteristics.

some postsecondary education (11 percent lower) for daughters whose mothers had completed primary school relative to those whose mothers had no schooling. Note that these hazards are cumulative across time periods. Thus, in survival terms, 51 percent of daughters whose mothers completed primary school had completed some postsecondary education, versus 35 percent of those whose mothers had no schooling. Panel B shows the modest advantage of daughters in father-absent households—an 8-point gap for daughters who enter postsecondary education. In survival terms, 75 percent of daughters in father-absent households completed secondary school and the matric, versus just 67 percent of those in father-present households.

Ethnic differences in school attainment are illustrated in Panel C. The probability that North Sotho females will leave school after matric is 15 points lower than that for Zulu daughters. This gap rises to 21 points for Zulu and North Sotho daughters who enter postsecondary education. Overall, 67 percent of North Sotho daughters complete some postsecondary schooling, versus just 35 percent of Zulu females.

Does Ethnic Membership Mask Regional and Institution-Level Forces?

The ethnic differences discussed above return us to the theoretical question of how household and institution-level forces may together shape female school attainment. The household factors on which we have focused certainly help

TABLE 7-3 School Supply and Distinguishing Features of North Sotho Communities[a]

	North Sotho Clusters [n = 16]	Other African Clusters [n = 113]	F value
Average number of secondary schools	1.1	0.7	4.14*
Percentage of clusters with tarmac roads	0%	24%	2.53†
Index of health care workers[b]	3.7	3.9	0.64
Percentage of clusters with resident doctor	13%	20%	1.11

[a]North Sotho communities are defined as those with more than 80 percent of households with North Sotho speakers. Overall multivariate analysis of variance is significant: $F = 2.65$, * $p < .05$, †$p < .10$.

[b]Count of whether the cluster has a midwife, family planning, and/or health worker in a local clinic.

explain which daughters are more likely to be enrolled and how far they persist through school. Yet even after taking into account a variety of family-level economic and social factors, ethnic effects remain strong and significant. What is it about ethnic membership—or the region in which a group predominates—that affects levels of female school attainment?

One argument is that the availability of secondary schooling may vary across provinces in ways that help explain these ethnic effects. We assessed this possibility by drawing on community-level data collected in each of the local communities from which sampled households were randomly drawn. Our subsample of the five major black groups includes 136 local clusters with complete data. We split these clusters between those where the share of North Sotho households equaled or exceeded 80 percent versus 20 percent or less. The former group is located mostly in the Northern Transvaal province, primarily within the old Lebowa homeland. Table 7-3 compares North Sotho and other clusters.

We found that the average number of secondary schools located in North Sotho communities equaled 1.1, compared with 0.7 per local cluster in the other black communities, a statistically significant difference. Interestingly, North Sotho communities have less infrastructure in terms of tarmac roads and health-care workers. But the greater supply of secondary schooling is clear as compared with the other black locales. Future research should examine such contextual differences more deeply, especially given that government policy and investments can address these institutional factors.

SUMMARY AND CONCLUSIONS

We have seen how low-income South African families are far from homogeneous. Elements of the household's economy, social resources and demands, and ethnic experience vary significantly and in ways that explain daughters' school attainment levels. After summarizing our basic findings, we speak to how this kind of evidence can inform stronger designs for the program interventions of governments and international agencies.

Our findings are generally consistent with claims made by researchers who employ the new family-economy model. Even when restricting our analysis to low-income African households, we find that the family's financial strength—indicated by household expenditures and access to local credit—is positively related to the likelihood that eldest daughters remain in school and advance their school attainment. One important finding is that mothers' linkage to the formal wage sector may suppress their daughters' school attainment, perhaps because of the associated increase in domestic labor demand placed on the eldest daughter.

Taken together, these findings confirm a basic family-economy process whereby resources and labor demands are associated with daughters' school attainment. Attainment appears to be linked to immediate and short-term labor demands, not necessarily to long-term optimization or human-capital investment, as neoclassical economists would have it. Thus far it seems that economic or structural interventions, such as income supplements, scholarships, or strategies for relieving female labor demand, might effectively boost girls' school attainment.

We also find that social resources and demands placed on daughters contribute to female school attainment. The positive influence of father absence is consistent with earlier findings in several African societies (Fuller et al., 1995a; Lloyd and Blanc, 1996). The way this influence operates inside households deserves more attention, through both survey and ethnographic research. The influence of mothers' school attainment on daughter's attainment is not surprising, but the finding is notable given that we are focusing on impoverished black families. Ethnic membership is consistently telling for North Sothos, independently of the influence of family-economy factors. We also document the expected negative effect of becoming pregnant on daughters' school attainment levels. And it appears that many young females return to school after giving birth, providing an opportunity for more focused policy initiatives and interventions inside schools. Given the rising rate of adolescent pregnancy in some African societies (Bledsoe and Cohen, 1993), efforts to delay the age of first and subsequent pregnancies for young females could effectively slow population growth in South Africa.

The strong influence of social resources and demands suggests that program interventions in some local regions and with some ethnic groups must focus on more than economic constraints and incentives. Where parents' own schooling levels are low, encouraging daughters to stay in school will be especially challenging. Influencing the attitudes of mothers alone may not be sufficient. When fathers are present in the household or rural labor demands are inextricably linked to daughters' social obligations, interventions might better be aimed at males at both the household and village levels.

Our analysis accents the higher school attainment levels found among North Sotho daughters, despite high rates of poverty and lower school attainment among older mothers. The more recent expansion of secondary education in North Sotho communities appears to be part of the key to understanding this advantage among young North Sotho females.

This finding highlights the sharp variations among regional and ethnic situations, even across low-income black communities. Families of the same ethnicity—be it Zulu, Tswana, or North Sotho—do share important individual and household-level attributes: language, family structure, and patterns of child socialization. But "ethnicity" in South Africa also manifests shared local institutional histories, thanks to the apartheid regime's migration controls and forced segregation of black groups under homeland administrations. The arid and rural Northern Transvaal province, where the former Lebowa homeland for North Sothos is situated, has a depressed regional economy, even relative to other poor regions. We saw earlier how per capita income is 2.5 times higher in KwaZulu/Natal than in the North. Among all North Sotho speakers, 83 percent live beneath the poverty line, versus 61 percent of Zulus. Father absenteeism is twice as high in the Northern Transvaal province, in part because of males' movement to stronger labor markets. Thus the economic context lowers the opportunity cost for females who remain in school. Job opportunities are few; many males are leaving the household. Females are left with the task of raising a growing number of young children, as population growth remains a point higher in the Northern Transvaal relative to KwaZulu/Natal—3.9 percent versus 2.8 percent per annum, respectively.

In addition to a shared economic context, particular ethnic groups have faced a distinct set of institutions over time. Demographers and anthropologists have tried to specify how changes in the institutional context are related to gains in maternal education, lower birth rates, and changed childrearing practices (Caldwell, 1986; LeVine et al., 1994a). But precisely how school, state, and church institutions act to legitimate female school attendance and novel fertility patterns remains a mystery. We do know that family demand for schooling is high in the Northern Transvaal province relative to other black communities. We reported earlier how a much higher percentage of North Sotho youths persist to grade 11 as a proportion of entering grade 1 pupils. Part of this advantage is attributable to the variable actions of local governments. For example, within schools that fell under the pre-1994 Lebowa administration, 54 percent of all youths persisted into grade 9, versus just 21 percent of black students attending schools run by the national education department (Verwey and Munzhedzi, 1994).[15] And prior research has revealed how school improvement efforts in the old Bophuthatswana *bantustan* have resulted in measurable gains in matric exam scores and literacy levels among young females (Education Foundation, 1993; Fuller et al., 1995b). It is the actions of local governments and institutions that make a difference.

Beyond secular action by the state, the Tswana and Sotho peoples of the Western and Northern Transvaal have been exposed to a common linguistic and religious history, one that may have affected female commitments to formal schooling over time. Of particular importance, missionaries from competing churches moved aggressively into the Transvaal during the mid-nineteenth century. Literacy came to be associated with one's faith and loyalty to the village church. To compete for members, churches continue to translate the Bible and other texts into indigenous languages (Hofmeyr, 1993). Mission and, eventually, government schools came to signal a new form of status for young women (see, e.g., Bozzoli, 1991).

We certainly have much to learn about how parents' beliefs and practices vary among households and in ways that contribute to daughters' school attainment levels. Clearly these micro household processes are rooted in parents' own schooling experience and the benefits of education they perceive. Yet our fundamental point is that the local economic situation and social institutions—contexts that differ across regions and ethnic groups in South Africa—further advance female school attainment.

International agencies continue to promulgate means by which female enrollment can be raised or fertility behaviors altered (e.g., Odaga and Heneveld, 1995). But in many African societies we have scarce empirical knowledge of variations in the actions of families that are situated within specific regional histories, institutional contexts, and ethnic experiences. Where institutional conditions vary beneficially—such as the greater supply of secondary schools in North Sotho communities—opportunities exist for policy makers to act with greater precision. But as long as development agencies and governments assume that universal factors constrain female school attainment, costly policies and school interventions may continue to yield disappointing results.

[15]In the larger Northern Transvaal province there are fewer than 3.0 residents for every one primary or secondary school student; this ratio is 3.7 in KwaZulu/Natal (calculated from data appearing in Verwey and Munzhedzi, 1994). Note that the Transvaal is now called Northern Province.

ACKNOWLEDGMENTS

The data analyzed in this chapter are from a household survey conducted in 1993-1994 by Francis Wilson and Pundy Pillay, University of Cape Town. Our work was supported by the World Bank with aid from the governments of Denmark, The Netherlands, and Norway. Special thanks go to Neeta Sirur at the World Bank for organizing the overall project. We are grateful to Yisgedullish Amde and Carlo del Ninno for their advice and essential help with data management. Caroline Bledsoe, Linda Chisholm, Barney Cohen, Duncan Thomas, and two anonymous reviewers provided very helpful comments on earlier drafts.

REFERENCES

Astone, N., and S. McLanahan
1991 Family structure, parental practices, and high school completion. *American Sociological Review* 49:359-382.

Becker, G.
1976 *A Treatise on the Family*. Cambridge: Harvard University Press.

Becker, G., and N. Tomes
1976 Child endowments and the quantity and quality of children. *Journal of Political Economy* 84:S143-S247.

Bledsoe, C., and B. Cohen, eds.
1993 *Social Dynamics of Adolescent Fertility in Sub-Saharan Africa*. Washington, D.C.: National Academy Press.

Bozzoli, B., with M. Nkotsoe
1991 *Women of Phokeng: Consciousness, Life Strategy, and Migrancy in South Africa, 1900-1983*. Portsmouth, N.H.: Heineman.

Bradshaw, Y., and B. Fuller
1996 Policy action and school demand in Kenya: When a strong state grows fragile. *International Journal of Comparative Sociology* 37:72-96.

Caldwell, J.
1976 Toward a restatement of demographic transition theory. *Population and Development Review* 2(3&4):321-366.
1986 Routes to low mortality in poor countries. *Population and Development Review* 12(2):171-214.

Caldwell, J., and P. Caldwell
1990 High fertility in sub-Saharan Africa. *Scientific American* 262(5):118-125.

Campbell, R.
1983 Status attainment research: End of the beginning or the beginning of the end? *Sociology of Education* 56:47-62.

Cochrane, S.
1979 *Fertility and Education: What Do We Really Know*? Baltimore, Md.: The Johns Hopkins University Press.

Coleman, J.
1988 Social capital in the creation of human capital. *American Journal of Sociology* 94:S95-S120.
1990 *Foundations of Social Theory*. Cambridge, Mass.: Belknap Press.

Comaroff, J.

1985 *Body of Power, Spirit of Resistance: The Culture and History of a South African People.* Chicago, Ill.: University of Chicago Press.

DiStefano, J.

1993 *The Demand for Primary Schooling in Rural Ethiopia.* Addis Ababa: United States Agency for International Development.

Easterlin, R., and E.M. Crimmins

1985 *The Fertility Revolution: A Supply-Demand Analysis.* Chicago, Ill.: University of Chicago Press.

Education Foundation

1993 Teacher qualifications and classroom effectiveness. *Edusource Data News* (December):5.

Erasmus, J.

1994 *A Human Development Profile.* Halfway House, South Africa: Development Bank of Southern Africa.

Fishlow, A.

1966 Levels of 19th century investment in education: Human capital formation or structural reinforcement? *Journal of Economic History* 26:418-436.

Fuller, B., and P. Clarke

1994 Raising school effects while ignoring culture? *Review of Educational Research* 64:119-157.

Fuller, B., J. Singer, and M. Keiley

1995a Why do daughters leave school in southern Africa? Family economy and mothers' commitments. *Social Forces* 74:657-682.

Fuller, B., P. Pillay, and N. Sirur

1995b *Literacy Trends in South Africa: Expanding Education While Reinforcing Unequal Achievement*? Cambridge, Mass., and Cape Town: Harvard University and University of Cape Town.

Glewwe, P.

1994 Student achievement and schooling choice in low-income countries: Evidence from Ghana. *Journal of Human Resources* 29:843-864.

Haveman, R., and B. Wolfe

1995 The determinants of children's school attainment: A review of methods and findings. *Journal of Economic Literature* 33:1829-1878.

Hill, M.A., and E. King

1993 *Women's Education in Developing Countries: Barriers, Benefits, and Policies.* Baltimore, Md.: The Johns Hopkins University Press.

Hofmeyr, I.

1993 *We Spend Our Years as a Tale That Is Told: Oral Historical Narrative in a South African Chiefdom.* Johannesburg: University of Witwatersrand Press.

Horan, P., and P. Hargis

1991 Children's work and schooling in the nineteenth-century family economy. *American Sociological Review* 56:583-596.

Hyde, K.

1993 Sub-Saharan Africa. Pp. 100-135 in A. Hill and E. King, eds., *Women's Education in Developing Countries: Barriers, Benefits, and Policies.* Baltimore, Md.: The Johns Hopkins University Press.

Isiugo-Abanihe, U.

1994 Demographic transition in the context of Africa's development. Pp. 61-73 in U. Himmelstrand, K. Kinyanjui, and E. Mburugu, eds., *African Perspectives on Development.* London: James Curry.

Kossoudji, S., and E. Mueller

1983 The economic and social status of female-headed households in rural Botswana. *Economic Development and Cultural Change* 31:825-838.

Lesthaeghe, R.

1989 *Reproduction and Social Organization in sub-Saharan Africa.* Berkeley, Calif.: University of California Press.

LeVine, R., S. LeVine, A. Richman, F.M. Tapia Uribe, and C. Sunderland Correa

1994a School and survival: The impact of maternal education on health and reproduction in the Third World. Pp. 303-338 in L. Chen, A. Kleinman, and N. Ware, eds., *Health and Social Change in International Perspective.* Boston, Mass.: Harvard University Press.

LeVine, R., S., Dixon, A., Richman, P., Leiderman, C., Keefer, and B., Brazelton

1994b *Child Care and Culture: Lessons from Africa.* New York: Cambridge University Press.

Lloyd, C.B., and A.K. Blanc

1996 Children's schooling in sub-Saharan Africa: The role of fathers, mothers, and others. *Population and Development Review* 22(2):265-298.

Lockheed, M., and A. Verspoor

1991 *Improving Primary Education in Developing Countries.* New York: Oxford University Press.

Loury, G.

1977 A dynamic theory of racial income differences. In P. Wallace and A. LeMund, eds., *Women, Minorities, and Employment Discrimination.* Lexington, Mass.: Lexington Books.

Mburugu, E.

1994 The persistence of high fertility in Africa and prospects for fertility decline. Pp. 74-83 in U. Himmelstrand, K. Kinyanjui, and E. Mburugu, eds., *African Perspectives on Development.* London: James Curry.

Odaga, A., and W. Heneveld

1995 *Girls and Schools in Sub-Saharan Africa: From Analysis to Action.* Africa Technical Paper Series 298. Washington D.C.: The World Bank.

Ogbu, J.

1978 *Minority Education and Caste: The American System in Cross-Cultural Perspective.* New York: Academic Press.

Project for Statistics on Living Standards and Development

1994 *Preliminary Abstract.* Cape Town: University of Cape Town, South African Development Research Unit.

Reconstruction and Development Programme

1995 *Key Indicators of Poverty in South Africa.* Pretoria: Office of the President.

Schneider, B., and J. Coleman

1993 *Parents, Their Children, and Schools.* Boulder, Colo.: Westview Press.

Schultz, T.P.

1990 Testing the neoclassical model of family labor supply and fertility. *Journal of Human Resources* 25:599-635.

Singer, J., and J. Willett

1993 It's about time: Using discrete time survival analysis to study duration and the timing of events. *Journal of Educational Statistics* 18:155-195.

Truscott, K.

1994 *Gender in Education.* Johannesburg: University of Witwatersrand, Education Policy Unit.

Tuma, N., and M. Hannan

1984 *Social Dynamics: Models and Methods.* New York: Academic Press.

United Nations

1995 *Women's Education and Fertility Behavior: Recent Evidence from the Demographic and Health Surveys.* Department of Economic and Social Information, Population Division. New York: United Nations.

Verwey, C., and E. Munzhedzi

1994 *Education in the Eastern Cape, Northern Transvaal, and KwaZulu/Natal* (3 volumes). Halfway House, South Africa: Development Bank of Southern Africa.

Walters, P., and D. James

1992 Schooling for some: Child labor and school enrollment of black and white children in the early twentieth century South. *American Sociological Review* 57:635-650.

Walters, P., and P. O'Connell

1988 The family economy, work, and educational participation in the United States, 1890-1940. *American Journal of Sociology* 93:1116-1152.

Whiting, B., and J. Whiting

1991 Adolescence in the preindustrial world. Pp. 814-892 in R. Lerner, A. Petersen, and J. Brooks-Gunn, eds., *The Encyclopedia of Adolescence.* New York: Garland.

World Bank

1995 *Priorities and Strategies for Education: A World Bank Review.* Washington D.C.: The World Bank.

8

Excess Fertility, Unintended Births, and Children's Schooling

Mark R. Montgomery and Cynthia B. Lloyd

INTRODUCTION

Consensus prevails as to the benefits of education: it is believed to promote economic development, speed the completion of the demographic transition, and enhance individual well-being. Where the determinants of education are concerned, however, no similar consensus has yet taken shape. The process by which individuals acquire education is exceedingly complex, involving their motivations and abilities, the goals and resources of their families, and the actions taken, or not taken, by the state. Among the many factors that may affect children's schooling, few have emerged in the literature as clearly decisive, and the role of demographic determinants has yet to be fully understood. In this chapter, we consider two demographic determinants of children's schooling: unintended and excess fertility within the family. Our analysis is empirical in nature and relies on Demographic and Health Survey (DHS) data for four developing countries. To our knowledge, this research is the first to combine data on children's schooling with data on excess fertility and the intendedness status of recent births. We show that in two of the four countries studied—the Dominican Republic and the Philippines—unintended and excess fertility have sizeable negative impacts on children's schooling. In the other two countries—Kenya and Egypt—we do not find such effects. It appears that these fertility effects can be important, but vary in strength according to socioeconomic context.

Our focus on fertility can be understood as follows. Developing-country parents, who face resource constraints in much of their behavior, may find their plans for children's schooling disrupted or compromised by the arrival of unintended births. Moreover, as the broader macroeconomic context changes, parents may find themselves situated in new and possibly unanticipated circumstances. In the light of these circumstances, current family size may be revealed to be excessive and may then present an obstacle to desired educational investments. Thus we consider two conceptually distinct measures of fertility: (1) *unintended fertility*, or the birth of children whom the mother reports were either unwanted at the time of conception or whose conception was reported to be mistimed; and (2) *excess fertility*, or the birth of a larger number of children than is implied by the mother's expressed family-size ideal. The essence of our approach is to compare the schooling achieved by children in families with and without such fertility.

For developing countries, the gap between desired and actual fertility is surprisingly large, with recent estimates suggesting that as many as one birth in five is unwanted (Bongaarts, 1990) and an even greater fraction unintended. As Bankole and Westoff (1995) demonstrate, in many middle-income developing countries, declines in desired family size now appear to be outpacing declines in fertility. The long-term educational implications of these trends deserve consideration.

Viewed from a broader perspective, our research addresses the individual welfare rationale that supports family planning programs. That rationale is based on the costs imposed by imperfect fertility control on women and their families. Our findings show that in some settings, at least, the rationale can be strengthened: effective family planning may improve the prospects for investment in children's human capital. It follows that if the fullest advantage is to be gained from public-sector investments in schooling, parents must have the means to limit their fertility to the levels they desire.

The remainder of the chapter is organized as follows. The next section provides a conceptual overview of the linkages among family size, excess fertility and unintended births, and human capital investments in children. It also reviews the rather meager literature that has addressed such questions. The third section presents a descriptive overview of the fertility and schooling environments in the four countries studied. The fourth section outlines the statistical model that motivates our empirical work; the results derived from that model are then given. The final section presents conclusions and suggestions for further research.

REVIEW OF CONCEPTS AND LITERATURE

Children with many or closely spaced siblings are often thought to be disadvantaged with respect to their schooling in comparison with other children. The disadvantages are believed to be due mainly to resource constraints, with children in larger families receiving smaller shares of total family resources. Economists have written about such issues under the rubric of the *quantity-quality tradeoff* (see, among others, Becker and Lewis, 1973; Hanushek, 1992; Parish and Willis,

1993). As used in this literature, the term *tradeoff* refers not to any fixed or mechanistic causal relationship between fertility and children's schooling, but rather to the often-found negative association between the two.

A tradeoff—a systematic negative association—between fertility and children's schooling is evident in many settings, but there are important exceptions to the general rule. In recent reviews, Lloyd (1994) and Kelley (1996) document a considerable range of empirical associations between fertility and children's schooling at the family level. The associations are usually negative, but they are not always statistically significant or quantitatively large, and positive associations appear as well (Hermalin et al., 1982; Parish and Willis, 1993; Montgomery et al., 1995a, 1995b; see also Diamond et al., this volume).

When the results of many studies are summarized, the relationship between fertility and children's education is seen to vary over time and among countries according to several factors: the stage of economic development, the role played by the state, the phase of demographic transition, and the nature of the family system (Lloyd, 1994). It appears that some threshold level of development must be attained before fertility comes to be strongly negatively associated with children's schooling. If the surrounding environment is one of few schools and few skilled jobs, parents will have neither the opportunity nor the incentive to invest in their children's education, irrespective of whether resources are to be spread over many children or only a few (Desai, 1995). Another consideration is the role played by the state in school provision and finance. In countries in which a high proportion of the money costs of schooling are borne by parents, parental resource constraints are more important in determining which children attend school than is the case in countries in which education is provided free by the state. If the benefits of schooling are substantial, then it is the former situation, with parents responsible for the money costs of schooling, in which one would expect a negative association between fertility and children's education to emerge. Finally, in family systems involving sibling chains of support or child fostering, parents can distribute the costs of schooling and childrearing among a network of relatives, thereby escaping the constraints imposed by their individual family budgets.

Consequences of Unintended and Excess Fertility

Economic models are built on the premise that fertility and children's schooling are jointly determined outcomes of a common set of exogenous determinants. According to this way of thinking—see Appendix A for an extended discussion—a negative association between fertility and schooling is only one of any number of associations that might emerge from family productive and reproductive strategies. Fertility is not, in itself, a causal determinant of children's schooling, nor is schooling a causal determinant of fertility. It is therefore not meaningful to ask how desired fertility might affect desired children's schooling. The question is ill defined; it confuses association with causation. It is appropriate, however, to ask how the exogenous *determinants* of desired fertility might affect desired schooling. When the issue is posed in these terms, there is a proper causal linkage to be considered.

In short, it is only the unintended or excess aspects of fertility that can act as causal determinants of children's schooling. An unintended birth imposes new and unanticipated demands on the resources that can be marshaled for schooling. Parents of unintended or excess children may be less able, and perhaps less willing, to increase the total resources devoted to their children or to reallocate resources among children on a particular child's behalf.[1]

To approach this issue more formally (see Appendix A for further discussion), let us imagine that parents make decisions so as to maximize a unitary utility function V(C, N, S, H), in which C refers to the level of parental consumption, N to the number of their children, S to the children's schooling, and H to the children's health or some other dimension of human capital investment.[2] Parents face a budget constraint and must restrict their total expenditures to no more than Ω, the level of their exogenous income. The decision problem yields a set of optimal or desired values C^*, N^*, H^*, S^*, where N^* represents the desired number of children. These optimal values yield utility level V^*.

Now suppose an unintended birth occurs, so that family size exceeds the optimal value N^*. Actual fertility is then $N = N^* + 1$. All else being equal, this additional birth must reduce parental well-being, causing actual utility to fall below V^*. How are we to gauge the magnitude of the impact? One approach is to ask what increment in income, $\Delta\Omega$, would be required to restore utility to V^*, that is, to just compensate the parents for the additional child. The required compensation will depend on numerous factors: the initial level of income Ω; the many childrearing prices and constraints faced by the parents; and the nature of the utility function V, in particular its curvature in the neighborhood of N^* with respect to the number of children.

This theoretical framework suggests an empirical model of the consequences of unintended fertility. In such an empirical model, the actual level of schooling S is a function not of actual fertility $N = N^* + U$, where U is unintended fertility, but rather of U itself,

---

[1]For the purposes of argument, we are here making a sharper distinction between unintended and intended fertility than may exist in the minds of the decision makers concerned.

[2]The simple model to be outlined here assumes that parents act as a unit in making decisions about family size and child investments. If mothers and fathers differ in their desires—and there is much evidence to suggest that this is often the case with expressed family-size ideals (see Lloyd, 1993, for a review)—the question arises of whether the couple strives for compromise, or one partner tends to override the wishes of the other. Likewise, the model abstracts from issues such as sibling chains of support, transfers of resources among the wider family, and child fostering.

$$S = X\beta + \gamma U + \varepsilon$$

This specification isolates the unintended, exogenous component of fertility. The coefficient γ associated with U thus measures the direct consequences of unintended fertility for children's schooling.[3] The set of other covariates X includes all exogenous factors (such as income Ω) that affect the desired level of schooling S^* and, likewise, the desired level of fertility N^*. Although not shown in this formulation, interactions of U and X could also enter the empirical model.

These concepts are easily generalized to the situation in which parents have, say, two life-cycle periods in which they can bear children. In period 1 they might desire to have N_1^* children and in period 2, N_2^* children. Associated with these fertility desires are the desired levels of schooling for the different sets of children, that is, S_1^* and S_2^*. (The subscripts on S^* refer to the period of the child's birth.) These educational investments are planned to take place in periods 2 and 3. Among other things, optimal choices about fertility and schooling depend on the anticipated sequence of parental incomes, Ω_1, Ω_2, and Ω_3.

Suppose that the parents succeed in having N_1^* births in period 1, but in period 2 have U_2 unintended births, so that $N_2 = N_2^* + U_2$. The unintended births may then affect the schooling of both older and younger children, as indicated in the following pair of equations:

$$S_1 = X_1\beta_1 + \gamma_{12}U_2 + \varepsilon_1$$

$$S_2 = X_2\beta_2 + \gamma_{22}U_2 + \varepsilon_2$$

Although the model as first written required that the effects of unintended or excess fertility be the same for all children in the family, differential effects among siblings, as shown in this expanded version, are perhaps more plausible. Going further, one might distinguish effects felt mainly by the unintended child herself (or himself) from those felt by other children in the family, as when an

[3]Rather little of the literature, unfortunately, has considered the consequences of unwanted fertility from this point of view. What is usually done is to estimate an equation of the form

$$S = X\beta_o + \gamma_o N + \varepsilon_o .$$

This specification is theoretically inappropriate, since children ever born, N, includes both the desired level of fertility N^* and U. It is also statistically inappropriate, given the likelihood of correlation between the choice variable N^* and ε_o. See Montgomery and Lloyd (1996) for a fuller discussion and an approach that uses the concept of measurement error in attempting to interpret results from this conventional framework.

older child is withdrawn from school to help care for a younger sibling whose conception was unintended.

The effects considered here may also be produced by changes in circumstances that render the parents' initially desired levels of fertility nonoptimal. Other than the arrival of an unintended birth, this is the primary reason for excess fertility as we have defined the term. Suppose that, anticipating life-cycle income levels of Ω_1, Ω_2 and Ω_3, parents initially desire to have N_1^* and N_2^* children. Imagine that they succeed in meeting exactly these fertility goals. Upon entering period 3, however, the parents encounter an unanticipated shortfall in their income. This shortfall in Ω_3 imposes new constraints on the remaining schooling investments they can afford and find it rational to make. Had the actual level of income been known in advance, the parents' desired fertility levels might well have differed from N_1^* and N_2^*. Our point is that although births N_1^* and N_2^* may have been fully desired at the time of their conception, later events may bring about revisions in desired family size and force a rethinking of educational investments. Viewing the situation in retrospect, the parents might well say in response to a survey question that the number of children they actually bore exceeded their ideal number. They would thus experience excess fertility even though, strictly speaking, no birth was unintended.

Consequences of Unintended or Excess Fertility

Remarkably little research has examined directly the consequences of unintended or excess fertility for developing-country families and children. This is surprising in view of the central role played by the elimination of such fertility in the rationale for family planning and in the emerging literature on unmet need. For example, much of the work on the health implications of birth spacing (see Montgomery and Lloyd, 1996, for a review) draws no distinction between intended and unintended fertility, although it can be assumed that very short birth intervals must generally be unintended.

Much of the research on the consequences of imperfect fertility control is concerned with the developed-country situation.[4] For instance, the vast literature on the consequences of teenage pregnancy and birth (see Brown and Eisenberg,

---

[4]Whatever the differences between the developed- and developing-country contexts, it seems that the incidence of unintended fertility is high in both. A recent Institute of Medicine study of unintended pregnancy in the United States (Brown and Eisenberg, 1995) documents that 57 percent of all pregnancies in recent years were unintended, that is, either unwanted at conception or mistimed. Evidently, even in a country that has achieved replacement-level fertility and in which abortion and birth control are readily available, the goal of full control over reproduction remains elusive for many women. These figures are based on current reports by women on the status of all pregnancies in the previous 5 years. Of the U.S. pregnancies that resulted in live births in 1988 to 1993, some 11 percent were unwanted and 33 percent mistimed.

1995, for a review) is dominated by studies of the United States. This literature has been concerned mainly with the consequences of teen births for the mothers, although a number of studies have examined effects on young children as well. Relatively few efforts have been made to distinguish intended from unintended births, as it has been assumed, quite plausibly, that the great majority of teen births in the United States are unintended.

A handful of studies in a variety of settings have documented negative effects for unwanted children, whether in terms of heightened mortality risks (Frenzen and Hogan, 1982, for Thailand), poor social development (Baydar and Grady, 1993; Baydar, 1995), poor psychological development (David et al., 1988), or greater risks of physical abuse and neglect (Zuravin, 1991).[5] Yet we are aware of only one study, from Finland, that explores the consequences of a child's wantedness for educational attainment (Myhrman et al., 1995). This study is based on a unique longitudinal design that began in 1966 with interviews of women who were then in their sixth or seventh month of pregnancy.[6] At the time of the first interview, the wantedness of each woman's pregnancy was ascertained. Some 63 percent of the pregnancies were reported to have been wanted at that time, 12 percent unwanted, and 25 percent mistimed. The study continued to monitor the women (all of whom gave birth) and their children, with assessments taking place in 1980-1981 and 1990, at which point the children were age 24. Myhrman et al. found that the children who were unwanted during pregnancy were subsequently less likely than their wanted counterparts to progress beyond the basic 9 years of education. The education of children who were mistimed fell between that of the other two groups. Among the young men surveyed in 1990, differentials in schooling by wantedness status were apparent only in larger families (those with three or more children). However, young women born into smaller families (two or fewer children) following an unwanted pregnancy had a particularly high risk of stopping after 9 years of compulsory schooling.

We know of no similar studies in the developing-country context. On occasion, however, ingenious efforts have been made to tease out the effects of unintended fertility by indirect means. In the case of India, Rosenzweig and Wolpin (1980) examined the educational consequences stemming from twin births, whose simultaneous arrival was clearly unintended. These consequences were negative, if not especially large, although one wonders whether an analysis focusing on unwanted fertility as well as spacing might have found more substantial impacts. In another interesting study, Rosenzweig and Schultz (1987) estimated levels of fecundability among Malaysian mothers, this being one of the

[5]For interesting recent research on unwantedness and investments in children's health in the Philippines using an approach that parallels our own, see Jensen et al. (1996).

[6]These children were born at a time when access to abortion was highly restricted in Finland; abortion had to be authorized by two physicians and could be granted only for medical reasons.

exogenous factors that might lead to unintended or excess births, and found a modest negative association between fecundability and children's schooling.

FERTILITY AND SCHOOLING IN THE STUDY COUNTRIES

The countries examined for this study—the Dominican Republic, Egypt, Kenya, and the Philippines—would seem to form an eclectic group, and one might wonder what features unite them. Four general criteria guided their selection. First, we required that several types of data be available: on the educational levels and enrollment of school-age children, on the fertility preferences of their mothers, and on access within the community to family planning and schooling. Surprisingly few DHS surveys gather this range of data, with data on children's schooling the most likely to be lacking. Second, these are countries in which the proportion of unwanted births is relatively high, in the range of 20-35 percent (Bankole and Westoff, 1995). Third, the study countries exemplify settings in which abortion is illegal.[7] And fourth, taken together, these countries represent each of the major regions of the developing world.

Fertility

In these four countries, total fertility rates (TFRs) for the 3 years before the respective DHS survey dates range from a low of 3.7 in the Dominican Republic to a high of 5.2 in Kenya, with the TFR for the Philippines being 4.1 and that for Egypt 4.7. In each of the surveys, women of reproductive age were asked about the intendedness of all pregnancies resulting in live births during the 5 years preceding the survey. Women were asked whether, at the time they became

[7]The illegality of abortion is a key consideration in our research. Where access to abortion is legal, conceptions that are most unwanted or most grievously mistimed will have a greater likelihood of ending in abortion. For example, in the United States, where abortion is legal, 51 percent of unintended pregnancies ended in abortion in 1987 (Brown and Eisenberg, 1995). Abortion induces a type of selection bias: the conceptions that presumably would have the most negative consequences never become births. In a setting in which abortion is illegal, by contrast, a greater percentage of such conceptions will be taken to term because of the risks and costs of illegal abortion. This reduces the selection bias, even if it does not entirely eliminate it, and permits the consequences of unintended conception to be more fully understood.

The penal codes in all four countries of this study prohibit abortion (United Nations, 1992, 1993, 1995). In the Dominican Republic, however, abortion is permitted to save the life of the mother. The grounds for this exception appear to be interpreted liberally, as abortion is reported to be widely performed in both public hospitals and clinics, and cases are rarely brought to the courts. In the Philippines, despite the severity of the law, abortion appears to be widely practiced and cases rarely prosecuted, although the surrounding climate is one of fear and shame. In Kenya, hospital-based studies show that illegal abortion is a growing health problem. Little information is available on the extent of illegal abortion in Egypt.

pregnant but before they gave birth, they wanted the birth then, later, or not at all. If a woman said she wanted the birth later, she was asked how much longer she would like to have waited.[8] These retrospective data provide the basis for our measures of unintended fertility. The measurement of excess fertility is based on the difference between cumulative fertility and the woman's report of her ideal family size, both being measured at the date of the survey.

Appendix B examines at some length the conceptual and empirical differences between measures of unintended and excess fertility. Our view is that although these measures have certain elements in common, each presents distinctive features. The differences between the two are sufficient, we believe, to justify separate analyses. Both measures suffer from incomplete information on timing, that is, on the dates at which the attitudes in question were held. For instance, no data were collected on the intendedness of births that occurred before the 5-year retrospective window adopted by the DHS. Thus, the wantedness status of children over age 5 cannot be assessed by the same means as that applied to younger children. Likewise, information on a woman's current family-size ideal is solicited by the DHS, but no inquiries are made about how long she has maintained that ideal or about the nature of the ideals that were previously held. Moreover, the attitudes measured are those of the women respondents. Independent questions were not asked of fathers, and it cannot be determined whether the views women express are uniquely their own or reflect a consensus forged between spouses (and perhaps involving others).

Table 8-1 presents summary statistics on the extent of unintended fertility among the births occurring in the 5 years before the DHS surveys. The percentage of such births that were unwanted at conception varies from 15 percent in the Dominican Republic to 22 percent in Egypt. Because of ex post rationalization, this is likely to be an underestimate of the actual level of unwanted childbearing at the time of pregnancy (see Bankole and Westoff, 1997, for longitudinal evidence from Morocco). However, the children still labeled as unwanted as of the survey date are those that were probably most intensely unwanted at the time of conception. Another 13 to 35 percent of births are reported to have been mistimed, with 8 to 24 percent mistimed by more than 2 years. The total percentage of recent births that were unintended ranges from 52 percent in Kenya, to 45 percent in the Philippines, to 38 in the Dominican Republic, to 35 in Egypt. Kenya, with the highest fertility overall, also has the highest percentage of unintended pregnancy.

Table 8-2 presents these data from another perspective, that of the women who might experience either unintended or excess fertility. A substantial percentage of women in each country (from 41 to 63 percent) had no births during

[8] No follow-up question on the preferred timing of mistimed births was asked in the Egyptian survey.

TABLE 8-1 Intendedness Status of Births in 5 Years Before Survey

Wantedness at conception	Dominican Republic (1991)	Egypt[a] (1988)	Kenya (1993)	Philippines (1993)
Number of births	4,216	8,716	6,115	9,152
Wanted at conception	61%	65%	49%	55%
Mistimed 2 years	16	13[b]	11	10
Mistimed >2 years	8		24	19
Unwanted	15	22	17	16
Total	100%	100%	100%	100%

n.a. = not available
[a]Based on ever-married women only.
[b]Desired time to next birth not asked.

TABLE 8-2 Incidence of Unintended and Excess Fertility Among Women

Variable	Dominican Republic (1991)	Egypt[a] (1988)	Kenya (1993)	Philippines (1993)
Number of women	7,318	8,911	7,540	15,029
Number of births in last 5 years (Percent)				
0	63	41	48	61
1	21	30	27	21
2	13	22	21	14
3	3	7	4	4
Of women with births in last 5 years				
At least 1 unwanted birth	18	28	20	21
At least 1 unwanted or mistimed by more than 2 years	28	n.a. [a]	48	40
For all women, ideal family size and fertility				
Number of births at survey > Ideal family size	22	52	30	20
Surviving children at survey > Ideal family size	19	42	25	16

n.a. = not available
[a]Only ever-married women interviewed; no data on desired time to next birth.

the preceding 5 years. Among those who did give birth, 18 to 28 percent had at least one unwanted birth; 28 to 48 percent had either one or more unwanted births or one birth mistimed by more than 2 years. From 43 to 59 percent of women (not shown) had at least one unintended birth. Egypt had the highest incidence of recent unwantedness and the Dominican Republic the lowest. Mistimed pregnancies were most prevalent in Kenya and least prevalent in the Philippines.

With regard to excess fertility, two measures are shown in Table 8-2, one based on children ever born and the other on surviving children.[9] Egypt displays the highest levels of excess fertility, with 42 or 52 percent of women reporting a number of children that exceeded their current family-size ideal. The figure for Egypt is more than double that shown for the Dominican Republic and the Philippines.

Schooling

Our analyses are focused on children of school age—those aged 6 or 7 to 18, with the lower end of the range depending on the normal age for starting the first grade of primary school. The DHS surveys gather limited information, through their household rosters, on current educational status. Unfortunately, no educational histories are available for children. Thus we cannot determine the ages at which children passed important educational milestones, and issues related to age at first enrollment, dropout and reentry, or grade repetition can be studied only indirectly.

To understand school enrollment and educational attainment in the four study countries, one must be familiar with certain structural aspects of their educational systems, such as school starting ages, grade-to-grade promotion policies, the duration of primary and secondary levels, and the critical transition points at which performance on national exams may limit opportunities for advancement. Each of the countries is distinctive with regard to such structural features.

Table 8-3 summarizes the main elements of the educational systems of the four countries, not only at the time of the DHS surveys, but also for the relevant school years of all children in the sample aged 6-18.[10] Egypt and Kenya have

[9]See McClelland (1983) for a discussion of the potential differences in these indicators of excess fertility. In our empirical work we employ the measure based on children ever born.

[10]In 1985, primary school in Kenya was expanded from 6 to 8 years. Because the DHS data were collected in 1993, all children aged 18 at the time of the survey (the oldest children in our sample) would have been 10 in 1985; this ensures that they would have been full participants in the transition to 8 grades. A reduction in the years of primary schooling in Egypt from 6 to 5 years came in 1989, the year after the 1988 DHS was conducted, thus allowing us to use the old system to analyze the full sample of children. Recent changes in the Dominican Republic's system have not been fully implemented, and it appears that two parallel systems are currently in place: the traditional system had an intermediate phase of 2 years before full secondary, whereas the reform plan has 4 years of secondary following 6 years of primary, with two additional years for university-bound students.

TABLE 8-3 National Educational Systems, Four Study Countries

Level	Dominican Republic (1991)	Egypt (1988)	Kenya (1993)	Philippines (1993)
Primary				
Starting age	7	6	6	7
No. of grades	6	6	8	6
Promotion from grade to grade	Teachers' evaluations, internally administered	Local exams at end of grades 2, 4, 6	Automatic	Cumulative rating system; pass grade = 75%, internally administered
Secondary				
Entry requirement	Primary completion (certificado de suficiencia)	Passing score on locally administered grade 6 exam	Passing score on national KCPE exam	Primary graduation certificate
No. of grades	Traditional Plan: 2 + 4 Reform Plan: 4 + 2	Preparatory: 3 Secondary: 3	4	4
Promotion from grade to grade	Teachers' evaluations, internally administered	Exam for basic education completed at end of grade 9; minimum score required for academic secondary	Automatic	Teachers' evaluations, internally administered
University placement	Secondary completion (bachillerato)	National exam	National exam	National exam
Total Grades Preuniversity	12	12	12	10

SOURCES: Postlethwaite (1992) and Kurian (1988).

starting ages of 6, whereas children do not normally begin primary school until the age of 7 in the Dominican Republic and the Philippines. Six grades of primary schooling characterize all the school systems except that of Kenya, where primary school lasts 8 years. Neither the Dominican Republic nor the Philippines imposes national exams during the primary and secondary years; to determine pass rates, they rely instead on internal exams administered separately within each school. The Kenyan system is rather different, allowing students to progress automatically from grade to grade until the end of standard 8, at which point students sit for a national exam that determines eligibility to enter secondary school. Roughly 44 percent of those completing primary school in Kenya are able to enroll in secondary school (UNESCO, 1994).[11] In Egypt, the critical transition points occur more frequently, in that local exams are administered at all schools in a district at the end of grades 2, 4, and 6. A national exam for basic education is administered at the end of grade 9 (the last year of the preparatory level). Results on this exam determine whether a student can proceed to the secondary level on an academic track or is eligible only for technical school. All systems except that of the Philippines have a total of 12 years of primary and secondary schooling; the Philippines is unusual in having only 10 years of schooling prior to university.

Current status data are used to show patterns of educational progress for each country.[12] The horizontal axes begin with the age at which children are meant to start grade 1 of primary school.[13] The children who are currently enrolled are divided into two groups: those whose age is appropriate to the grade (labeled "okay") and those who are over age because of either a late start or grade repetition ("behind").[14] Students who have been but are not currently enrolled in school are labeled "dropped."

---

[11]This figure is based on the ratio of the number of students enrolled in the first grade of secondary school (1992) to the number of students in the last year of primary school (1990). This figure is likely to be an overestimate. Data for 1991 are not yet available (UNESCO, 1994).

[12]Figure 8-1, which compares children of different ages at a particular point in time, reflects both secular trends and life-cycle changes. Although we would like to use the data to depict a profile of school participation for the current cohort of school-age children, we know that patterns of school participation had been changing over the decade preceding the DHS surveys. As overall enrollment rates rise, we would expect to see the trends reflected in declining proportions of children never in school at younger ages. Interestingly, among our sample of countries, this pattern is clearly apparent only in Egypt. Indeed, the picture for the Dominican Republic suggests a deteriorating situation, with 6 percent of those aged 18 never having attended school, but as many as 14 percent of those aged 11. This deterioration is confirmed by a recent World Bank (1995) assessment.

[13]School participation can begin before the first grade of primary school in preprimary, nursery, or kindergarten. The prevalence of preschool attendance varies from country to country, as does its content. Because so little is known about preschool, it has been excluded here so that all the figures can be presented on a comparable basis.

[14]This approach follows that used by Lloyd and Blanc (1996) in their analyses of children's schooling in Africa. Children are classified as behind grade level if their number of grades com-

In Figure 8-1a, we compare Egypt and Kenya; both countries have a normal starting age of 6 for the primary level. The patterns reveal a striking contrast. In Kenya, starting ages are flexible, with children continuing to enter primary school until age 11.[15] Late entry is evidently the major factor causing children to be behind grade for their age. With 8 grades of primary schooling and automatic promotion from grade to grade, dropout becomes significant only when children reach the end of primary school and sit for the national Kenyan Certificate of Primary Education (KCPE) exam. Given the limit on places in the first form of secondary, only the top-scoring 40 percent of Kenyan students can continue into secondary school. On the positive side of the ledger, relatively few students have never been to school.

In Egypt, a heavily bureaucratized school system enforces a strict age of school entry. Students who have not gained a place in school by age 7 are therefore unlikely to have the opportunity to attend later. As a result, enrollment in primary school is exceptionally high by age 7 (87 percent enrolled, in comparison with 61 percent in Kenya at the same age), but begins to drop off by age 9. The percentages never enrolled are noticeably higher than in Kenya, and dropout begins to occur at a steady rate at age 10, when students sit for a series of standard exams at the end of grades 2, 4, 6, and (most important) 9. Relatively few students appear to be behind grade for their ages, suggesting that those who are not able to keep up are more likely to drop out.

Figure 8-1b compares the Philippines and the Dominican Republic. In the Philippines, almost all children enter school eventually, and most have entered by age 9. Most children are able to complete the 6 primary grades, but participation begins to fall off during the 4 years of secondary. Late entry and repetition do not appear to be important problems. By contrast, late entry is evidently common in the Dominican Republic, with children behind grade representing almost half of all enrolled students aged 11-16.

Table 8-4 shows the distribution of children in each of our samples by educational status at the time of the survey and summarizes their performance on

---

pleted is less than the number of years that would have been completed if they had started school within 2 years of the recommended starting age in the country according to UNESCO (1994) and attended continuously from that age onward. Specifically, a child is behind grade level if completed years of education < current age – (recommended starting age + 2). The 2-year adjustment is made because children in any given grade may be observed at one of two ages (for example, a child starting school at age 6 will turn 7 during first grade) and coupled with an additional adjustment to produce a conservative estimate of the proportion of children behind grade level given possible age and grade misreporting. Thus in a country with a school starting age of 6, enrolled children who had completed grade 1 by age 8 would be classified as "at grade level."

[15]In Kenya, the preschool sector is large and growing. One reason for the high enrollment in preschool may be that it is increasingly a requirement for admission to primary school (Appleton, 1995). In our sample, 40 percent of those aged 6 in Kenya were in nursery school, 25 percent of those aged 7, 12 percent of those aged 8, and 4 percent of those aged 9.

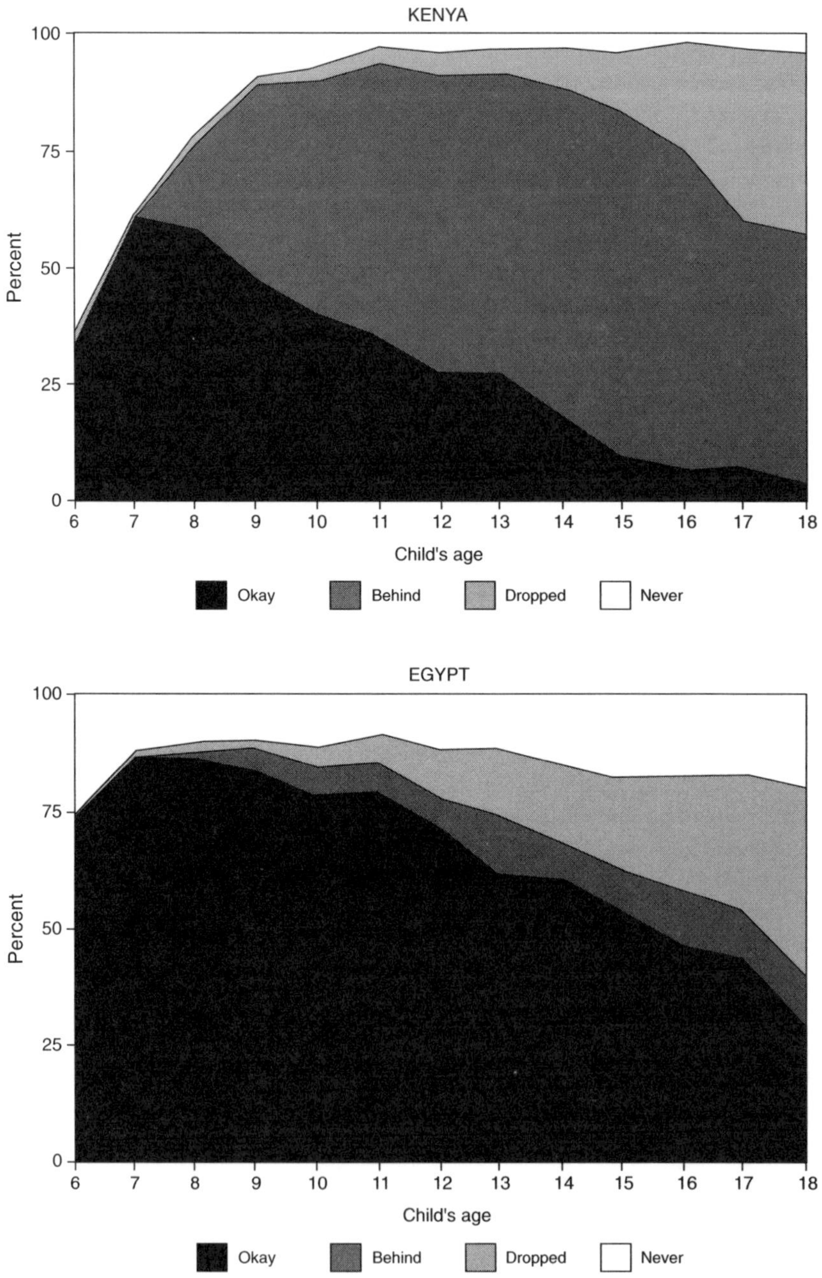

FIGURE 8-1a Children's educational progress by age in Kenya and Egypt (enrollment in preschool not included).

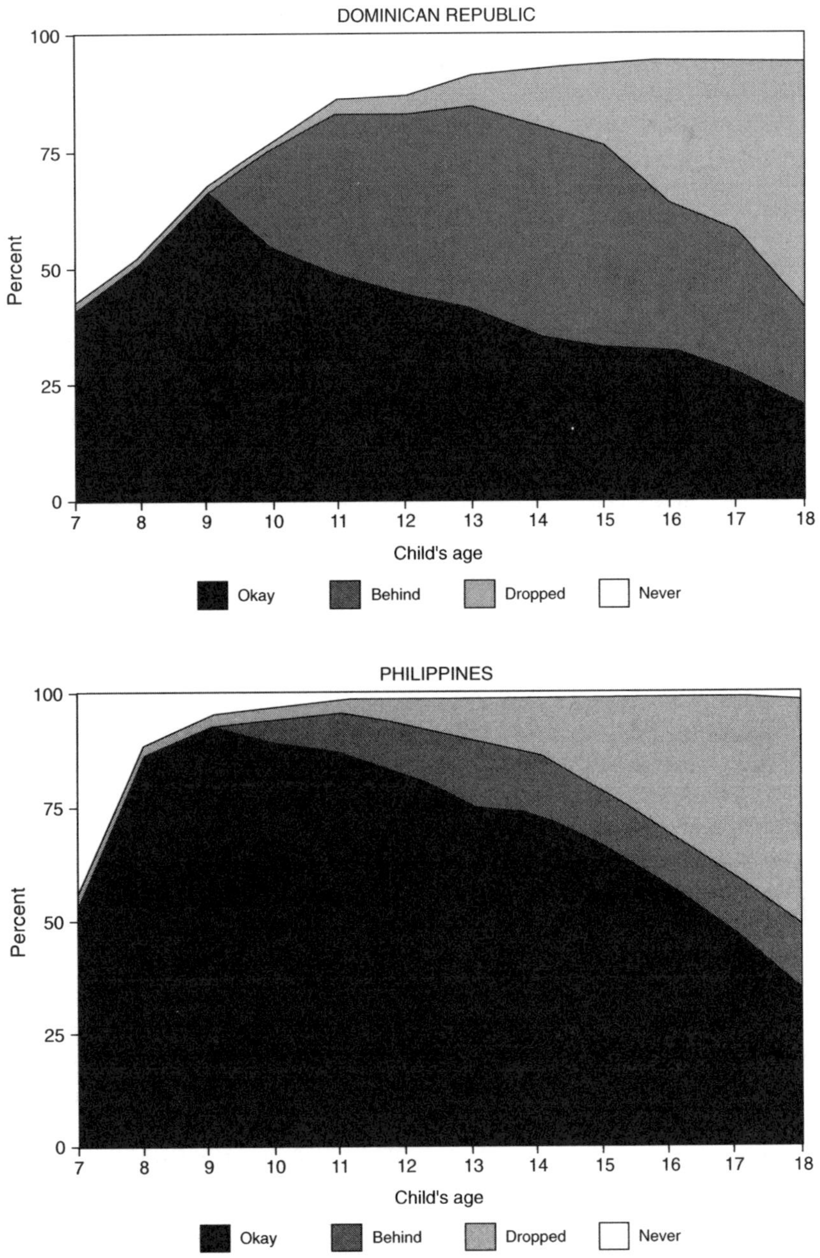

FIGURE 8-1b Children's educational progress by age in the Dominican Republic and the Philippines (enrollment in preschool not included).

TABLE 8-4 Education and Fertility Measures: Samples of School-Age Children

Characteristic	Dominican Republic (1991)	Egypt (1988)	Kenya (1993)	Philippines (1993)
Number of children[a]	5,475	13,521	8,765	14,296
Educational status measures (percent):				
Never attended	20	12	17	8
Dropped out	8	10	5	10
Enrolled but behind schedule	25	6	43	8
Enrolled, on schedule	48	72	35	74
Total	100	100	100	100
Years completed (mean)	3.4	4.1	2.8	4.5
Percent Completing 1 Year Secondary Schooling, Among Those in Relevant Age Group[b]	46	66	10	72
Unwanted and excess fertility measures (percent):				
1 unwanted sibling born in last 5 years	9	22	17	15
2 or more unwanted siblings born in last 5 years	3	8	7	4
At least 1 sibling unwanted or mistimed by more than 2 years	14	36	38	27
In family with excess fertility	57	83	72	53

[a]Age range 7-18 for the Dominican Republic and the Philippines, 6-18 for Egypt and Kenya.
[b]Age groups: 14 and above for the Dominican Republic and the Philippines, 13 and above for Egypt, 15 and above for Kenya.

two indicators—mean grades of schooling completed and percentage completing 1 year of secondary school. The latter is a critical transition point in all countries. Interestingly, the Dominican Republic has the highest percentage of children never in school (20 percent). Egypt and the Philippines have the highest percentages currently enrolled and on schedule (72 and 74 percent, respectively).

Unintended and Excess Fertility in the Families of School-Age Children

The lower portion of Table 8-4 summarizes unintended and excess fertility in the samples of school-age children; Tables 8-1 and 8-2 presented similar figures for children born in the past 5 years and for women. The summary statistics in

Table 8-4 represent the incidence of such fertility from the perspective of the children whose educational attainment we are investigating. Note that the general rankings of the study countries resemble those shown in the previous tables, with the Dominican Republic and the Philippines having the lowest levels of both unintended and excess fertility and Kenya and Egypt the highest. In all four countries, well over 50 percent of school-age children reside in families with excess fertility. The incidence of unintended fertility is considerably lower, although it should be borne in mind that this measure is restricted to events occurring in the past 5 years.

In summary, the study countries offer considerable diversity with respect to levels of fertility overall, the extent of unintended and excess fertility, and the levels and age patterns of schooling. With this background, we now turn to a discussion of the methods applied to determine whether unintended and excess fertility affect children's schooling.

MODEL SPECIFICATION AND ESTIMATION

To understand the implications of unintended and excess fertility for children's schooling, one must first ask who experiences such fertility. Our analysis is therefore set forth in terms of a two-equation system, in which one equation specifies the likelihood of unintended or excess fertility, and the second equation (or set of equations) focuses on the consequences of such events for children's schooling. In thinking along these lines, we are mindful of the possibility that unmeasured factors may at the same time affect exposure to the risk of unintended fertility and the levels of investment in children's schooling. Such unmeasured "common causes" could make it appear as if unintended fertility itself affects schooling, even if no such causal relationship exists. This possibility has been an important theme in the literature on consequences of teenage pregnancy in developed countries, motivating the use of longitudinal data and the application of a variety of appropriate statistical techniques, such as sister comparisons. Unfortunately, the data available to us are cross-sectional and provide only a single measure of each of the key variables—children's schooling, excess fertility, and recent unintended fertility. This fundamental data constraint must be kept firmly in mind as our statistical methods are developed and applied in this section and the next.

Our system is represented in latent-variable form in the equations below:

$$U^* = Z\beta^1_u + FP\beta^2_u + \varepsilon_u \tag{8.1}$$

$$S^*_i = X_i\beta_s + \gamma U + \varepsilon_{i,s} \qquad i = 1, N \tag{8.2}$$

In this system, U^* represents the parents' propensity either to (1) have an unwanted or mistimed conception leading to a birth in the 5 years before the survey or (2) report excess fertility, as measured by the difference between the number of births at the time of the survey and the woman's ideal family size. We specify separate U^* equations for these different indicators. Note that women who experienced no unanticipated events in the past 5 years, whether they had no births or only intended births, are treated identically in this estimation, an approach that is consistent with our theoretical framework.[16] Note, too, a fundamental measurement difficulty: because the angle of vision on the past provided by DHS data is only 5 years, we risk grouping women who had an unintended event before the 5-year window of observation with those who did not. The likely consequence is to dilute the estimated effects (Wolfe et al., 1996).

The propensity for unintended or excess fertility U^* is determined by a set of exogenous factors, denoted by Z, and by access to family planning services, FP. Using the DHS service availability surveys that complement the individual-level surveys, we assembled a number of measures of access to family planning and reproductive health services. These access variables are assumed to influence the likelihood of unintended or excess fertility, but not otherwise to influence children's schooling. Thus, the family planning access measures serve as excluded or instrumental variables in the equation system.

The second set of equations, with latent dependent variables S_i^*, has to do with the schooling of children in the family. Their schooling may be affected by the occurrence of an unintended birth or excess fertility (denoted here by U without an asterisk), as well as by a set of child-specific, family-specific, and community-specific variables X_i. As just mentioned, the family planning access measures are excluded from X_i. The schooling propensity for child i has an observed counterpart in either a binary indicator of school enrollment or an ordered index of educational attainment.

Figure 8-2 may help explain the essentials of our approach, showing how the analyses and implications may differ for unintended as compared with excess fertility. The time line in the figure depicts the 5-year window of the DHS surveys, the window within which data on intendedness were gathered. Child 1, shown in the upper portion of the figure labeled "Unintended," reached the minimum starting age for school before the date of the DHS survey and therefore must have been born before the 5-year window opened. Although this child's educational status is known, at least as of the survey date, the circumstances of his or her conception are not known. Child 2, by contrast, was born within the 5-year window, and in the case shown in the figure is reported to have been unintended. The educational consequences of this unintended birth may be evident if child 1 is affected, but because child 2 is still too young to have attended school, the consequences for him or her cannot be determined. Thus when we study the

[16]In this approach, we ignore the case of women who desire a birth but are unable to have one.

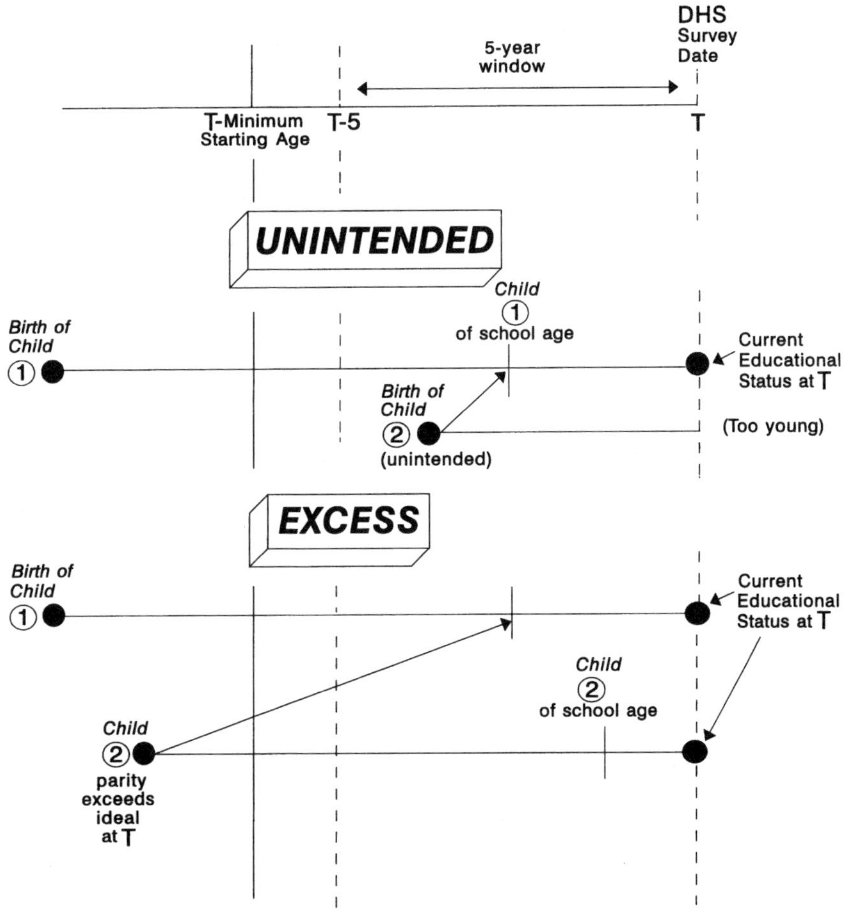

FIGURE 8-2 DHS data on children's schooling, unintended and excess fertility.

educational consequences of unintended fertility using DHS data, we are necessarily considering *cross-sibling* effects. For both children, these potentially negative consequences can be summarized only using the educational status data gathered at the time of the DHS survey, which reflect the cumulative effects of delays in school entry, repetition of grades, temporary withdrawal, and premature dropout up to the time of the survey. The longer-term effects of having an unintended sibling cannot be assessed because the window of observation is only 5 years.

Situations involving excess fertility, one example of which is depicted in the lower panel of Figure 8-2, are somewhat different. The family-size ideals measured in the DHS refer to an ideal as of the survey date. In the case shown in the figure, the parity of child 2 exceeds the survey date ideal, and in a sense it is this child who brings about a situation of excess fertility for the family as a whole. Of course, the mother is not asked to single out and thereby label child 2 in her survey response on ideal family size. If child 2 is old enough to have attended school as of the survey date—this is the case shown in the figure—the educational consequences of excess fertility may be evident for both children. That is, where excess fertility is concerned, we can consider both *own* and *cross-sibling* effects. The situation is greatly complicated, however, by the possibility of change over time in family-size ideals. For example, the parities of both child 1 and child 2 might initially have been below the family-size ideal, but the ideal itself might then have declined in the interim between the birth of child 2 and the survey date. These possibilities cannot be explored using DHS data; the required information on the timing of events and attitude change is not available.

Data Construction

The estimation of equation (8.1) is based on individual data from women of reproductive age, supplemented by service availability data for their communities collected in each DHS sample cluster. To estimate equation (8.2), we constructed a sample of the school-age children (those aged 6-18) of these women. To link a child's educational status (recorded in the household roster) with information on fertility (collected from the mother), we had to match children from the birth histories to their records in the household roster using the mother's identifier code. We recognize that these are selective samples, yet they nontheless display educational distributions that are similar to those of all children aged 6-18.[17]

Estimation and Endogeneity Bias

If the disturbance terms ε_u and $\varepsilon_{i,s}$ of the above equations are jointly normally distributed, the system can be viewed as a joint probit, ordered-probit system. The probit equation is equation (8.1), having to do with the incidence of unin-

[17]Children who did not live with their mothers at the time of the survey could not be matched and had to be excluded from the analysis; the DHS collects no data on the schooling of children living outside the household. Thus our sample of children is not representative of all children in the population aged 6-18, but, strictly speaking, only of children of reproductive-age women who still live with their mothers. If children who do not live with their mothers are more likely to come from families with unintended or excess fertility, and these children are also less likely to be enrolled at any age, the educational attainment in our samples is likely to be biased upward. However, the profiles of current school enrollment by age for our samples are almost identical to the profiles generated from the full household samples of children (results not shown). This provides some assurance that our sample displays similar schooling patterns to those found in the population.

tended or excess fertility; the ordered-probit equation is equation (8.2), which is estimated using ordered indices of educational attainment.[18]

A full implementation of the statistical model presents challenges in several dimensions. The main difficulty concerns the possibility of correlation between the disturbance terms in the fertility equation (8.1) and the children's schooling equation (8.2). If it were not for this correlation, the system could be neatly separated into two equations and the children's schooling model then considered on its own. It is quite important, therefore, to test for such cross-equation correlation before embarking on an ambitious exercise in joint estimation.

We carried out such endogencity tests using generalized residuals from the fertility equation (Hausman, 1978; Guilkey et al., 1992; Bollen et al., 1995). The results, summarized in Appendix C, provide no evidence of cross-equation correlation in either the Dominican Republic or Kenya. There is a suggestion of endogeneity bias in the results for the Philippines and clear statistical evidence of bias, although this is not readily interpretable in substantive terms, for Egypt.

With these results in mind, the next section presents the findings from models that do not incorporate corrections for endogeneity bias. For the Dominican Republic and Kenya, we are on solid statistical grounds in doing so; the approach is less defensible for the Philippines, and the case of Egypt will require additional research.

RESULTS

We now proceed to the multivariate analyses. Three measures of unintended and excess fertility are considered: (1) the occurrence of no, one, or two or more unwanted births in the 5 years preceding the DHS survey; (2) the occurrence of at least one unwanted birth or at least one badly mistimed birth, where the birth in question was desired more than 2 years after it occurred; and (3) the presence of excess fertility, defined earlier as having more births at the survey than the ideal family size reported by the woman. Many alternative measures and combinations of measures, including interactions with the child's sex, were examined in

[18]In specifying the full system, we should in principle allow for additional family-level effects that induce a correlation in educational outcomes among children. We have not fully implemented that approach in the present analysis, but intend to do so in future work. Such a system can be estimated using the method of Gaussian quadrature (Guilkey and Murphy, 1993; Hedeker and Gibbons, 1994). We have explored this approach for the schooling equations alone and found that unmeasured family effects account for 25-35 percent of the overall disturbance variance. The family variance components are highly significant. The structural coefficient estimates, however, changed remarkably little when we estimated the random-effects models, nor were their estimated standard errors much affected. We therefore choose to present here the simple models without random effects.

preliminary analyses.[19] We restrict our attention to these three measures because they seem to capture the main empirical features of interest.

The incidence equation—equation (8.1), in which the dependent variable is a measure of unintended or excess fertility—is estimated separately using each measure of unintended or excess fertility. These dependent variables are yes-no dummy variables for which we employ a probit model, with the exception of the first measure, indicating 0, 1, or 2+ unwanted births, for which we use an ordered-probit model.

With regard to measures of children's educational attainment, we have likewise restricted our attention to two dependent variables. The first represents the grades of schooling completed. For this variable we adopt the ordered-probit estimation method, a choice that allows us to capture in a flexible manner the irregular features of a years-of-schooling distribution. A second dependent variable is also defined—a dummy variable taking the value 1 if a child has completed any years of secondary schooling. To study this variable, we must limit the admissible age range of the children who enter into the analysis. The lower end of this age range is defined such that given first entry to primary school at the appropriate starting age and steady progression thereafter from grade to grade, the first year of secondary school should have been completed.

Incidence of Unintended and Excess Fertility

Given that the fertility equation of our system is estimated with three dependent variables for four countries, we choose to present here a summary qualitative assessment of the findings rather than the extensive details. Table 8-5 displays the main features of the results for each country.

As can be seen, in three of the four countries the likelihood of unintended and excess fertility is significantly reduced by the schooling of the woman. This finding is indicative of one of the important ways in which education affects fertility. Other things being equal, it is the children of less-educated mothers who

---

[19]In addition to the measures discussed in the text, we also explored measures based on the woman's reports of unintended or excess fertility taken in conjunction with her report of her spouse's views about the desirability of having more children. These measures added little of substantive interest. We suspect that having the spouse's own views, rather than the woman's report on them, might have made a difference. We also explored interactions between our measures of unintended and excess fertility and the sex of the school-age child, seeking to determine whether the impact of such fertility differs for the education of girls and boys. These interactions did not prove to be significant. We considered an alternative measure of excess fertility, defined by the difference between the number of surviving children and the family-size ideal. This measure behaved in much the same way as the difference between the number of births and the family-size ideal. The DHS surveys also gathered information on the ideal spacing between births. We examined these reports and compared them with the spacing actually achieved, as represented in the respondent's birth histories. We found that substantial proportions of women have had two or more births whose spacing violated their current ideal. These spacing variables may merit further work.

TABLE 8-5 Incidence of Unintended or Excess Fertility: Summary of Results

Characteristic	Dominican Republic	Egypt	Kenya	Philippines
Woman's education	Negative and significant	Negative and significant	Positive and significant to mixed	Negative and significant
In union	Positive and significant	Positive and significant	Positive and significant	Positive and significant
Spouse's education	Mixed and weak	Weak and negative	Mixed and weak	Weak to positive
Standard of living	Negative and significant	Weak and not significant	Positive at low levels, then negative	Negative and significant
Urban residence	Positive and significant to mixed	Not significant	Nairobi negative and significant; otherwise not significant	Weak and mixed

are more likely to bear the consequences of unintended or excess fertility. Kenya provides the exception to the rule, and we find this exception intriguing. It may be that the Kenyan woman who labels a particular conception as unwanted or who says that her current number of children is greater than her ideal is in some respects atypical in a social setting that has historically emphasized spacing rather than numbers as the key dimension of fertility control. In preliminary work focused specifically on detailed measures of spacing (not reported here), both the determinants and the consequences of mistimed fertility in Kenya appeared to differ from fertility described as unwanted or excessive.

Returning to Table 8-5, we find the expected result that being in union (married or living with a partner) is associated with a higher incidence of unintended or excess fertility. No doubt this association is due mainly to the elevated risk of exposure to conception in general. The education of the spouse, a variable defined in the DHS as referring to either the current or the most recent spouse/partner, shows a somewhat erratic relationship to fertility, being in some cases positive, but usually weak. A standard-of-living index, defined as the summation of a number of socioeconomic items,[20] is generally associated with reduced

[20]The standard-of-living index varies from 0 to 9. Each household is assigned a score of 1 for each of the following items: access to clean drinking water; access to water within the household; access to water within 30 minutes of the household; access to some toilet facility; access to a flush toilet; nondirt flooring; and possession of refrigerator, a television, and a bicycle.

incidence of both unintended and excess fertility. The effects are weakest in Egypt, but then Egypt is the case in which the education of the spouse exerts the strongest effect, and the spouse's education variable may in this case function as the better measure of living standards. Residence in an urban area (different coefficients were estimated for residence in towns, small cities, and the capital city) exhibits somewhat modest but usually negative effects on unintended and excess fertility.

Not shown in Table 8-5, but of great importance on both substantive and scientific grounds, is the role of access to family planning services in reducing unintended and excess fertility. To explore the effects of access, we incorporated in the models the numerous indicators of access that are available in the DHS family planning and health services questionnaires. These indicators are not at all standardized across countries, and in one case (Egypt) the service questionnaires were fielded only in rural areas. (For Egypt, we devised additional measures of access for urban areas by aggregating individual measures of knowledge of family planning method sources up to the community level.) The results clearly indicate that access to family planning services is a statistically important influence on unintended and excess fertility. This finding supports our research strategy, in which access measures are employed as instrumental variables. But it is less clear what dimensions of access matter in which settings, and we are not yet able to offer any summary assessments that could help guide program interventions. This is a high-priority area for future research.

Effects of Unintended and Excess Fertility

We now come to the heart of the matter—the effects of unintended and excess fertility on children's schooling. These effects are summarized in two ways: first with respect to an index of the number of grades of schooling completed, and second with an analysis that focuses on attainment of at least 1 year of secondary schooling for children in the relevant age range. The first analysis is conducted using the method of ordered probit, which, as will be shown, allows us to capture the main features of the distribution of completed schooling; the secondary schooling analysis employs simple probits.

We should repeat here the caution issued above regarding the statistical endogeneity of unintended or excess fertility. We have tested for this and found no cause for concern in the cases of Kenya and the Dominican Republic. For the Philippines the situation is less clear, and standard tests clearly indicate the presence of cross-equation correlation in Egypt. Thus, less confidence should be placed in the results for the latter two countries.

Table 8-6 presents estimates of a baseline model for all four countries in which no measures of unintended or excess fertility are included. This table establishes a set of benchmarks against which the models including fertility can be assessed. The coefficients shown here are not greatly affected by the inclusion of the fertility measures, and after Table 8-6 we do not again report their estimates.

The findings in Table 8-6 reaffirm the central role played by the mother's education in furthering the educational achievements of her offspring. Likewise, we see evidence that the education of the spouse is also important. The coefficients on spouse's education (recall that the variable refers to current or most recent spouse) do not in general display the strength of the mother's education, although Egypt in some ways presents an exception. The standard-of-living indices function much as expected (the squared term needs to be taken into consideration in interpreting these coefficients, as does the range of the index, which runs from 0 to 9), with higher values of the index being associated with greater educational attainment for children. Urban residence is associated with greater educational attainment in most cases, particularly if the family lives in the capital city, but there are examples of weak or inconsistent results, such as for the Philippines.

For three of the four countries (Kenya is the exception), community-level measures of travel time to the nearest primary and secondary school are available. In some cases, the community informant could not supply an estimate (this occurred for both primary and secondary schooling in the Philippines and for secondary schooling in the Dominican Republic and Egypt). We therefore included dummy variables indicating knowledge of travel time, together with the estimated time itself. These access-to-schooling measures fall well short of what would be ideal, but regrettably, the DHS surveys collect no additional information on schools. It is interesting that in the Philippines and Egypt, longer travel times are associated with reductions in educational attainment. The effects are statistically significant, but within the range of travel times in the data, of only modest substantive importance.

The coefficients from these ordered-probit and probit models require some translation if they are to be understood in substantive terms. To aid in this interpretation, we present Figure 8-3, which summarizes the implications of the years-of-schooling model for children's educational attainment and may facilitate cross-country comparisons. Figure 8-3 shows, for each year of schooling, the predicted proportion of children who would achieve that year or more. To generate the curves, we apply the coefficient estimates of Table 8-6 to a hypothetical child aged 18, whose education should be complete or nearly so. The left-most curves indicate the countries with the lowest levels of educational attainment—Kenya and the Dominican Republic—with the Philippines and Egypt showing higher levels of attainment.

Table 8-7 presents our estimates of the consequences of unintended and excess fertility. The results are striking and, in some respects, unexpected. In the Dominican Republic and the Philippines, unintended and excess fertility are associated with clear reductions in the educational attainment of children. In Egypt and Kenya, by contrast, no such effects appear. At first glance, this pattern

TABLE 8-6 Baseline Estimates of Children's Schooling Models

Characteristic	Dominican Republic: Years of Schooling (ordered probit)	Dominican Republic: Any Secondary (probit)
Children's Characteristics		
Girl	.353*	.370*
(z statistic)	(12.16)	(5.46)
Age	.540*	–7.277
	(2.49)	(–.49)
Age, squared	.001	.520
	(.05)	(.55)
Age, cubed	–.000	–.012
	(–.87)	(–.61)
Parental Characteristics		
Mother, primary schooling	.540*	.494*
	(10.99)	(3.94)
Mother, secondary schooling	.973*	1.098*
	(14.66)	(6.30)
Mother, higher schooling	1.209*	1.474*
	(14.38)	(5.19)
Mother, age	.008*	.016*
	(2.86)	(2.21)
Currently in union	–.001	–.091
	(–.02)	(–1.01)
Spouse, primary schooling	n.a.	n.a.
Spouse, secondary schooling	.254*	.246*
	(5.59)	(2.15)
Spouse, higher schooling	.344*	.457*
	(5.22)	(2.13)
Standard of living index	.240*	.145
	(6.53)	(1.53)
Index, squared	–0.00	.010
	(–.10)	(1.03)

Egypt		Kenya		Philippines	
Years	Secondary	Years	Secondary	Years	Secondary
–.267	–.275	.165*	.199	.261*	.455*
(–14.57)	(–6.80)	(6.97)	(1.92)	(15.00)	(9.81)
2.179*	19.569*	1.241*	37.29	1.792*	.217
(20.40)	(4.37)	(9.01)	(.59)	(12.70)	(.02)
–.142	–1.194	–.044	–2.219	–.081	.036
(–15.34)	(–4.09)	(–3.65)	(–.58)	(–6.92)	(.06)
.003*	.024*	.001	.044	.002*	–.002
(13.58)	(3.85)	(1.96)	(.58)	(4.89)	(–.12)
.183*	.238*	.355*	.507*	n.a.	n.a.
(8.46)	(5.07)	(12.57)	(3.99)		
.251*	.774*	.719*	.848*	.268*	.426*
(5.64)	(4.82)	(16.39)	(4.16)	(11.9)	(7.22)
.216*	.952*	n.a.	n.a.	.281*	.676*
(3.06)	(3.52)			(8.79)	(6.29)
–.001	.001	.019*	.048*	.007*	.008
(–.32)	(.32)	(8.96)	(4.22)	(3.85)	(.15)
.074*	.147*	-.089	.217	.076	.177
(2.05)	(2.20)	(-2.43)	(1.25)	(1.85)	(1.80)
.323*	.346*	n.a.	n.a.	n.a.	n.a.
(14.60)	(7.57)				
.443*	.914*	.264*	.336*	.217*	.471*
(12.46)	(9.19)	(8.56)	(2.61)	(9.52)	(7.88)
.479*	.620*	n.a.	n.a.	.254*	.577*
(10.07)	(5.03)			(8.26)	(6.18)
.352*	.224*	.154*	–.025	.271*	.251*
(11.09)	(3.28)	(6.49)	(–.24)	(16.55)	(5.79)
–.025	–.005	–.003	.025*	–.016	–.006
(–6.15)	(–.54)	(–.77)	(2.03)	(–8.59)	(–1.19)

TABLE 8-6 Continued

	Dominican Republic	
Characteristic	Years of Schooling (ordered probit)	Any Secondary (probit)
Cluster characteristics		
Town	–.072	–.055
	(–1.25)	(–.40)
Small city	.063	.115
	(1.58)	(1.26)
Capital city	.210*	.226
	(3.74)	(1.77)
Travel time to primary school known	n.a.	n.a.
Primary travel time (minutes)	.000	.003
	(.031)	(1.01)
Travel time to secondary school known	n.a.	n.a.
Secondary travel time (minutes)	–.001	–.001
	(–1.89)	(–.78)
χ^2 (d.f.)	5,785 (18)	620 (18)
p-value		0.00
N	5,428	1,798

n.a. = not available

* denotes significance at the 5 percent level.

	Egypt			Kenya		Philippines	
	Years	Secondary		Years	Secondary	Years	Secondary
				–.002	.327	–.020	.176*
				(–.02)	(.83)	(–.74)	(2.43)
				.323*	–.236	–.033	–.079
	.379*	.486*		(3.24)	(–.54)	(–1.46)	(–1.34)
	(6.13)	(3.80)					
				.094	.742*	.016	.243*
				(1.45)	(3.32)	(.44)	(2.06)
	n.a.	n.a.		n.a.	n.a.	.218	–.220
						(1.24)	(–.40)
	.018*	.022*		n.a.	n.a.	–.010	–.001
	(4.85)	(2.95)				(–10.4)	(–.66)
	.235*	.308*		n.a.	n.a.	–.011	.214*
	(3.78)	(2.40)				(–.27)	(2.21)
	–.015	–.017		n.a.	n.a.	–.001	–.001
	(–11.19)	(–6.26)				(–3.84)	(–2.13)
	13,657 (18)	1,373 (18)		11,817 (14)	266(14)	20063 (19)	1286 (19)
	0.00	0.00	0.00	0.00	0.00	0.00	0.00
	13,481	5,154		8,763	1,500	14,290	4,481

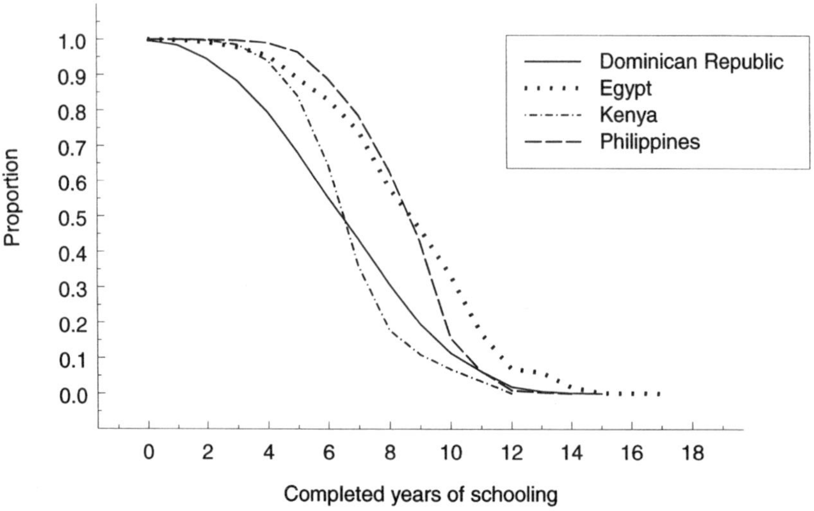

FIGURE 8-3 Predicted proportion with given years of schooling or more: Baseline model results for a child at 18 years of age.

of results is disconcerting: Why should the countries with the lowest levels of unintended and excess fertility show the greatest impact of such fertility on education? We believe at least six factors may account for this pattern of results.

First, it may be that in an environment in which parents are generally more effective in controlling the timing of births and achieving their desired number of children, an unintended birth is perceived to be less likely, so that when it occurs, it may be more disruptive to family-building strategies. Note that the Dominican Republic and the Philippines are the lowest-fertility countries in the group. The point applies better to the case of the Dominican Republic, where some 34 percent of women use modern contraceptive methods, than to the case of the Philippines, in which only 15 percent use such methods.

Second, it is reasonable to expect that the disruption occasioned by an unintended birth may be greater where three conditions obtain: the returns to education are perceived to be considerable, the (direct) costs of education are also considerable, and there exist reasonably strong preferences for equalizing educational investments across children. In such an environment, parents might feel compelled to make across-the-board adjustments, so to speak, when faced with an unanticipated birth. (On these points, see Appendix A.)

Third, recall that the reports of unintended and excess fertility are those of women rather than their spouses. In the case of Egypt, women are said to cede much decision-making authority to their spouses, and in such settings a woman's own views of whether a birth was wanted or fertility is excessive might have little to do with household resource allocation. If the man were to declare a birth unwanted, the implications might be quite different.

Fourth, a closely related point is that in none of these countries is there available a measure of the *intensity* of preferences, that is, of the degree of motivation to avoid excess family size or unintended births. It is plausible that in Egypt and Kenya, countries still in the early stages of demographic transition, such motivations may often be superficial or clouded by ambiguity and second thoughts.

Fifth, in all countries the possibility of random, nonsystematic measurement error in preferences deserves consideration.[21] Such errors would tend to bias the estimated effects downward, and it may be that the measurement error variance is itself a function of a country's stage of demographic transition.

Finally, a point that bears in particular on the case of Kenya, we have not fully explored measures of birth mistiming. In a society in which birth spacing has been a dominant concern, with the possibility of and desires for limiting fertility a more recent development, the impact of poor spacing deserves further attention.

How important in substantive terms are the effects of unintended and excess fertility? To address this question, we consider the years-of-schooling estimates for the Dominican Republic and translate the parameter estimates into predicted years of schooling for a hypothetical child aged 18. (Of the two countries where effects were found, we choose the Dominican Republic case because these results are better justified in statistical terms than are those for the Philippines.) The calculations used here apply to unwanted fertility, but the nature of the results would be similar had we chosen to illustrate the estimated consequences of excess fertility. We generate three predictions—one for the case in which no unwanted birth occurred, another in which one such birth occurred, and a third in which two such births occurred. The range in predictions then illustrates the role of this particular covariate, other things being held constant. To provide a sense of relative strength, we then compare the predictions with those generated by the single strongest socioeconomic covariate in our models—mother's education.

The comparison in substantive terms can be seen in Figures 8-4 and 8-5. Figure 8-4 graphs the results when unwanted fertility is varied as just described, and Figure 8-5 carries out the analogous exercise for mother's education. These estimates do not include the indirect effects of mother's education that operate through unintended fertility, only the direct effects. To understand the figures, it may be helpful to focus attention on grade 6, which is the end of primary schooling in the Dominican Republic. The predicted proportion of children achieving at least this level of schooling is .56 in the case of no unwanted births, .48 in the case of one unwanted birth, and just .39 in the (extreme) case of 2 or more

[21]We thank John Casterline for this observation.

TABLE 8-7 Selected Coefficients on Measures of Unintended or Excess Fertility

	Dominican Republic		Egypt	
Measure of Unwanted or Mistimed Fertility	Completed Years	Secondary Schooling	Completed Years	Secondary Schooling
Model I				
One unwanted birth in last 5 years (z value)	–.280* (–5.22)	–.249 (–1.66)	.000 (0.02)	.009 (0.18)
Two or more	–.550* (–6.16)	–.340 (–1.22)	–.032 (–0.92)	–.121 (–1.50)
χ^2_2 p-value	.00	.12	.64	.29
Model II				
At least one unwanted birth or birth mistimed by 3 or more years	–.322* (–7.22)	–.245 (–1.89)	–.023 (–1.15)	–.049 (-1.09)
Model III				
Number of births > Ideal family size at survey	–.219* (–6.87)	–.259* (–3.49)	.031 (1.12)	–.088 (–1.21)

*Significant at p<.05.

unwanted births, a total difference of some 17 percentage points. This is a substantively important difference. Similar results can be derived from the other measures of unintended and excess fertility. Had we chosen the Philippines for our example, the differences would not have been quite as large (and recall the potentially contaminating role of statistical endogeneity in those results).

To be sure, the difference produced in children's education in the Dominican Republic by varying the incidence of unwanted childbearing (in a 5-year period) is not as large as what would be generated by variations in the educational level of the mother. Figure 8-5 shows that the predicted proportion of children having 6 or more completed years of schooling ranges from .39 in the case when mothers have no schooling to .75 when they have postsecondary schooling. The conceptual experiment in this figure, however, involves a great range for mother's education (from none to postsecondary), and it is not obvious what policy instruments could effect such a change.

Kenya		Philippines	
Completed Years	Secondary Schooling	Completed Years	Secondary Schooling
.006	.139	–.033	–.081
(0.20)	(1.01)	(–1.33)	(–1.24)
–.073	–.126	–.129*	–.190
(–1.49)	(–0.56)	(–2.99)	(–1.76)
.30	.46	.01	.12
–.058	.058	–.075*	–.141*
(–2.29)	(0.48)	(–3.69)	(–2.62)
–.008	–.256	–.124*	–.203*
(–0.29)	(–1.81)	(–6.73)	(–4.17)

CONCLUSIONS

Our empirical results suggest that in the middle to latter phases of a fertility transition, the positive effects of mother's education on children's education are likely to be reinforced by reductions in the incidence of unintended or excess fertility. The consequence is a "virtuous circle" linking mothers and their children. The children of women who are able to avoid unintended fertility benefit in terms of their schooling; one assumes that as adults, they will be better equipped to manage their own fertility and to make appropriate provision for the children of the next generation. This phase of the fertility transition is exemplified by the cases of the Philippines and the Dominican Republic, where the TFR lies between 3.7 and 4.1. The full extent of these effects cannot be estimated with DHS data given the 5-year window of observation. These longer-term effects are potentially greater than those estimated here.

At an earlier phase of the fertility transition, as illustrated here by the case of Kenya with a TFR of 5.2, women with more education are among the first to

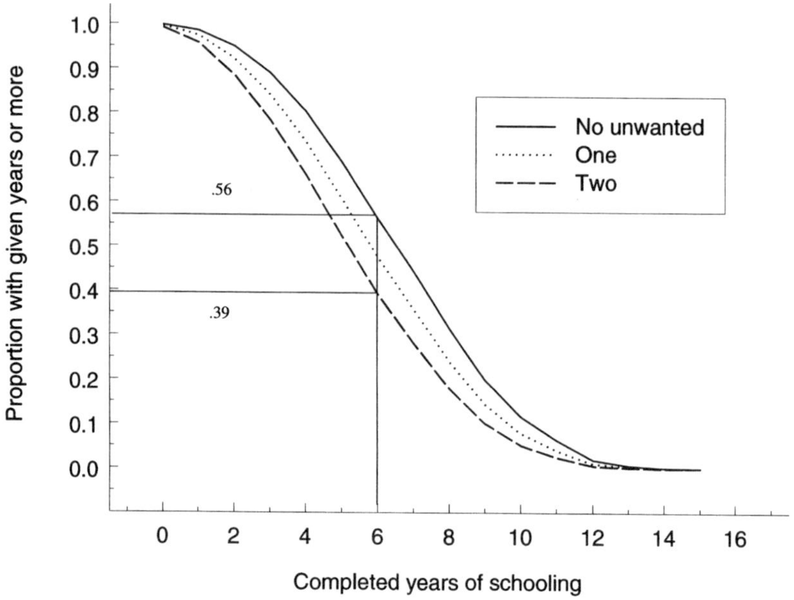

FIGURE 8-4 Unwanted fertility and completed schooling: Dominican Republic estimates.

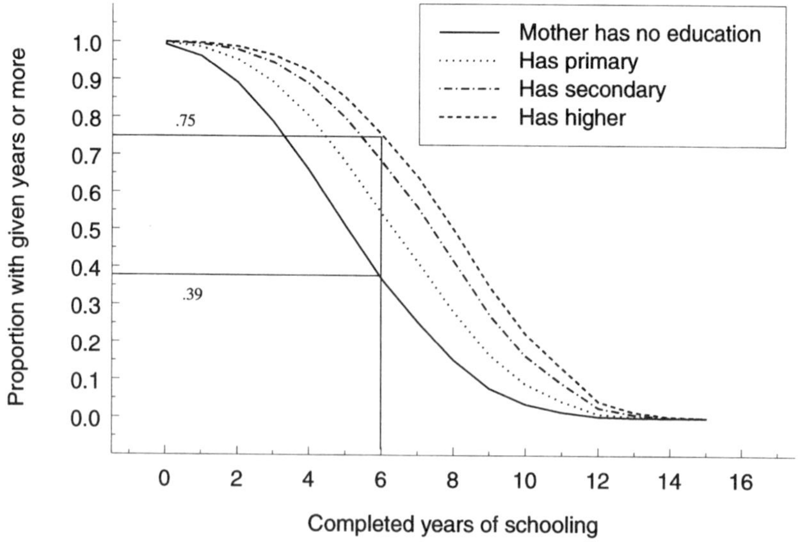

FIGURE 8-5 Mother's education and completed schooling: Dominican Republic estimates.

reduce their family-size desires, a change that induces an initial positive association between mother's education and unintended and excess fertility. In a setting where birth spacing has traditionally been important, but family-size preferences remain high, a child's schooling appears to suffer, if it suffers at all, only when siblings are mistimed. The gap between actual and desired fertility does not otherwise seem to hinder children's schooling. This result is consistent with research suggesting that the relationship between fertility and education may become significant and negative only after certain development and demographic thresholds have been passed. Also, in Kenya as in much of sub-Saharan Africa, there are possibilities for meeting unanticipated childrearing costs through sibling chains of support and networks of relatives. Furthermore, the direct costs of schooling may be sufficiently low, in this early phase of transition, that an unintended birth can be accommodated without serious disruption to planned investments. In Egypt, where the fertility transition is in a more intermediate phase (a TFR of 4.7 at the time of the 1988 survey), our results are not easily interpreted, although again the direct costs of schooling may not be sufficiently high for an unintended birth to present difficulties.

One implication of these findings is that as the transition reaches its later phases, differences among women in the ability to meet, yet not exceed, their reproductive goals may be an important factor generating social inequalities among their children. Access to family planning services for women of all socioeconomic levels is important, and our findings underscore the continuing need for investment in family planning services for the disadvantaged.

ACKNOWLEDGMENTS

We gratefully acknowledge the support of the Rockefeller Foundation through its grant to the Population Council, "Interrelationships Between Fertility and Child Investment: New Research Frontiers." Edmundo Paredes and Jie Wang provided invaluable research assistance throughout the project. We also acknowledge, with thanks, comments from Dennis Ahlburg, John Bongaarts, John Casterline, Deborah DeGraff, Jane Guyer, and two anonymous reviewers.

REFERENCES

Appleton, S.

1995 *Exam Determinants in Kenyan Primary School: Determinants and Gender Differences.* Washington, D.C.: Economic Development Institute, World Bank.

Bankole, A., and C.F. Westoff

1995 *Childbearing Attitudes and Intentions.* DHS Comparative Studies No. 17. Calverton, Md.: Macro International, Inc.

Bankole, A., and C.F. Westoff

1997 The Consistency and Validity of Reproductive Attitudes: Evidence from Morocco (unpublished manuscript).

Baydar, N.
1995 Consequences for children of their birth planning status. *Family Planning Perspectives* 27(6):228-234.
Baydar, N., and W. Grady
1993 *Predictors of Birth Planning Status and Its Consequences for Children.* Seattle, Wash.: Battelle Public Health Research and Evaluation Center.
Becker, G., and H.G. Lewis
1973 On the interaction between the quantity and quality of children. *Journal of Political Economy* 81(2 Part II):S279-S288.
Behrman, J.
1988 Intrahousehold allocation of nutrients in India. *Oxford Economic Papers* 40:32-54.
Bollen, K.A., D.K. Guilkey, and T.A. Mroz
1995 Binary outcomes and endogenous explanatory variables: Tests and solutions with an application to the demand for contraceptive use in Tunisia. *Demography* 32(1):111-131.
Bongaarts, J.
1990 The measurement of wanted fertility. *Population and Development Review* 16(3):323-334.
Brown, S., and L. Eisenberg, eds.
1995 *The Best Intentions: Unintended Pregnancy and the Well-Being of Children and Families.* Committee on Unintended Pregnancy, Division of Health Promotion and Disease Prevention, Institute of Medicine. Washington, D.C.: National Academy Press.
Casterline, J., A. Perez, and A. Biddlecom
1996 *Factors Underlying Unmet Need for Family Planning in the Philippines.* Research Division Working Paper. New York: The Population Council.
David, H., Z. Dytrych, Z. Matejcke, and V. Schuller, eds.
1988 *Born Unwanted: Developmental Effects of Denied Abortion.* New York: Springer Publishing.
Desai, S.
1995 When are children from large families disadvantaged? Evidence from cross national analyses. *Population Studies* 49(2):195-210.
Frenzen, P.D., and D.P. Hogan
1982 The impact of class, education and health care on infant mortality in a developing society: The case of rural Thailand. *Demography* 19(3):391-408.
Guilkey, D.K., and J.L. Murphy
1993 Estimation and testing in the random effects probit model. *Journal of Econometrics* 59:301-317.
Guilkey, D.K., T.A. Mroz, and L. Taylor
1992 *Estimation and Testing in Simultaneous Equations Models with Discrete Outcomes Using Cross Section Data.* The Evaluation Project Working Paper Document #IM-01-01. University of North Carolina at Chapel Hill.
Hanushek, E.
1992 The trade-off between child quantity and quality. *Journal of Political Economy* 100(1):84-117.
Hausman, J.
1978 Specification tests in econometrics. *Econometrica* 46(6):1251-1271.
Hedeker, D., and R.D. Gibbons
1994 A random-effects ordinal regression model for multilevel analysis. *Biometrics* 50:933-944.
Hermalin, A., J. Seltzer, and C.-H. Lin
1982 Transitions in the effect of family size on female educational attainment: The case of Taiwan. *Comparative Education Review* 26(2):254-270.

Jensen, E., D. Ahlburg, and M. Costello
1996 *The Impact of Wantedness and Family Size on Child Mortality and Health-Care Allocations Within Filipino Families.* Williamsburg, Va.: The College of William and Mary.

Kelley, A.
1996 The consequences of rapid population growth on human resource development: The case of education. In D. Ahlburg, A. Kelley, and K. Mason, eds., *The Impact of Population Growth on Well-Being in Developing Countries.* Berlin: Springer-Verlag.

Kurian, G.T., ed.
1988 *World Education Encyclopedia.* New York: Facts on File Publications.

Lightbourne, R.E.
1985 Individual preferences and fertility behaviour. In J. Cleland and J. Hobcraft, eds., *Reproductive Change in Developing Countries: Insights from the World Fertility Survey.* Oxford: Oxford University Press.

Lloyd, C.B.
1993 *Family and Gender Issues for Population Policy.* Population Council Research Division Working Paper No. 48. New York: The Population Council.
1994 Investing in the next generation: the implications of high fertility at the level of the family. In R. Cassen, ed., *Population and Development: Old Debates, New Conclusions.* Washington, D.C.: Overseas Development Council.

Lloyd, C.B., and A.K. Blanc
1996 Children's schooling in sub-Saharan Africa: The role of fathers, mothers, and others. *Population and Development Review* 22(2):265-298.

McClelland, G.H.
1983 Family-size desires as measures of demand. In R. Bulatao and R. Lee, eds., *Determinants of Fertility in Developing Countries. Volume 1: Supply and Demand for Children.* New York: Academic Press.

Mensch, B., M. Arends-Kuenning, A. Jain, and M. Garate
1995 *Meeting Reproductive Goals: The Impact of the Quality of Family Planning Services on Unintended Pregnancy in Peru.* Population Council Research Division Working Paper No 81. New York: The Population Council.

Montgomery, M.R., and C.B. Lloyd
1996 The effects of family planning programs on maternal and child health. In D. Ahlburg, A. Kelley, and K. Mason, eds., *The Impact of Population Growth on Well-Being in Developing Countries.* Berlin: Springer-Verlag.

Montgomery, M. R., A. Kouamé, and R. Oliver
1995a *The Tradeoff Between the Number of Children and Child Schooling.* Living Standards Measurement Study Working Paper No. 112. Washington, D.C.: The World Bank.
1995b *The Tradeoff Between the Number of Children and Their Schooling: Evidence from Côte d'Ivoire and Ghana.* Population Council Research Division Working Paper No. 80. New York: The Population Council.

Myhrman, A., P. Olsen, P. Rantakallio, and E. Laara
1995 Does the wantedness of a pregnancy predict a child's educational attainment? *Family Planning Perspectives* 27(3):116-119.

Parish, W., and R. Willis
1993 Daughters, education and family budgets: Taiwan experiences. *Journal of Human Resources* 28(4):863-898.

Postlethwaite, T.N., ed.
1988 *The Encyclopedia of Comparative Education and National Systems of Education.* Oxford: Pergamon Press.

Rosenzweig, M., and T.P. Schultz
1987 Fertility and investments in human capital: Estimates of the consequences of imperfect fertility control in Malaysia. *Journal of Econometrics* 36:163-184.

Rosenzweig, M., and K. Wolpin
1980 Testing the quantity-quality fertility model: The use of twins as a natural experiment. *Econometrica* 48(1):227-240.
1993 Maternal expectations and *ex post* rationalizations. *The Journal of Human Resources* 28(2):205-229.
UNESCO
1994 *Statistical Yearbook.* Paris: UNESCO.
United Nations
1992 *Abortion Policies: A Global View. Volume 1: Afghanistan to France.* New York: United Nations.
1993 *Abortion Policies: A Global View. Volume 2: Gabon to Norway.* New York: United Nations.
1995 *Abortion Policies: A Global View. Volume 3: Oman to Zimbabwe.* New York: United Nations.
Varian, H.R.
1984 *Microeconomic Analysis.* Second edition. New York: W.W. Norton & Company.
Westoff, C.F., N. Goldman, and L. Moreno
1990 *Dominican Republic Experimental Study: An Evaluation of Fertility and Child Health Information.* Columbia, Md.: Institute for Research Development/Macro Systems, Inc.
Wolfe, B., R. Haveman, D. Ginther, and C.B. An
1996 The 'window problem' in studies of children's attainments: A methodological exploration. *Journal of the American Statistical Association* 91(435):970-982.
World Bank
1995 *Staff Appraisal Report, The Dominican Republic.* Second Basic Education Development Project. Report No. 14963-DO. Washington, D.C.: The World Bank.
Zuravin, S.J.
1991 Unplanned childbearing and family size: Their relationship to child neglect and abuse. *Family Planning Perspectives* 23(4):155-161.

APPENDIX A
A PARENTAL UTILITY MAXIMIZATION MODEL FOR FERTILITY AND CHILDREN'S SCHOOLING

In this appendix, we develop a formal decision model in which parents choose the number of their children and the level of educational investment in each child, taking into account the implications of alternative choices about children for their own consumption levels. The model is primarily a vehicle for illustrating in a formal manner the theoretical points made in the main text. It is therefore a highly simplified representation of the decision problem. In particular, the model is set in a one-period decision framework, in which both fertility and education choices are made at the outset of the reproductive life cycle. A more realistic and interesting approach, as discussed in the main text, would be to allow for multiple decision periods, so that parents would have the opportunity to learn about the educational abilities of their children and might adjust subsequent fertility and consumption in light of the accumulated information. Such dynamic decision models are extremely complex to analyze, however, and as our purpose is mainly to illustrate key points, we do not pursue this generalization here.

There are conceptual benefits to be gained from a formal mathematical approach, even if this representation is understood to be no more than a stylized and simplified depiction of the decision problem. Perhaps the principal benefit is in showing that parental desires—as expressed in their wanted fertility levels, their desired pattern of educational investments in children, and their preferred level of own consumption—are jointly determined by a common set of exogenous factors. These factors include the level of parental income, the prices and related resource constraints parents face, and the fixed features of parental preferences. We therefore think of wanted fertility and wanted education as being joint outcomes of a common decision process: they each depend on the exogenous determinants, but *do not* depend, in any causal sense, on each other. The level of wanted fertility is not a causal determinant of the level of wanted children's schooling, nor is the level of wanted schooling a causal determinant of wanted fertility.

In this framework, it is not meaningful to ask how wanted fertility affects wanted levels of children's education, nor is it appropriate to put the question the other way. The dimensions of wanted fertility and wanted children's education are closely associated, to be sure, but this association is not, in itself, a causal one. Rather, the association reflects the joint dependence of fertility and education on the exogenous causal determinants mentioned above. Where *unwanted* fertility is concerned, however, one can ask about the causal consequences. This is because unwanted fertility can be regarded as an exogenous shock that displaces parental consumption and human capital investment strategies from what would otherwise have been optimal.

In a more complex, dynamic decision framework, one could investigate the consequences of unwanted fertility (or other exogenous shocks) during the reproductive life cycle on subsequent fertility and subsequent child investments. These consequences might well depend on the level and age pattern of the wanted births that had already occurred at the time of the exogenous shock. Such earlier births (likewise, earlier child investments) would function as predetermined constraints (or sunk costs) that could limit the scope and nature of any post-shock adjustments on the part of parents. Moreover, in a dynamic decision problem in which the spacing and arrival of wanted births is not fully controllable by parents, it becomes conceptually appropriate to ask how the timing of wanted births affects subsequent fertility, child schooling, and parental consumption. Likewise, one can ask how imperfectly predictable factors, such as a child's educational abilities, might affect the parents' fertility as these factors become known.

Given that this chapter is mainly empirical in nature and based on cross-sectional data sets, we have chosen not to pursue the theoretical possibilities afforded by dynamic modeling. The empirical concerns are indeed difficult to address. If lagged, predetermined values of ex ante choice variables are to be included in the empirical model, a means must be found to protect the estimates against the effects of persistent omitted variables, which would be expressed first in the lagged values of the choice variables and again in the current values being modeled. Thus, demanding data requirements must be met to permit consistent estimation of such models. Longitudinal data are required, at a minimum, and the DHS data used here simply do not meet these requirements. With richer data, one could begin to ask a richer set of causal questions.

Elements of the One-Period Model

We begin by separating the one-period parental utility function into two factors. The first factor, denoted here by U, measures the utility that parents derive from the number of children and their education. We follow Behrman (1988) in using the constant elasticity of substitution (CES) specification, that is,

$$U = \left(\sum_{i=1}^{n} s_i^{\rho} \right)^{1/\rho}$$

in which i is a subscript for child i, and s_i is the education of that child. Here n is the total number of children. The parameter ρ of this subutility function serves to index the degree of parental aversion to inequality in the distribution of resources among their children. It ranges from $-\infty$ to 1, with the case of $\rho = 1$ representing no aversion to inequality and, at the opposite end, the case of $\rho \to \infty$ representing no tolerance of inequality, that is, Leontief preferences.[22]

[22]This specification has one awkward feature: if $s_i = 0$, then child i provides no utility benefits to the parents. In other words, there is a utility return to increasing the number of children only if the

In addition to U, the utility of the parents is affected by their own consumption C. We assume that the full utility function can be expressed in a Cobb-Douglas form,

$$V = UC^{a}$$

where the parameter α gives the subjective weight parents attach to their own consumption. The full parental utility function is therefore a composite in which a CES factor, having to do with child services, is nested within a Cobb-Douglas function in which the two arguments are the child services aggregate U and parental consumption C.

The budget constraint for this problem allows for both discretionary and exogenous components of expenditure on children. Each child is assumed to require a fixed amount w in childrearing expenditures; in addition, a child-specific net price p_i is associated with each unit of education s_i. The rationale for making the net price of education child-specific is to account for differences across children in the expected future benefits of schooling. We could accomplish the same goal by elaborating the model in the time dimension, with the nature of the future benefits made explicit, but the current specification should suffice for the purposes of illustration.

The budget constraint can then be expressed as

$$\sum_{i=1}^{n} p_i s_i + wn + C = \Omega$$

where Ω is total parental income.

Solving the Utility Maximization Problem

The utility maximization problem can now be divided into discrete stages that correspond to the alternative numbers of children that parents could contemplate having. For any given number of children n, parents face the task of optimally dividing their discretionary income, $\Omega - wn$, between child services U and their own consumption C. The Cobb-Douglas specification for the full utility function implies that with n given,

$$C = \frac{\alpha}{1+\alpha}(\Omega - wn),$$

---

additional children receive a strictly positive amount of schooling. In future work, we will study more general specifications that do not impose this requirement.

and what remains of household resources is then available to be distributed among the n children for their schooling.

The properties of the CES framework (see Varian, 1984, for details) imply that each child will receive

$$s_i = \frac{p_i^{(r-1)}}{\sum_i^n p_i^r} Y ,$$

in education, where $r = \rho/(\rho - 1)$ and $Y = (\Omega - wn)/(1 + \alpha)$ is the total amount of discretionary income available for schooling. We refer to this as the schooling demand equation, where by demand we mean demand that is conditional on a particular fertility level n. The conditional indirect utility derived from child services is then

$$U^*(n) = \left(\sum_i^n p_i^r \right)^{-1/r} Y .$$

We can now summarize the overall parental utility derived from n children as

$$V^*(n) = \left(\sum_i^n p_i^r \right)^{-1/r} \alpha^\alpha (1+\alpha)^{-(1+\alpha)} (\Omega - wn)^{1+\alpha} .$$

This is a conditional indirect utility function, giving maximum parental utility as a function of the number of children, which is itself a choice variable. Using this expression, the task that remains is to search over discrete values of n to find the optimal value—the level of fertility that maximizes parental utility. In the main text, we refer to the optimal value of n as *wanted fertility*. Since n is discrete, no analytic expression for wanted fertility is available, but for given parameter values, it is straightforward to find the level of wanted fertility by numerical means.[23]

Let n^* denote the level of wanted fertility. The wanted level of children's education, which will in general differ across children, is then determined by substituting n^* for n in the denominator of the schooling demand equation above. Likewise, the optimal level of parental consumption is given as $C = \alpha/(1 + \alpha)(\Omega - wn^*)$. Since n^* is a function only of the set of exogenous factors (Ω, p, w, ρ, α), wanted schooling and consumption are also fully determined by these factors. It is in this sense that wanted fertility and schooling are jointly determined.

[23]Note that the expression applies to values of $n \geq 1$.

Some Properties of the Solution

As Behrman (1988) demonstrates in a related context, parental aversion to inequality has a potentially important role to play in allocating educational investments among a set of children. This role emerges in situations in which the net price of schooling, p_i, differs across children, so that there is an economic incentive to invest differentially. The extent to which such differential investment takes place depends on ρ, the utility parameter that expresses whether parents are indifferent to inequality ($\rho = 1$) or would tend to resist allocating resources in an unequal manner ($\rho < 1$), other things being equal. When parents are wholly indifferent to inequality, educational resources are concentrated in the child whose net price of schooling p_i is lowest. When they resist such a concentration of resources, by contrast, educational investments tend to be spread more equally among children, although the child with the lowest net price will generally continue to receive more in the way of parental investment (apart from the extreme case of Leontief preferences).

The discrete nature of fertility also influences patterns of child investment. To see this, consider the comparative statics of the response to a change in parental income Ω. Suppose that Ω is reduced. In addition to reducing their own consumption, parents faced with lower income have the option to adjust to the situation in two ways that affect their children: on the extensive margin, by reducing the desired number of children, and on the intensive margin, by leaving the number of children unchanged and reducing educational investments. For certain combinations of parameters, as income Ω falls, parents will adjust first by cutting back on children's schooling. After a certain point, however, income will be low enough that parents will find it necessary to reduce fertility. A one-child reduction in fertility frees an amount w in exogenous childrearing expenses. Once that fertility reduction has been made, a portion of the freed w can be used to increase children's schooling, that is, to increase it relative to what it was before the fertility reduction took place. Thus, if we were to graph the relationship between Ω and children's schooling, the graph could exhibit a sawtooth pattern whose shape would reflect both the intensive and the extensive margins of adjustment. A similar pattern could characterize the parental response in own consumption as Ω varies. As far as we are aware, these potentially complex responses have not been much studied, whether from a theoretical or an empirical perspective.

Parental Responses to Unwanted Fertility

The conceptual approach developed here can be used to study the consequences of unwanted fertility for parental consumption and children's educational investments. As above, let n^* denote the level of wanted fertility. If an unwanted birth occurs, actual fertility is then $n' = n^* + 1$. Returning to the expressions above concerning children's education, we can determine the education response to unwanted fertility by inserting n' in the demand equation where n^* had appeared; we can do likewise for parental consumption. The implied adjustments in education and consumption will depend on a number of factors: the level of exogenous childrearing costs w, the child-specific net prices for education p_i, the level of income Ω, and so on.

The full welfare cost for parents can be summarized in terms of *compensating variation*, that is, in terms of the additional level of income Ω that would be required to leave the parents as well off with n' children as they would have been with the number of children they actually wished to have, or n^*. It is possible to calculate the required compensation by using the conditional indirect utility function $V^*(n)$ shown above. This compensation can then be interpreted as a summary measure of parental motivation to avoid unwanted fertility. Alternatively, it can be interpreted as the monetized welfare costs (again from the parents' point of view) that are imposed by unwanted fertility.

APPENDIX B
MEASUREMENT OF UNINTENDED AND EXCESS FERTILITY

In the main text, we focus on two distinct concepts—excess fertility and unintended fertility. As noted, the former is measured by the extent to which a woman's cumulative fertility exceeds her expressed ideal family size at the time of the survey. Reports on ideal family size are elicited by the following DHS question: "If you could go back to the time you did not have any children and could choose exactly the number of children to have in your whole life, how many would that be?" Unintended fertility, by contrast, is typically measured with reference to the 5-year window of time ending at the survey. Within that window, the intendedness of each birth is determined by asking the mother to think back to her feelings at the time she was first pregnant with the child and to report whether she wanted the pregnancy at that time. If the pregnancy was wanted, she is asked whether it was wanted then or later.

Concerns about the measurement of unwantedness have focused primarily on the problem of ex post rationalization. Rationalization is a potential problem when respondents who already have children are asked questions about desired or ideal family size or about the unwanted status of specific surviving children (McClelland, 1983). In particular, the questions on unintended fertility are asked on a child-by-child basis, and in answering them, the woman may feel that she is being required, in effect, to affix a label to each child. Yet a child whose conception was unwanted might have grown up to become a loved and much "wanted" member of the family. The woman might therefore feel some reluctance to label the child's conception as unwanted, and the approach might produce underreports of unwanted conceptions. (No similar bias would be expected to distort estimates of birth timing.) The DHS questions were worded so as to minimize ex post rationalization, and there is some evidence from experimental studies in Peru and the Dominican Republic (Westoff et al., 1990) that the emphasis on feelings at the time of conception helps reduce the problem. The fact that substantial numbers of women report excess fertility and unwanted births appears to be ample proof that family-size desires represent considerably more than rationalization.

Another form of rationalization could lead to biases in the opposite direction. Rosenzweig and Wolpin (1993) have conjectured that women may be overly optimistic at the time of pregnancy about the endowments of their unborn children. They suggest that retrospective reporting of unwantedness at the time of pregnancy may produce an overestimate rather than an underestimate of the actual level of unwantedness prior to birth. The possibilities for ex post revisionism, regardless of the direction of the possible bias, are what make the kind of longitudinal data available in the Finnish survey ideal for the study of the consequences of unwantedness.

Apart from considerations of recall error and ex post rationalization, a woman's reports on the intendedness of a particular child's conception should not change over time. Such reports are based on the memory of feelings held at a particular fixed point in the past. We do, however, expect to observe changes over time in measures of excess fertility for an individual woman, even if her actual fertility remains unchanged. A woman's desire for children, as expressed in her ideal family size, can be altered by changes in economic, marital, or health circumstances, or by the receipt of new information or knowledge, even if her underlying preferences are held constant (McClelland, 1983). Thus a woman could report her last birth as being wanted at the time of conception and during the same survey interview report excess fertility in the present. She might do so if, in the interim, she faced deteriorating economic conditions, gained new skills in the labor market that increased the opportunity costs of childbearing, absorbed new ideas about the advantages of small families from the media, or lost a husband through death or divorce. Similarly, a woman who reports not having wanted a particular pregnancy in the past could report no excess fertility in the present for a variety of reasons, including an improvement in her own or her community's economic circumstances that allows her to afford more children than previously, the arrival of a new husband who is eager for her to have children with him, or a change in government policies. It is therefore quite difficult to determine from the survey questions themselves whether a woman is inconsistent in her responses. The fact that a woman currently views her family size as excessive does not necessarily mean that any particular child was unwanted at the time of conception, nor does it mean that any particular child is unwanted now. Excess fertility indicates only that the woman now sees her family size as being too large in relation to current ideals.

Of course, if fertility ideals and intentions are wholly transitory, their measurement as of a particular point in time will not provide a reliable guide to either past or future behavior. Recent evidence from Peru suggests that desired fertility is reasonably stable in the short run (Mensch et al., 1995). In this study, over 80 percent of women reinterviewed after 3 years provided consistent responses to a question about future fertility intentions. When responses to the question about future childbearing desires from the 1991-1992 DHS were compared with responses to the same question in the 1994 follow-up survey, 72 percent of women gave the exactly the same response. Of those who did not want more in 1994 but had wanted more in 1991-1992, roughly half had had a child in the interval or had experienced a marital disruption; thus an additional 7-8 percent gave consistent answers. Therefore, roughly 80 percent of women gave consistent answers between the two surveys. This provides some evidence to suggest that women's fertility desires do not change wholesale over 3 years. Casterline et al. (1996) examined changes in the Philippines over a shorter reinterview period—6 weeks—and also found considerable evidence of stability.

Although Bankole and Westoff (1995) consider recent births, the aggregate measures of unwanted fertility reported elsewhere in the literature are not based on reports on the wantedness status of particular births, but rather on measures of ideal family size (Lightbourne, 1985) or the desirability of the next birth (Bongaarts, 1990). In the terms we have employed, the Lightborne measures are measures of excess fertility. Bongaarts (1990) compared such excess fertility measures with alternative, forward-looking measures based on the desirability of a next birth. He found strong correlations between these two alternatives, but much weaker correlations between the desire for a next birth and the wantedness status of recent births. Evidently, the alternative measures must tap different concepts; in addition, they are differentially affected by changing events and by recall or misreporting error.

To obtain a sense of the empirical overlap between measures of excess and unintended fertility, we examined the DHS data from our four study countries. We investigated whether women who say they currently have excess fertility also report as unwanted at conception those recent births whose parity exceeds the mother's current ideal. The proportion of such recent births reported to be unwanted at the time of conception ranges from 35 percent in the Philippines to 65 percent in the Dominican Republic.

In light of the above discussion, it should be clear that such differences in the fertility measures can be interpreted in various ways. One possibility among many is that ideal family size may have declined over the 5 years preceding the survey (Bankole and Westoff, 1995), perhaps as economic circumstances changed. Thus some children who were wanted prior to their birth may now be found in a family that is larger than their mother would view as ideal under her present circumstances.

In summary, it appears reasonable to proceed with the excess and unintended fertility measures, each taking a place in the analysis. These measures are fundamentally different in character, and as just shown, they are sufficiently different empirically to warrant separate consideration.

APPENDIX C
ENDOGENEITY TESTS USING GENERALIZED RESIDUALS IN SCHOOLING EQUATIONS

APPENDIX C Endogeneity Tests Using Generalized Residuals in Schooling Equations

Measure of Unwantedness	χ^2 on family planning access in incidence equation (p-value)	Generalized residual coefficient, years equation (z stat.)	Generalized residual coefficient, secondary school equation (z stat.)
Dominican Republic			
0, 1, or 2+ unwanted births in last 5 years	23.6 (0.07)	0.022 (0.15)	0.354 (0.79)
Any unwanted births or births mistimed by 3 or more years	17.6 (0.29)	–0.109 (–0.66)	0.752 (1.50)
Number of births exceeds family-size ideal	31.0 (0.01)	0.170 (1.08)	0.100 (0.57)
Egypt			
0, 1, or 2+ unwanted births in last 5 years	50.5 (0.00)	–0.173* (–3.23)	–0.327* (–2.37)
Any unwanted births or births mistimed by 3 or more years	61.2 (0.00)	–0.175* (–2.68)	–0.384* (–2.21)
Number of births exceeds family-size	85.9 (0.00)	–0.141 (–1.94)	–0.447 (–1.98)

APPENDIX C Continued

Measure of Unwantedness	χ^2 on family planning access in incidence equation (p-value)	Generalized residual coefficient, years equation (z stat.)	Generalized residual coefficient, secondary school equation (z stat.)
ideal			
Kenya			
0, 1, or 2+ unwanted births in last 5 years	21.8 (0.02)	–0.238* (2.57)	0.218 (0.46)
Any unwanted births or births mistimed by 3 or more years	17.5 (0.06)	–0.172 (–1.26)	0.093 (0.12)
Number of births exceeds family-size ideal	27.2 (0.00)	–0.162 (–1.89)	0.438 (0.71)
Phillippines			
0, 1, or 2+ unwanted births in last 5 years	27.0 (0.04)	–0.059 (0.71)	–0.129 (0.20)
Any unwanted births or births mistimed by 3 or more years	29.3 (0.02)	–0.202* (-2.18)	–0.001 (–0.01)
Number of births exceeds family-size ideal	34.7 (0.01)	0.324* (3.17)	0.440 (1.22)

*Significant at $p < .05$.

9
Women's Education, Marriage, and Fertility in South Asia: Do Men Really Not Matter?

Alaka Malwade Basu

INTRODUCTION

The quest for pathways in the relationship between female education and fertility in developing countries has run the gamut of the proximate determinants proposed by Davis and Blake (1956). Some of these proximate determinants, such as the length of breastfeeding or of postpartum abstinence, have been found to be related to education in the direction of potentially increased fertility. These findings have led to much speculation in the literature on the surprising magnitude of those variables which act in the direction of reducing fertility, since the net impact of education on fertility is generally negative.[1] Thus, for example, given that birth intervals are often shorter for educated women, we are impressed by the role of modern contraception, which seems not only to compensate for the resultant increase in fecundity, but also to reduce fertility to levels lower than those seen with longer birth intervals.

Now that the negative relationship between female education and fertility has been clearly established, further research on this issue, at least in demography, seems to consist of doing more of the same, albeit with bigger and better data sets. The uniformity is particularly striking in the way some of the proximate determinants of fertility are conceived and interpreted. While such uniformity of definition and analysis is understandable in the case of single-component

[1]The finding that educated women want lower family sizes and seem to be better able to achieve such lower fertility is remarkably universal in a range of fertility surveys and smaller studies across the world (for a review, see Jejeebhoy, 1995; see also Diamond et al., this volume).

variables such as intercourse frequency,[2] it seems unnecessary to reduce other variables to such mechanical numbers.[3]

In particular, a narrow perspective continues to characterize the demographer's treatment of marriage as an intermediate variable in the relationship between socioeconomic factors and fertility. The timing of marriage (and in more sophisticated versions, the start of a sexually active life) is taken as the only way the fact of marriage affects fertility, whether natural or controlled. This is especially the case for studies on Asia.[4] That is, most analyses that use marriage as an intermediate variable to study fertility are concerned with the question of differentials in when women marry, and not at all with the question of whom they marry.[5]

In addition, because female education continues to have a strong relationship with fertility even when the standard household variables (of income, occupation, and so on) are controlled, the explicit conclusion in the literature is that educated women have a single-handed role in their lower fertility. This conclusion in turn is taken to suggest that women's autonomy is important to fertility decline (a proposition first put forth by Dyson and Moore, 1983). This latter conclusion is

---

[2]Even here, however, the imaginative researcher can be concerned with more aspects of this variable than the simple presence or absence of a particular act of sexual intercourse.

[3]This is not to say that demographic research is unaware of the many aspects of a single variable. Breastfeeding in particular has now undergone detailed scrutiny, and we know it cannot be related to fertility in terms of simple measures such as its duration; we must also note whether it is total or partial, disciplined or available on demand, and so on.

[4]Mainstream demography has long been interested in the interrelationships among different *forms* of marriage (polygyny in particular) in sub-Saharan Africa and a few local communities elsewhere; in addition, there is a small literature, focused on the developed world, on the implications of marriage dissolution and reformation for fertility. But for Asia, where marriage is relatively stable and universal (and perhaps *because* it is seen to be stable and universal), the only measure of variation deemed interesting is that of its timing.

[5]There are too many studies with this focus on the relationship between female education and age at marriage to make it possible to provide a few representative references. See, for example, the scores of references to the relation between education and the age at marriage in a recent comprehensive review by Jejeebhoy (1995). This book itself also addresses the intermediate role of marriage almost entirely in the context of its timing. There is, admittedly, increasing awareness of one other dimension of marriage in semi-anthropological demographic research specific to Asia: the question of whether modernization or education or other factors associated with lower fertility are also associated with an increase in "love" versus "arranged" marriages (see, for example, Jeffery and Jeffery, 1993; Caldwell, 1996). But this notion of love marriages has yet to catch on in the standard demographic literature, as the brief reference to it in Jejeebhoy's review suggests.

In the literature on sub-Saharan Africa, there is also an acknowledgment of the impact of education on the *kind* of marriage women enter into—in particular the impact of female education on polygynous marriages. In addition, there is some interest in the effect of education on interspousal factors, such as the age gap between husbands and wives. Such analyses, if extended to look more carefully at the husbands of educated women, and especially in regions outside Africa as well, should move the debate in demography on the relation between female education and marriage much further.

buttressed by the several studies that do indeed find educated women have more freedom in decision making and action on a range of domestic and extradomestic matters (see, for example, Basu, 1992; Vlassoff, 1996; Morgan and Niraula, 1995; and the reviews in Jejeebhoy, 1995, and Sathar, 1996). But from this conclusion (that educated women have greater autonomy as well as lower fertility), an implicit conclusion that has much less empirical basis is drawn: that educated women have greater reproductive autonomy than uneducated women. And a further implicit conclusion follows: that there is somehow an intrahousehold conflict in reproductive preferences that is resolved in the woman's favor when she is educated and therefore has greater autonomy in reproductive decision making.

Marriage is brought into this framework in a somewhat confusing way. There is a direct effect of later marriage on natural fertility, of course, simply because of the reduced period of exposure to the risk of pregnancy and childbearing. But later marriage is also believed to reduce the demand for children through the woman's increased premarital exposure to the kind of culture and ideas that encourage lower fertility. In addition, later marriage is believed to make it easier to achieve these lower fertility goals through increased access to and autonomy in using birth control information and services. At the same time, these are all things that education is believed to do directly as well, so that the educational effect through later marriage is primarily in reducing the period of exposure to potential childbearing. Jejeebhoy (1995) concludes that in this sense, the delayed marriage associated with women's education has an "unintended" impact on fertility in that educated women do not delay marriage as a means of reducing their fertility.

This chapter attempts to isolate only one strand of the female education-marriage-fertility relationship. It argues that aspects of marriage other than its timing are relevant to fertility. Quite apart from whether educated women marry early or late is the question of the kind of men educated women marry. Are these the kind of men whose reproductive goals need to be changed or overruled by their educated wives? That is, is reproductive autonomy an essential ingredient of the education-fertility relation? The chapter suggests that it is not. The marriage market ensures that educated women will find the kind of husbands who share their reproductive preferences and that intrahousehold gender inequalities in daily life need not imply gender inequalities in reproductive goals.

Analyses of the female education-fertility relation that focus only on the timing of marriage and therefore its effects on the attitudes and abilities of the woman assume that while there is something special about the educated woman, there is nothing special about the educated man. This chapter argues that there is something special about the educated man who marries an educated woman, even if there is much less to distinguish the educated man in general than the educated woman. Merely by marrying an educated woman, this man is saying something about himself; he is not just a random educated man who then has his attitudes and preferences molded by his educated spouse.

This hypothesis is not inconsistent with the empirical finding that the wife's education has a much clearer relation to fertility than does the husband's education. The special feature of the husband of the educated woman is not his education, but rather other characteristics that standard surveys have not attempted to capture.[6]

WOMEN'S EDUCATION AND THE MARRIAGE MARKET

Assume four categories of marriageable individuals: less-educated men, more-educated men, less-educated women, and more-educated women, represented, respectively, by A, B, C and D. At a very broad level of generality, A and B can marry from among C and D. But in reality, given their relative numbers and norms about marriage in South Asia, groups A and D are much more restricted in their spousal options than are groups B and C.

What are these relative numbers? Assume for the moment that A + B = C + D. That is, assume that there are roughly equal numbers of marriageable men and women. Given the difference in age at marriage in countries such as India, this assumption is not strictly true—there should be more women than men. But given the sex differential in mortality that also exists in this region, it may be fairly correct to assume that the total number of women of marriageable age is about the same as the total number of men that group of women can potentially marry, that is, men aged about 5 years older than these women.

It requires a much greater stretching of the facts, however, to assume that the numbers of men and women in the two educational categories are also about equal. Given the differential emphasis placed on the schooling of boys and girls in many parts of the developing world, it is more likely by far that B is a much larger group than D, and A is probably a much smaller group than C. Any table on the sex differential in educational attainment of the population in South Asia should make this quite obvious. For example, Table 9-1 is based on the sample households in the National Family Health Survey in India. The gender differences in education are obvious from this table. For example, while 22.5 percent of men aged 20-25 are illiterate, and 11.7 percent have studied beyond high school, the corresponding figures for women aged 15-19 (these men's potential spouses) are 43.8 percent and 1.7 percent. Men aged 25-29 show a similar dissimilarity to women aged 20-24.

[6]Perhaps it is the *kind* of education that matters more for men than for women. A general measure such as "years of schooling" may be able to discriminate much better among women than among men.

TABLE 9-1 Educational Levels of Marriageable Men and Women: India

Sex	Age	Illiterate	Literate: Up to primary school (%)	Middle and high school (%)	Above high school (%)
Men	20-24	22.5	21.7	44.0	11.7
Women	15-19	43.8	21.4	33.0	1.7
Men	25-29	28.8	23.4	35.3	12.4
Women	20-24	52.3	18.3	22.8	6.6

SOURCE: Internal Institute of Population Sciences, 1995.

Thus, in every population of equal numbers of marriageable men and women, there are significantly fewer less-educated men than less-educated women, and a larger number of more-educated men than more-educated women.

Why do these relative numbers matter? They matter because they severely restrict the marriage market for two categories of individuals—less-educated men and more-educated women. They do so because of the norm of hypergamy in much of South Asian society (see Basu, 1998). In a general way, the system of hypergamy refers to the practice of women marrying men of higher ritual and social status than themselves. This is not simply a matter of preference. It is an injunction that is set forth in the scriptures themselves and that dictates marriage rules on the subcontinent even today. For example, the ancient Hindu lawgiver Manu states, "If a virgin makes love with a man of a superior caste, the king should not make her pay any fine at all, but if she makes love with a man of the rear castes, he should have her live at home in confinement" (Doniger, 1991:191). And again, "According to tradition, only a servant woman can be the wife of a servant; she and one of his own class can be the wife of a commoner; these two and one of his own class for a king; and these three and one of his own caste for a priest" (Doniger, 1991:44).

In the present context, marrying "up" by women requires that they marry men at least as educated and preferably more so. The education of girls may in fact increase the chances of their finding such high-status grooms. Indeed, on this aspect of hypergamy, South Asia is perhaps not unique at all. Around the world it seems to be as common for women to marry men more educated than themselves as it is for them to marry men older than themselves.

Yet this phenomenon is not exactly the same as the positive assortative mating with respect to education hypothesized by Becker (1981) and characteristic of most societies in the developed world (see, for example, Epstein and Guttman, 1984; Warren, 1966; Layard and Zabalza, 1979; Schirm, 1986). In the South Asian case, it applies to women, but may not apply to men. In turn, this difference implies that men in group B can choose their partners from among women in group C or D (since they are barred only from marrying women more educated than themselves, not those less educated), while men in group A are restricted to women in group C. Similarly, women in group C can marry men in group A or B, but women in group D are restricted to men from group B.[7] These restrictions are fortunate in at least one respect because they mean that in principle everyone can find a potential spouse: the larger numbers of less-educated women can turn to more-educated men to make up for the shortage of less-educated men, and the larger numbers of more-educated men can turn to less-educated women to make up for the shortage of more-educated women.

Does this phenomenon happen in practice at more than an anecdotal level? That is, does it happen in statistically significant numbers? Tables 9-2 and 9-3 (again from the Indian National Family Health Survey) certainly suggest that it does. The data in Table 9-2 show that virtually none of the sampled women with more than a high school education have married men with no education,[8] whereas the data in Table 9-3 show that a substantial number of the sampled men (though fewer in the southern states, where the gender gap in education is less pronounced) with more than a high school education have married illiterate women. Moreover, the vast majority of sampled women with more than a high school education have married men who also have more than a high school education,[9] while far fewer than half the sampled men who have gone beyond high school have wives who have done the same.

Looking only at more-educated brides and grooms, that is, at members of groups B and D, it is thus obvious that men have a much wider field than women. The main thesis of this chapter is that the way they play this field has a bearing on the relationship between female education and fertility. While the majority of more-educated women marry more-educated men, there are two kinds of more-

---

[7]Indeed, the anthropological literature from South Asia is rich in descriptions of the marriage squeeze that occurs when marriages are hypergamous for any characteristic, not just education. In general, this hypergamy squeezes the marriage market for higher-status women (as measured by income, education, caste, or any other feature) and lower-status men, explaining to some extent the prevalence of dowry in the upper-status groups and of bride-price in the lower-status groups (see, for example, some of the readings in Uberoi, 1993).

[8]The disaggregated National Family Health Survey data indicate that the few educated women who do marry uneducated men are almost all in the southern part of India. In addition, they are all in rural areas, that is, areas where there is a lower premium on education, and other socioeconomic factors, such as income, employment, caste, or landholding, substitute for education among men in the marriage market.

[9]Kerala, both urban and rural, is a little different in this regard. Relatively larger numbers of women with more than a high school education have married men less educated than themselves. This new phenomenon has been attributed to the rising unemployment of educated men in the state, so that employment rather than education has become the preferred feature of hypergamy (Rajan et al., 1996).

TABLE 9-2 Educational Level of Husbands Relative to Wives: India, 1992-1993

	Husband's Education Level (%)		
Education of Wife	Illiterate	Up to middle school	Above middle school
Illiterate	28.4	56.9	14.7
Up to middle school	4.0	59.0	37.0
Above middle school	0.3	10.0	89.7

SOURCE: International Institute of Population Sciences, 1995.

TABLE 9-3 Educational Level of Wives Relative to Husbands: India, 1992-1993

	Wife's Education Level (%)		
Education of Husband	Illiterate	Up to middle school	Above middle school
Illiterate	92.5	7.2	0.3
Up to middle school	64.3	33.7	3.0
Above middle school	24.0	33.0	43.0

SOURCE: International Institute of Population Sciences, 1995.

educated men—those that marry more-educated women and those that marry less-educated women. The hypothesis here is that those who do the former are a select group who themselves have low reproductive goals, so that controlling family fertility requires no extraordinary effort on the part of their more-educated wives. There is no conflict of wills involved, and there is little spousal difference in the returns to childbearing.

Likewise, those more-educated men who marry less-educated women are themselves more likely to have the same high-fertility goals as their wives and as their less-educated male counterparts. Thus again higher fertility results from the spousal partnership, rather than women's low-fertility intentions being crushed by overbearing husbands with high-fertility desires.

THE POSSIBILITY THAT THERE ARE TWO KINDS OF EDUCATED HUSBANDS

How do we know that there are two kinds of more-educated men? That is, how can we assume that educated men who marry educated women are not a random sample of all educated men, but a group selected in some way? If they were a random sample, we could indeed infer that a strong relation between female education and fertility and a relatively weak one between male education and fertility reflects the primary or even sole impact of the woman's education on reproductive behavior, with men's reproductive goals being immaterial or even contrary to women's, as is often implied in the literature.

The notion that educated men who marry educated women are in some way different from educated men who marry uneducated women makes intuitive sense; marriage is too important a life event in most societies to be left to random circumstances. Conscious decision making is involved, and both the individuals concerned (or, more commonly, their families) have a list of preferred characteristics, whether these preferences are dictated by norms, ambitions, or tastes. The nature of these preferred characteristics in turn tells us much about the individual or family that holds these preferences. Thus the educated man (or his family) who marries an educated woman is saying something about his preferences, given that he has a pool of educated and uneducated women from which to choose. We may note that the preferences of the educated woman in the marriage market are less transparent in this regard, given that she is effectively barred from choosing her partner from the larger pool of uneducated as well as educated men.

It thus follows that the educated man who marries an educated woman is displaying a different set of preferences from those of the educated man who marries an uneducated woman, a difference that cannot be accounted for by their relative levels of education. A field inquiry seeking to discriminate between these two sets of men would therefore not get very far by focusing on their education; information about other aspects of their lives and personalities is necessary.

Since intuition is not an acceptable form of evidence in academic (and especially demographic) research, more empirical and measurable means of demonstrating that there are indeed two kinds of educated husbands are needed. This chapter proposes two possible lines of evidence. The first focuses on identifying some of the specific ways in which educated men who marry educated women differ from those that marry less-educated women, even before they get married. That is, what relevant background characteristics could distinguish these two sets of men? The second focuses on demonstrating a similarity between educated women and their husbands, assuming it is possible that the lower fertility of educated women is not an outcome of their ability to reject the different reproductive goals of their husbands, but an outcome of having husbands who think like them.

To begin with the first line of evidence, the fact that male education itself has only a weak relationship with fertility is not surprising. In most parts of the developing world, and especially in contemporary South Asia, families are well aware of the returns to schooling and increasingly are even embarrassed about illiteracy, especially in males (see, for example, Jeffery and Jeffery, 1993). In addition, the education of sons faces no cultural or attitudinal inhibitions. I have yet to come across a survey in which the bulk of respondents did not reply "as much as possible" when asked to what extent they would like to educate their sons. The bounds of this possibility are set primarily by resource availability, so that male education levels are a proxy for the schooling facilities and financial resources available to households, rather than for the household attitudes and values that female education more often reflects.[10] Educational differentials in men thus capture little more than their resource differentials. Moreover, we know from a mass of research on historical and contemporary populations that economic factors can explain fertility declines only imperfectly. Thus if the male is the unit of analysis and we want to relate male characteristics to fertility, we need markers other than education to identify the bundle of values and attitudes that make up the "modern" world view.[11]

In principle, it should be quite straightforward to collect empirical information on differentials among educated men. The trouble is that most data sets have not gone beyond searching for other proxies for education to capture such differentials. Thus income, occupation, and some background family characteristics (such as caste in the Indian context) are the kinds of things measured by most large surveys, whereas what we need is some information about differences in the world views of different kinds of educated men. Do some educated men (and, by extension, their families) live by a different set of values and have a different set of attitudes toward life from those of other educated men? Is this what makes them gravitate toward educated women when the time comes for them to marry?

As already mentioned, if a family can afford to educate its sons, it does so;

---

[10]Female education does also partly reflect resources and services. But the use of these resources and services is much more conditioned by norms and values than is the case for males.

[11]That some form of "modernization" or, more accurately, "westernization" inspires the transition to lower fertility is now acknowledged in the literature to be as important as, and often more important than, changes in affordability occasioned simply by changing incomes. Indeed, even those changes in the costs and benefits of childbearing caused by changed incomes are usually mediated by changes in attitudes and aspirations. If this were not the case, increases in income would lead to a rise in the demand for children.

there is no larger principle involved. But in marriage, men are expressing more than their financial constraints; they are expressing a preference. Therefore, one way of differentiating among educated men is by looking at their marriage partners. But then, of course, one must ask whether the husbands of educated women are different because they were always different, or have become different through spousal influence.

Fortunately, information on premarital differences in world views requires no specialized survey instruments. One does not need to devise psychological tests of modernization to identify the educated man who will prefer an educated wife. One can of course ask young unmarried men about their preferred spousal characteristics. But such a measure would suffer from the same kinds of potential biases as any attitudinal questions asked in the impersonal style of a survey.

This chapter suggests a much simpler measure of modernization. If one assumes (quite reasonably) that female education is as much an outcome as a determinant of modern attitudes and values, one potential way of classifying educated men (and their families) according to these attributes would be to look at the investment made in the education of their sisters.[12] The latter cannot logically be the result of the educated women these men marry, unless their sisters are very much younger than they. If one can thus demonstrate that educated men who marry educated women come from backgrounds that are relatively modern to begin with, one must give less credence to theories that explain the lower fertility of educated women in terms of their own characteristics alone.

Most data sets in demography already routinely collect some background information on all household members. From this information it should be possible to measure the educational levels of the girls and women in the husbands' natal families and to relate these levels to those of the wives of these men.[13] If such a relationship does indeed exist, it will provide strong empirical support for the thesis that there are two kinds of educated men. The hypothesis is that households in which both sons and daughters receive an education are qualitatively different from those in which only the sons are sent to school (or remain in school for any length of time), and that the men who marry educated women are more likely to belong to the former group.

---

[12]Alternatively, one could look at the education of their mothers. But in a society in which female education is a recent event, this indicator might not be discriminatory enough. Moreover, the education of mothers may reflect the attitudes of the grandparents of the husbands more accurately than those of their parents.

[13]One can foresee several problems with getting these tabulations, of course. For example, given the nature of existing data sets, one would be able to look at the educational levels of sisters only when the families are joint. In addition, one could look only at the education of the unmarried sisters of the husband, since his married sisters would be living elsewhere. But these problems may not exist in all data sets, and in any case, future research on this issue would merely need to add some questions to the standard household survey instrument to eliminate these potential biases.

TABLE 9-4 Educational Level of Husbands' Sisters According to the Education of Their Wives: India, 1992-1993

	Education of Sisters of Husbands[b] (%)		
Education of Wives[a]	Illiterate	1-6 years of school	7+ years of school
Illiterate	71.4	17.6	11.0
1-6 years of school	35.0	35.0	30.0
7+ years of school	6.4	19.1	74.5

NOTES: Sample Size = 186. Includes only those households that recorded the presence of wives as well as sisters in the household survey.

[a]Includes women aged 20-29 who are the wives, daughters-in-law, or sisters-in-law of the household head.

[b]Includes women aged 15-24 who are the sisters and daughters of the household head.

SOURCE: Computed from Indian National Family Health Survey data.

Table 9-4 lets us look for such a relationship in the results of the Indian National Family Health Survey. The table plots the educational distribution of the available daughters and sisters (that is, the agnates of the respondents' husbands) against the education of the wives, sisters-in-law, and daughters-in-law of the household (that is, the in-marrying women) to see whether educated women marry into homes in which female education is already valued.[14]

Table 9-4 is primarily indicative since the data have many limitations (see note 13); nevertheless, the results are strongly indicative. Educated women are much more likely to marry into homes in which the daughters are also educated. Compare, for example, Tables 9-2 and 9-4. While only 28 percent of the husbands of illiterate women in Table 9-2 are illiterate themselves, as many as 71 percent of the sisters-in-law of the illiterate women are illiterate (Table 9-4). On the other hand, while 90 percent of the husbands of women with 7 or more years of schooling have 7 or more years of education themselves, 74 percent of the

[14]By restricting the age ranges of the two categories of women—those marrying into the family and those born in it—Table 9-4 manages to exclude the daughters of the married women from the set of women born into the family before the woman entered it; a woman aged 20-29 is extremely unlikely to have a daughter aged 15-24.

sisters-in-law of these educated women are also as educated as the women. That is, sex differentials in education are much higher in the families of the men who marry less-educated women.

This finding in turn suggests that the families of the educated men that choose to marry educated women are qualitatively different from the families of the educated men that choose less-educated or illiterate wives. This finding is not simply one more demonstration of the existence of positive assortative mating for education. For one thing, while it is true that the more educated the woman, the more educated her spouse, it is not similarly true that the more educated the man, the more educated his spouse. Instead, from the husband's perspective, the assortative mating occurs for his sisters' and his wife's education. That is, the more educated are his sisters, the more educated is his wife. The resultant implications for fertility could receive further support from analyses that would try to estimate the relationship between the woman's fertility and the education of her sisters-in-law, controlling for the woman's own education. According to the present hypothesis, this relationship would be stronger than that between her husband's education and her fertility.

In other words, what we see here is a case of educational hypergamy for women (that is, women tending to marry men more educated than themselves), but a continuing social homogamy for spouses (that is, a tendency for spouses to belong to similar social backgrounds). This combination of educational hypergamy and social homogamy is not unique to the Indian case used to illustrate the present discussion; instead it seems to be a feature of most societies in most parts of the world (see, for example, Bozon, 1991, for France).[15]

When the data needed to study husbands' background are not available (and even when they are), the second possible line of evidence mentioned above—the similarities between educated women and their husbands (and by extension, the similarities between less-educated women and their husbands, whether educated or not)—can strengthen the case for stating that the husband is an important intermediate variable in the relationship between female education and fertility. This is a difficult research undertaking given the trend in academic and policy circles to focus on intrahousehold conflict, treating any convergence of interests as incidental at best and a result of bulldozing at worst. Even on a narrowly demographic matter such as reproductive goals, the assumption in the literature is that there must be an interspousal difference in interests.

---

[15]The implications of social homogamy for fertility may explain some findings from unrelated parts of the world. For example, Mascie-Taylor (1986) reported for a British sample that as educational heterogamy increased, so did fertility. Given that the woman's education in Britain would be more straightforwardly a function of her economic and social class than it is in South Asia, this finding may reflect the socioeconomic heterogamy of the high-fertility couples. Their analogue in the South Asian case would be educated women married to educated men with uneducated or poorly educated sisters.

Two examples will illustrate the point. The first is a stylized representation of the situation in the developing world from an influential World Bank publication on the virtues of female education (King and Hill, 1993:vi):

> A poor family has six children. The mother never attended school, was married at age 15 and remains illiterate. Her husband earns most of the family's meager income and decides how it is spent. Since his own economic security depends on his sons' ability to support him in his old age, he insists that the boys go to school while the girls remain at home to do chores. . . .

Summers (1993:vi) provides a second example:

> A poor family has three children. The mother went to school for five years and is able to read and do arithmetic well enough to teach school in the village. As her last birth was extremely difficult, she and her husband adopted family planning. She now has more time and resources to spend on her family. Hoping for a better future for her children, she insists that they all go to school and practice their reading every night. . . .

How real is this characterization? In the first family, is it only the man that wants many children and especially many sons? If the wife had her way, would fertility necessarily decline? And in the second family, are there fewer children, and do they all go to school, only because the wife wishes this? Despite the hypothesizing and the rhetoric, there is really very little evidence in the literature to support these contentions.

The trouble is that while the literature posits that education leads women to have a smaller need or desire for children or a better ability to achieve their low-fertility desires, it is generally silent on male preferences, except by implication. When we say that female education is necessary for fertility decline, are we saying that:

- In the case of low female education, women want fewer children than men, but cannot articulate or execute their wants?

or

- Women with low education want more children than men, while those with high education want as few children as men, and such convergence of wants is necessary for fertility to decline?

or

- In the case of low female education, both men and women want more children than they do in the case of high female education? (This is not to imply that husbands and wives have similar fertility goals altruistically, although that is not as impossible as the literature on intrahousehold conflict would have us believe; it could just be that their fertility goals are similar because their socio-economic and external circumstances are similar.)

What about the empirical evidence on spousal differences in reproductive goals? Given the amount of hypothesizing on this matter that is implicit in the literature on intrahousehold disparities, it is surprising that there is so little actual information available on this question from the field. Most of the few surveys that have concerned themselves with differences in reproductive preferences between spouses have had to rely on the reporting of only one spouse, usually the wife. This is, of course, partly a matter of convenience given the tradition in demographic research to focus on the woman in data collection and analysis. But the result is that we have no sound basis for assuming that husbands think differently from wives in the area of reproductive goals.

Indeed, in an extensive review of the literature, Mason and Taj (1987) found little evidence of gender differences in fertility goals. A search of the more recent literature on this subject, especially the few studies in which both husbands and wives were interviewed, finds little reason to alter this conclusion (see, for example, Ezeh, 1993; Bankole, 1992; Jeffery and Jeffery, 1993; Stycos, 1996).

One can of course think of several reasons for this finding of a similarity in husband-wife reproductive preferences that are compatible with couples having different goals in reality. First, as Mason and Taj (1987) discuss, most of the available literature may refer to populations that are already undergoing a fertility transition, and it is in pretransition societies that one would expect to find the greatest gender differentials. Second, since the review measured net differences between the average family-size goals of husbands and wives, as opposed to the proportion of individual couples in which husbands and wives had differing goals, there may have been a tendency for subgroups with a difference in one direction to be balanced out by those that differed in the other. If that is the case, it is not clear how important differences in fertility goals are in aggregate reproductive behavior. Third, family-size ideals may be a reflection of behavior, rather than predating and/or determining behavior. But this supposition does not apply to younger cohorts who have yet to attain their desired family sizes. Fourth, family-size goals may be similar between spouses because both spouses have accepted and are stating the preferences of the more powerful spouse. This kind of dominance is difficult to detect by the ordinary survey method and is understandably inferred from other kinds of evidence and theories about intrahousehold relationships. Fifth, and this is a more charitable variant of the fourth interpretation, there may be a convergence of fertility goals between husband and wife as the two influence and are influenced by each other, not necessarily through pressure, but through persuasion and constant exposure to one another's views and beliefs.

There is also a sixth and most plausible possibility: that husbands and wives do indeed enter a marriage with similar attitudes toward reproduction and family size. This possibility is not at all incompatible with great intrahousehold gender inequality. That is, it is quite plausible that husbands and wives do have similar, independently generated fertility goals because their motivations and background circumstances are similar.

In any case, it is not at all clear theoretically why male and female reproductive goals should differ. Moreover, if they should, there are as many theories that would lead one to expect higher fertility goals in women as there are theories that would imply lower fertility goals in women. For example, the literature on the status of women and fertility that rationalizes the high fertility of women with low autonomy in terms of their need for sons to provide risk insurance and old-age security does not suggest that these women are so fertile only because their husbands and mothers-in-law override their wishes. At the same time, when this literature addresses the limited access of women to contraception and their limited ability to be heard in the matter of reproductive decision making, the inference is that they would have fewer children if only their families were more receptive to the idea.

In theory, however, it makes much more sense for the husband of the low-autonomy (or, in this context, poorly educated) woman himself to want many children because the conditions under which women are limited in their life choices are the very ones that should increase men's own need for sons to provide risk insurance and old-age security. Similarly, when the wife is in the position of supporting herself or being supported by her daughters in an emergency, she (or her daughters) is also in a position to support the husband when the need arises, so that the interests of both spouses are well served by fewer children. That is, all theories about the low-status woman's need for several children are consistent with her husband's and household's need for several children as well.

I would therefore rewrite the earlier quotations from King and Hill (1993) and Summers (1993) as follows:

> A poor family has six children. Their mother never attended school, was married at age 15, and remains illiterate. Her husband earns most of the family's meager income and decides how it is spent. Since their economic security depends on their sons' ability to support them in their old age, both parents insist that the boys go to school, while the girls remain at home to do chores.

and

> A poor family has three children. The mother went to school for five years and may or may not teach in the village school (the link between female education and employment being much more complex than that implied in the original quote). Hoping for a better future for their children and themselves, both parents insist that they all go to school and practice their reading each night.

FEMALE EDUCATION, MARRIAGE, AND REPRODUCTIVE MOTIVATION

If it is true that the educated men who marry educated women are qualitatively different from the educated or uneducated men who marry uneducated women, if an important part of this difference lies in the lower fertility goals of the former, and if these lower-fertility goals are shared by the men's educated wives, the question of the reasons for these lower goals still remains. Why do educated women and their husbands want fewer children? These common motivations are not the focus here, but some possibilities are nevertheless worth reviewing briefly.

If it is true that educated wives and their husbands both desire fewer children than do uneducated wives and their husbands, it cannot also be true that the woman's control over reproduction or over her husband (or mother-in-law) is the critical issue. It is the couple's control over life in general that makes both husbands and wives interested in controlling fertility. Indeed, contrary to the common wisdom, the woman's control over any aspect of life—sexual, reproductive, or otherwise—need not follow from her education even if her education is associated with low fertility (see, for example, several of the papers in Jeffery and Basu, 1996). Continued intrahousehold hierarchies are quite compatible with fertility decline even in the face of rising female education, and in fact seem to be characterizing recent fertility declines in much of Asia today (see, for example, Greenhalgh, 1985; Basu, 1995).

I would suggest that an important determinant of intentional fertility decline associated with female education is an increase in the family's or, more narrowly, the husband-wife team's united ability to manipulate the environment, rather than an increase in such ability in the woman alone. Female education is partly a proxy for this joint ability, since it is a proxy for the husband's characteristics that cannot be measured by his education. In addition, the wife's education is a facilitator of this ability because there are now two individuals who can appreciate and reinforce each other's understanding that low fertility is one way to satisfy the new aspirations and wants resulting from their education (as well as their exposure to the mass media, of course). As Freedman (1979) and others have pointed out, one should not underestimate the value of such changing aspirations in general and increased material aspirations in particular, independently of change in the objective conditions of life, in motivating fertility control. In addition, female education allows households as a whole to better exploit the opportunities that open up because of education, an exploitation that often hinges on smaller family size.

For example, although an educated woman may not have much direct control over whether she grinds her spices on the grinding stone or in an electric grinder, her education and her exposure to the mass media tell her clearly that the electric grinder is more convenient (and more fun), and that one way of affording an electric grinder is to have one less child for whom school fees must be paid. If, in addition, the woman has fewer but more-educated children, they can provide her with a television to watch during the time she saves by having an electric grinder. In India (and in South Asia in general), the woman's education has also reinforced her awareness that to effect such transfers from children to parents, one needs sons, not daughters, and that with daughters, in fact, the transfers are all in the opposite direction. This kind of reasoning ability may explain why educated women want fewer children than do uneducated women, but are not much more indifferent than are uneducated women to the sex composition of these fewer children. For example, in the all-India survey of the Operations Research Group (1991), only 1.5 percent of educated women were indifferent to the sex composition of their children, although the minimum number of sons wanted was, at 1.6, lower than it was for illiterate women at 2.0. The husband of this educated woman will, as is argued in the last section, already have similar low-fertility desires (except perhaps that the electric grinder is replaced in his imagination by a motorcycle).

Another important determinant is likely to be the hypothesized relation between parents' and children's education. If the mother's education increases the possibility of her daughters' education, the overall proportion of children being educated is higher in families with educated wives, thereby increasing the costs and decreasing the immediate benefits of children—another rationale for reduced fertility. In addition, if the literature on the impact of mass schooling on fertility has any basis (see, in particular, Caldwell, 1980, and Bongaarts, 1996), then at the macro level, too, there should be a fertility impact as larger proportions of children are sent to school—even if these larger proportions are merely a mechanical outcome of the greater probability that the daughters of educated mothers will be sent to school.

Yet rising material aspirations and greater investments in the education of daughters are but two of the ways the more ambitious partnership that characterizes the couple in which the wife is educated can provoke a fertility decline. Other ways include the differential impact of changes in the broader economy (couples with some education may be more likely to benefit from such changes if they have fewer children, or may even have more to lose with high fertility than do uneducated couples); access to modern views about family size in general; changing aspirations for one's children; the prestige of education being able to compensate for the loss of status associated with low fertility in uneducated families; the higher incomes that reduce the need for children as security; and the reduced fatalism about life in general and fertility control in particular that brings conscious birth control within the calculus of human choice. The important point is that none of these changes hinge on the ability of the educated wife to override the wishes of an ignorant or conservative husband; merely by marrying her, this husband has already demonstrated that he can be as modern as she is.

SOME IMPLICATIONS

The policy implications of this chapter do not tally exactly with those derived from a framework in which women's education is connected to fertility decline purely or even largely through its effects on women's control over their lives and their reproductive performance. Control over reproduction is not implied if the men who marry educated women also have low fertility goals themselves. This is not to make the case that women's control over reproduction is not a desirable goal—it is—but to clarify that such control is not a necessary condition for fertility decline because there is often no conflict of reproductive goals to begin with, even given the lower-fertility preferences of educated women. Such women are likely to be married to men who share their fertility preferences even if they do not otherwise discard the trappings of patriarchy. That is, patriarchal family structures are not necessarily inconsistent with fertility decline (on this, see also Weinstein et al., 1994).

Given the impact of education on knowledge about and aspirations for a better (or at least different) material life, even in the face of unchanged autonomy in domestic or reproductive decision making,[16] female education remains a major goal of antinatal policy. Whatever their origins, educated women do clearly have lower fertility preferences, and a convergence of reproductive preferences between spouses should undoubtedly make it easier for fertility to decline than if one partner alone must impose fertility control. In addition to conscious policy, however, the goal of female education may also be easier to attain as female educational levels rise further and increase the demand for educated wives from the brothers or other relatives of these women, and as uneducated women now find themselves increasingly excluded from marriage with desirable grooms.

ACKNOWLEDGMENTS

I am grateful for many suggestions for improving the paper from participants, from Kaushik Basu, and from two anonymous referees. I am also grateful to Annabel Perkins for research assistance.

REFERENCES

Bankole, S.A.
1992 Marital partners' reproductive attitudes and fertility among the Yoruba of Nigeria. Ann Arbor, Mich.: University of Michigan. (mimeographed)

Basu, A.M.
1992 *Culture, the Status of Women and Demographic Behavior; Illustrated with the Case of India*. Oxford: Clarendon Press.
1995 The many routes to a fertility transition: Fertility decline and increasing gender imbalances in Tamil Nadu, India. Ithaca, N.Y.: Cornell University. (mimeographed)
1998 Anthropological insights into the links between women's status and demographic behavior: The notions of hypergamy and territorial exogamy. In A.M. Basu and P. Aaby, eds., *The Methods and Uses of Anthropological Demography*. Oxford: Clarendon Press.

---

[16]But, as stated at the beginning of this chapter, education may also actually increase female autonomy and undoubtedly frequently does; the main point is that this is not necessary for a negative education-fertility relationship to exist.

Becker, G.
1981 *A Treatise on the Family*. Cambridge, Mass.: Harvard University Press.

Bongaarts, J.
1996 Remarks made at National Research Council Workshop on Female Education and Fertility in Developing Countries. Washington, D.C. February 29-March 1, 1996.

Bozon, M.
1991 Mariage et mobilite sociale en France. *European Journal of Population* 7(2):171-190.

Caldwell, J.C.
1980 Mass education as a determinant of the timing of fertility decline. *Population and Development Review* 6(2):225-255.

Caldwell, B.
1996 Female education, automony, and fertility in Sri Lanka. Pp. 288-321 in R. Jeffery and A.M. Basu, eds., *Girls' Schooling, Women's Automony, and Fertility Change in South Asia*. New Delhi, India: Sage Publications.

Davis, K., and J. Blake
1956 Social structure and fertility: An analytic framework. *Economic Development and Cultural Change* 4:211-235.

Doniger, W.
1991 *The Laws of Manu*. New Delhi: Penguin.

Dyson, T., and M. Moore
1983 On kinship structure, female autonomy and demographic behavior in India. *Population and Development Review* 9(1):399-440.

Epstein, E., and R. Guttman
1984 Mate selection in man: Evidence, theory and outcome. *Social Biology* 31(3-4):243-278.

Ezeh, A.C.
1993 The influence of spouses over each other's contraceptive attitudes in Ghana. *Studies in Family Planning* 24(3):163-174.

Freedman, R.
1979 Theories of fertility decline: A reappraisal. *Social Forces* 58(1):1-17.

Greenhalgh, S.
1985 Sexual stratification: The other side of "growth with equity." *Population and Development Review* 11(2):265-314.

International Institute for Population Sciences
1995 *National Family Health Survey (MCH and Family Planning): India, 1992-93*. Bombay: International Institute for Population Sciences.

Jeffery, R., and A.M. Basu, eds.
1996 *Girls' Schooling, Women's Autonomy, and Fertility Change in South Asia*. New Delhi, India: Sage Publications.

Jeffery, P., and R. Jeffery
1993 Killing my heart's desire: Education and female autonomy in rural North India. In N. Kumar, ed., *Woman as Subject*. Calcutta: Bhatkal and Sen.

Jejeebhoy, S.J.
1995 *Women's Education, Autonomy and Reproductive Behaviour: Experience from Developing Countries*. Oxford: Clarendon Press.

King, E., and M.A. Hill, eds.
1993 *Women's Education in Developing Countries: Barriers, Benefits, and Policies*. Baltimore, Md.: The Johns Hopkins University Press.

Layard, R., and A. Zabalza
1979 Family income distribution: Explanation and policy evaluation. *Journal of Political Economy* 87(5, part 2):S133-S161.

Mascie-Taylor, C.G.
1986 Assortative mating and differential fertility. *Biology and Society* 3(4):167-170.
Mason, K.O., and A.M. Taj
1987 Difference between women's and men's reproductive goals in developing countries. *Population and Development Review* 13(4):611-638.
Morgan, S.P., and B.B. Niraula
1995 Gender inequality and fertility in two Nepali villages. *Population and Development Review* 21(3):541-561.
Operations Research Group
1991 *Family Planning Practices in India: Third All-India Survey.* Baroda: Operations Research Group.
Rajan, S.I., M. Ramanathan, and U.S. Mishra
1996 Female automony and reproductive behaviour in Kerala: New evidence from the recent Kerala Fertility Survey. Pp. 269-287 in R. Jeffery and A.M. Basu, eds., *Girls' Schooling, Women's Automony, and Fertility Change in South Asia.* New Delhi, India: Sage Publications.
Sathar, Z.A.
1996 Women's schooling and autonomy as factors in fertility change in Pakistan: Some empirical evidence. Pp. 133-149 in R. Jeffery and A.M. Basu, eds., *Girls' Schooling, Women's Automony, and Fertility Change in South Asia.* New Delhi, India: Sage Publications.
Schirm, A.
1986 Assortative mating when individuals differ by many traits. Paper presented at the annual meeting of the Population Association of America, San Francisco.
Stycos, J.M.
1996 *Men, Couples and Family Planning: A Retrospective Look.* Population and Development Program Working Paper. Ithaca, N.Y.: Cornell University.
Summers, L.H.
1993 Foreword. Pp. v-vii in E.M. King and M.A. Hill, eds., *Women's Education in Developing Countries: Barriers, Benefits, and Policies.* Baltimore, Md.: The Johns Hopkins University Press.
Uberoi, P., ed.
1993 *Family, Kinship and Marriage in India.* Delhi: Oxford University Press.
Vlassoff, C.
1996 Against the odds: The changing impact of schooling on female autonomy and fertility in an Indian village. Pp. 218-234 in R. Jeffery and A.M. Basu, eds., *Girls' Schooling, Women's Automony, and Fertility Change in South Asia.* New Delhi, India: Sage Publications.
Warren, B.D.
1966 A multiple variable approach to the assortative mating phenomenon. *Eugenics Quarterly* 13(4):285-290.
Weinstein, M., T.H. Sun, M.C. Chang, and R. Thornton
1994 Co-residence and other ties linking couples and their parents. In A. Thornton and H. Lin, eds., *Social Change and the Family in Taiwan.* Chicago, Ill.: University of Chicago Press.

10

Fertility and Education: What Do We Now Know?

Parfait M. Eloundou-Enyegue

INTRODUCTION

The preceding chapters in this volume have examined various associations between education and fertility. This chapter addresses the broad question of what these associations mean in light of current scholarship. The title of this chapter poses essentially the same question as that of a classic review by Cochrane (1979): *Fertility and Education: What Do We Really Know?* Presumably, such a similarity in the question posed reflects a similarity of preoccupation. In both cases, the objective is apparently to summarize the existing evidence on education-fertility relationships. Both works also reflect a critical stance and imply an invitation to transcend superficial interpretations and seek deeper understanding. Perhaps as important is a common rhetorical flavor. While apparently calling for literal answers, both works could usefully be addressed by focusing on their raison-d'être: Why, in spite of countless empirical studies on the subject, may one still entertain doubts about the meaning of education-fertility connections? And does such soul searching indicate a lack of scientific progress? Such questions are unavoidable today in view of the knowledge gains that can be assumed to have occurred in the decades since Cochrane's review. Accordingly, they constitute the focus of the present discussion.

Specifically, this chapter addresses the persistent difficulty of deriving general conclusions from existing studies on education and fertility. Because most of these difficulties—including those of definition; functional form; and the interactive, contextually variable, multifaceted, and cross-generational nature of relationships—are well known, the emphasis is not on their enumeration, but on their integration within a systematic analysis of historical changes in the education-fertility discourse.

The main argument developed throughout is that the persistence of interpretive difficulties—and the resulting ambiguity in the education-fertility discourse—arises largely from an uneven growth in the four pillars that sustain this discourse: policy agenda, theory, methodology, and empirical evidence. On the one hand, the volume of empirical evidence has greatly expanded in the last two decades as the result of steady progress in research technology and the increased availability of large data sets. On the other hand, this empirical expansion has uncovered new complexities (interactions, nonlinearities, and contextual variability), some of which remain unexplained because of a lag in theoretical development. Furthermore, this accumulation of evidence has been accompanied by an even more rapid raising of methodological standards (notably, a greater demand for data and statistical tools that address issues of temporal sequence, unobserved heterogeneity, and endogeneity). The result has been dissatisfaction with much of the earlier evidence that fails to conform to these high standards. Finally, new policy demands have encouraged the study of additional linkages, including reverse, indirect, and intergenerational influences between education and fertility.

In short, it has become more difficult to assess what education-fertility associations mean because the body of evidence has grown at once too complex in comparison with existing theories and too crude in light of current methodological standards and heightened policy demands. Together, these trends have resulted in a paradoxical situation in which the education-fertility discourse has become more diffident as the facts accumulated and analytical methods have improved. To state the point differently, the current uncertainty does not reflect a lack of scientific progress, but a lag in the progress achieved on certain fronts, including theoretical arguments and actual methodological practices.

The rest of the chapter develops this argument by reviewing and comparing the progress achieved on the policy, theory, methodology, and empirical fronts. This evolution is summarized in Table 10-1, which distinguishes three time periods, ending in the mid-1970s, mid-1980s, and mid-1990s, respectively.[1]

Until the mid-1970s, the key policy objective of education-fertility research was to assess how one's education affects an individual's fertility. In fact, studies focused even more narrowly on the effects of the formal schooling of women on their fertility. The theoretical expectation, derived from modernization and microeconomic theories, was a negative effect. Consistent with this policy emphasis and theoretical expectation, analysis methods consisted of recursive mod-

[1]Clearly, this is an arbitrary breakdown. Because history does not proceed in orderly decennial jumps, this historical discontinuity must be viewed only as a didactic necessity. Similar didactic considerations require overstating the consensus on the definition of key concepts, notably theory and methodology.

TABLE 10-1 Education and fertility research in developing countries: Changes in underlying policy issues, theory, methodology, and empirical evidence.

Time Period	POLICY Key issue(s) / connection(s)	THEORY Expected relation	METHODOLOGY Statistical tools	EVIDENCE Findings / Interpretation
Before Mid-**1970s**	HIGH FERTILITY **Education** → **Fertility**	Negative	Simple correlations Multiple regression	Few studies; findings generally negative *"...Parental education in LDC's reduces fertility, this much is clear from both cross-national and intra-country cross-sections ..." (Simon, 1974, quoted in Cochrane, 1979).*
Mid-**1970s** **to** Mid-**1980s**	HIGH FERTILITY **Education** — *Demand* / *Supply* / *Fertility regulation* → **Fertility**	Negative on demand Positive on supply Positive on fertility regulation	Multiple regression / Path analysis	More findings; findings more mixed *"Education does not affect fertility directly, but acts through many variables [including] the biological supply of children, the demand for children by husbands and wives, and the regulation of fertility ..." (Cochrane 1979:7).*
Mid-**1980s** **to** Mid-**1990s**	HIGH FERTILITY / CHILDREN'S WELFARE WOMEN'S STATUS / LABOR FORCE QUALITY/ SOCIAL STRATIFICATION **Education** ⇄ **Fertility** ⇄ **Child schooling**	Depends on link and on path	Event history analysis	Many, mixed findings; larger set of research questions *Education and fertility outcomes affect each other, both within and across generations. They may also result from the same decision processes. Both these reciprocal influences and endogenous processes vary in direction and magnitude, depending on context.*

els featuring fertility as the dependent and education as the independent variable. These analyses relied on cross-sectional data on either individuals or countries. The empirical evidence at the time was rather limited in both volume and geographic coverage, most data being drawn from the more industrialized nations. By and large, this evidence indicated negative associations between education and fertility. Thus, there was a good match among (1) the scope and precision of the policy question addressed (whether education reduces fertility), (2) confidence in the use of methodology based on regression and cross-sectional analysis to answer this question (despite some qualifications), (3) the scope and precision of prevailing theories (education should reduce fertility), and (4) the nature of the available evidence (findings showed negative relationships most of the time). Because of this match, the education-fertility discourse was relatively unequivocal.

During the next decade (1975-1985), several developments occurred. First, policy demands required better specification of the education benefits that affect fertility, as well as processes through which these benefits operate. Second, more data became available (mainly through the World Fertility Surveys [WFS]), some of which indicated atypical cases in which education had no or a positive effect on fertility (see also Diamond et al., this volume). These atypical patterns suggested the possibility that education may have differing effects on the various proximate determinants of fertility and on the demand for children. It therefore became necessary to distinguish the effects of education on, say, nuptiality, contraceptive use, and fertility demand. Accordingly, while statistical analysis still ran in one direction, there was greater emphasis on the paths through which education effects operate. Overall, the discourse became more qualified and acknowledged differences depending on paths and context.

Since 1985, aided by the Demographic and Health Surveys (DHS), evidence has continued to accumulate. At the same time, the policy agenda has progressively expanded to include the reciprocal effects of fertility on education, as well as intergenerational links between education and fertility. That is, high fertility is no longer the unique policy issue sustaining education-fertility research. Instead, this research is increasingly motivated by policy concerns related to women's educational attainment, the welfare of children, labor force quality, economic inequality, and social stratification. Along with these changes in substantive focus, research methods have also improved. For the most part, these advances address previously recognized but unresolved methodological issues of temporal order, endogeneity, contextual variation, and heterogeneity. As a side-effect however, these advances confirm the need to correct for potential biases before inferring causal connections. Therefore, they cast doubt on the reliability of earlier results that are based on less refined methods. Together, these substantive and methodological developments further complicate the set of links that require explanation, even as they suggest caution against hasty and broad generalizations.

The remainder of this chapter is organized as follows. The next section reviews alternative interpretations of education-fertility associations. The following four sections examine in turn what were referred to earlier as the four pillars of the discourse on education and fertility: policy agenda, theory, methodology, and empirical evidence. The final section presents a summary, conclusions, and recommendations for future research.

ALTERNATIVE INTERPRETATIONS OF EDUCATION-FERTILITY ASSOCIATIONS

Correlation is a necessary but not sufficient criterion for causation. In the absence of other evidence, researchers finding a negative statistical association between education and fertility generally suspect one of several explanations: causation, heterogeneity, reverse causation, or endogenous association. As Table 10-2 suggests, these alternative interpretations differ along two key dimensions: (1) whether education is viewed as a choice and (2) whether education is viewed as having a causal influence on fertility. The first interpretation, referred to here as causal, emphasizes what Carter (this volume) terms "the productive aspect of education" and neglects individuals' active choices in determining the level and content of their educational outcomes. In this view, schooling is largely an exogenous influence that transforms individuals and confers some attribute that modifies fertility preferences and/or one's capacity to actualize preexisting preferences. A few researchers have extended the analysis to examine the specific benefits that are responsible for the effect of schooling on fertility. For instance, working in the context of South Africa, Thomas (this volume) concludes that "the impact of comprehension skills . . . may be important in affecting family decision making." In a similar vein, Oliver (1997, cited by Glewwe, this volume) indicates that literacy but not numeracy contributes to reduce fertility.

Conversely, one may recognize that individuals do make deliberate choices about their schooling, sometimes overcoming major obstacles.[2] However, such schooling choices need not involve a conscious anticipation of fertility implications, nor do the distinctive characteristics of the educationally driven necessarily shape fertility outcomes. In essence, individuals decide how much, when, and what type of schooling to obtain, but later experience unexpected fertility consequences of these schooling choices. Although exposure to schooling is a choice, this interpretation is still causal in the sense that the schooling experience affects fertility independently.

---

[2]Such obstacles exist wherever schooling opportunities are limited by a lack of schooling infrastructure, limited family resources, or active discriminatory policies, as was the case for South African blacks during the apartheid regime, when "state policies actively sought to limit the education opportunities of blacks" (Thomas, this volume, citing Samuel, 1990).

TABLE 10-2 **Alternative interpretations of education-fertility associations.**

EDUCATION IS VIEWED AS A CHOICE	EDUCATION IS VIEWED AS HAVING A CAUSAL INFLUENCE ON FERTILITY: **Yes**	EDUCATION IS VIEWED AS HAVING A CAUSAL INFLUENCE ON FERTILITY: **No**
No	**I. Causal** E → F The experience of schooling, an exogenous outcome, changes individual values, attitudes, knowledge, opportunities, or behavior in ways that affect fertility.	**III. Heterogeneity** X → E; X → F Exogenous determinants of education outcomes also determine fertility outcomes. Individuals who elect to pursue schooling are different from others in ways that will also have a bearing on fertility outcomes. **IV. Reverse causation** E ← F The unintended initiation of childbearing interrupts or disrupts school continuation.
Yes	**II. Causal** [E] → F Individuals self-select themselves into educational attainment, and lower fertility occurs as a by-product. Characteristics that determine self-selection into educational attainment have no bearing on fertility	**V. Endogeneity** X → [E , F] Individuals make fertility and schooling investments *simultaneously*, and a tradeoff is involved in that dual choice (e.g.,"fertility-schooling tradeoff ").

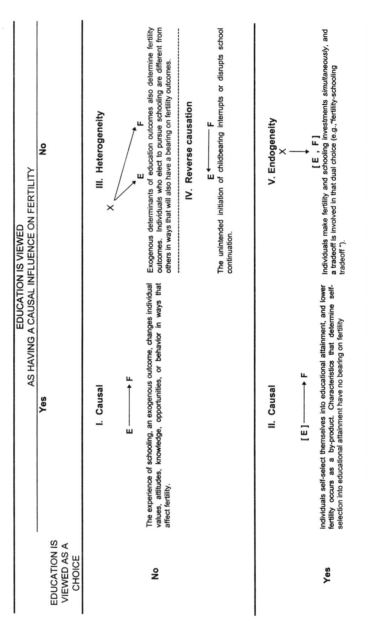

NOTES: E and F indicate education and fertility outcomes, respectively. Bracketed letters indicate that the outcome reflects largely individual choice.

A third possibility is that schooling in itself does not cause fertility outcomes. Rather, the educated differ from the noneducated in meaningful ways that have a bearing on their later fertility. Educated individuals may come from distinct social or family backgrounds, and this explains subsequent differences in fertility behavior (see Thomas, this volume). Educated individuals may also tend to have educated spouses with distinctive fertility preferences. Hence this assortative mating, rather individuals' education per se, may explain differences in fertility outcomes (see Basu, this volume). Should one correlate individual education with fertility without considering these distinctive characteristics, a spurious association will be observed. This association should disappear with adequate controls. In practice, however, it is difficult to control for all distinctive factors, whether because corresponding data were not collected or because some factors are inherently difficult to measure.

Fourth, without data on the timing of fertility and schooling events, an equally tenable interpretation is that educational attainment results from, rather than causes, fertility. The initiation of childbearing might disrupt or interrupt schooling. Ultimately, therefore, late childbearers who successfully avoid the economic and social burdens of childbearing are more likely to achieve higher levels of schooling. This interpretation is referred to as reverse causation.

A final possibility is endogeneity. In the fertility-schooling literature, parents' decisions about fertility and their investments in the human capital of individual children are simultaneous and involve a tradeoff—a choice of high fertility ipso facto implying a lesser amount of resources per child (Becker and Lewis, 1973; Hanushek, 1992). This dual decision is viewed as a rational choice influenced by the prevailing socioeconomic environment. In particular, Lloyd (1994) argues that four contextual factors are likely to be important in that respect: stage of economic development, the role of the state, the phase of the demographic transition, and the nature of the family system. In this context, an association between education and fertility does not mean that one affects the other in a causal sense, but simply that the two decisions are simultaneous and interdependent.

Table 10-2 thus illustrates the possible ambiguity in the meaning of education-fertility associations. Depending on assumptions and evidence on the timing of fertility and schooling, randomness in the distribution of schooling outcomes, and the relatedness of schooling and fertility choices, one can infer causation, unobserved heterogeneity, reverse causation, or endogeneity. While a different typology may be offered, the key point here is that, a priori, any given association between education and fertility can be interpreted as having several equally plausible meanings. Without additional evidence, a fair arbitrage among these meanings is difficult. Furthermore, these various interpretations are not necessarily mutually exclusive. For example, Thomas' analysis (this volume) concludes that "a small part of the correlation [between maternal education and fertility] can be attributed to the role of the family and community resources, a larger part to the role of husband's schooling, and part to the acquisition of cognitive skills. An indeterminate fraction of the correlation is associated with unobserved heterogeneity. . . ."

As this research indicates, the ultimate question therefore is not whether an association reflects a causal influence, heterogeneity, reverse causation, or endogenous choices. Rather, it is how much each of these processes contributes to the association. Such fine distinctions, it must be added, are not meant solely to satisfy researchers' penchant for complication, but in fact bear on the identification of effective policies in the areas of education and population.

Thus far, this section has focused narrowly on the issue of interpreting the results of a single study. However, a full analysis must also summarize the diversity of findings in the education-fertility literature. Throughout the chapter, the first issue is referred to as a question of interpretation, while the second is termed a question of generalization. As indicated earlier, the objective of the discussion is not so much to reveal what education-fertility associations mean as it is to analyze why difficulties of interpretation and generalization have persisted over the years, despite considerable research attention. To answer this question, we examine historical changes in the four foundations of the scientific discourse on education and fertility noted earlier: policy agenda, theory, methodology, and empirical evidence.

AN EXPANDING POLICY AGENDA

Research questions circumscribe findings. Therefore, a possible starting point in evaluating education-fertility findings is to explore the underlying policy agenda and its evolution over time. If one defines a research agenda as the set of policy questions that, at a given time, are deemed worthy of research attention, the trend has clearly been toward expansion. As shown in Table 10-1, the policy focus has shifted progressively from an exclusive concern for whether one's education affects one's fertility to a larger set of questions, including whether one's fertility affects one's educational attainment, whether parents' fertility affects their children's schooling outcomes, and whether the schooling experience of children affects their fertility. As noted earlier, this evolution in research themes reflects a growing concern of population policy with issues of women's status and educational attainment, child welfare, labor force quality, economic inequality, and social stratification.

Prima-facie evidence for this agenda expansion can be found in a comparison of Cochrane's (1979) review and the agenda for the workshop that generated this volume. While posing the same question as the workshop (What is known about the connections between education and fertility?), Cochrane's assessment focused entirely on the effects of one's education on one's fertility, while the workshop explored a broader set of linkages.[3] To be sure, this classic relationship still held center stage during the workshop, but a few presentations addressed the reverse relationship (see Fuller and Liang, this volume), as well as links across generations (see Montgomery and Lloyd, this volume). Additional evidence for this substantive expansion may be found in a comparison of publication dates for key studies or reviews. For instance, Cochrane's (1979) review, which focuses on the effects of one's education on one's fertility, precedes by 15 years a similar review of the effects of parents' fertility on child schooling (Lloyd, 1994). To date, no comparable review has been done for the effects of child schooling on parents' fertility, even though such analyses are warranted by rapid changes in schooling costs throughout the developing world. This remark aside, the fact of an expansion in research focus is hardly disputable.

Granted that the research agenda has indeed broadened to incorporate reverse and intergenerational influences, what drove this expansion, and what are its ultimate implications for our understanding of the relationships between education and fertility? Shifts in research agenda result from intricate political processes that are difficult to reduce to a few isolated causes. Nonetheless, the following societal changes in developing countries and sociological changes within the field of demography are likely to have played important roles.

One key societal change concerns women's rising levels of educational attainment. It makes little scientific sense to search for fertility effects on women's schooling in low-education societies where schooling precedes childbearing with little or no overlap in the life course of most women. Following recent gains in the duration of females' school enrollment in most developing countries, the overlap between schooling and childbearing years has increased, making it possible that the initiation of childbearing may compromise further schooling. This development should promote research on the socioeconomic consequences of adolescent fertility. In addition to trends in female schooling, ideological changes are also worth mentioning. To be considered worthy of research attention, a dependent variable must reflect a socially valued outcome. Therefore, to the extent that societies increasingly value women's education and their participation in the labor market, this should promote research on the determinants of female schooling.[4]

Along with these societal transformations, the contours of demography have expanded. While formal demography restricts analysis to the three cardinal processes of fertility, migration, and mortality, a wider range of outcomes (including schooling) may be studied under the umbrella of population studies

[3]Because of this expansion, there is a growing distinction between "education-fertility" research, which takes fertility as the dependent variable, and "fertility-schooling," in which education outcomes are the dependent variable.

[4]A recent article by Presser (1997) also highlights such shifts in policy agenda, although the author argues that this new policy emphasis on issues of gender equity (evident, for instance, at the 1994 International Conference on Population and Development) has yet to translate into a strong feminist research agenda in demography.

(McNicoll, 1992; Preston, 1993). Therefore, as the distinction between formal demography and population studies has blurred, research on schooling increasingly becomes a legitimate area of inquiry within demography. This rapprochement of formal demography and other social sciences is likely to continue and remain beneficial for both camps, especially in education-fertility research. In that symbiosis, social sciences improve demographic analyses of education's effects on fertility by clarifying the meaning and measurement of education, drawing attention to important control variables, or contributing complementary theoretical perspectives or special methods of data collection or analysis (Bogue, 1993; Crimmins, 1993; Carter, this volume). While the social sciences complement demographic analysis, formal demography can reciprocate by contributing powerful tools to the analysis of schooling outcomes. In particular, life-table methods may be usefully applied to research on educational attainment. Such applications are likely to grow in popularity when longitudinal data on schooling become available.

In summary, three main factors contributed to an expansion of the policy agenda sustaining education-fertility research, in a direction that gives greater emphasis to the effects of fertility on schooling both within and across generations. These three factors are the rising levels of female enrollment, changing ideological climates in developing countries, and the blurring of the distinction between formal demography and population studies.

A THEORETICAL LAG

If one overlooks nuances among empirical generalizations, frameworks, principles, and formal theories, a theory can be defined as a "systematic explanation for observed facts" (Babbie, 1989:46). Generally, theories are expected to play both predictive and explanatory/organizing roles in the course of normal science. In their predictive role, theories focus empirical investigations by generating relevant and testable hypotheses. In their explanatory role, they help organize findings from different studies into a cumulative body of knowledge. Fulfilling this second role, however, requires that the scope and precision of theory exceed the scope and precision of findings (Kuhn, 1970). Unfortunately, this requirement is not currently met in education-fertility research, in which empirical findings have clearly outgrown the scope and precision of existing theories.

With regard to scope, empirical studies have increasingly covered a wider variety of settings and highlighted the contextual dependency of the education-fertility relationship, whether this relation is examined within or across generations (see Diamond et al., this volume; Jejeebhoy, 1995; Lloyd, 1994). However, existing theories do not typically consider, let alone explain, these contextual variations. Implicitly the (questionable) assumption is that the content and meaning of education vary little across countries (see Glewwe and Carter, this volume). With regard to precision, empirical studies yield quantitative estimates of education's effects, specifying when those effects are nonlinear or interactive, and in fact showing that their size and functional form vary substantially with the socioeconomic context and the aggregate educational level of a society (see Diamond et al., this volume; Singh and Casterline, 1985). In contrast, the theories that are supposed to explain these precise, quantitative, interactive, and context-dependent findings afford only hypotheses that are vague, verbal, monotonic, and context-invariant (Burch, 1996; Eloundou-Enyegue and Stokes, 1997).

Such limitations in the scope and precision of theories restrict the extent to which one can integrate findings from different studies and build a cumulative body of knowledge, unless results happen to be uniform or follow an obvious pattern. When such uniformity is lacking, better theory is needed to reconcile seemingly disparate findings, or alternatively to refute ostensible similarities. By separating analysis of the effects of education into effects on demand, supply, and fertility regulation, various frameworks may explain why the effects of education on fertility outcomes are nonlinear. However, the effects of education on these proximate factors are themselves likely to be nonlinear and context dependent, and such variations also require explanation. For instance, discussions at the workshop outlined the need to investigate how education-fertility relations may depend on the stage of development, educational transition, or fertility transition.

Context dependency is also important in studying the effects of fertility on schooling, both within and across generations. For instance, the quantity-quality tradeoff provides a common argument for expecting an inverse relationship between sibship size and child schooling (Becker, 1981; Kaplan, 1994). However, the nature of this tradeoff seems to vary across contexts, and the patterns of these variations need to be understood. A meta-analysis of existing studies suggests that the tradeoff depends on the level of development, state policies, the culture of the family, and the phase of the demographic transition (Lloyd, 1994). Although these empirical generalizations represent a major advance, the ultimate step is to develop contextual theories that can generate quantitative hypotheses on the effects of specific contextual variables on the quantity-quality tradeoff and optimal fertility and parental investment choices (Eloundou-Enyegue and Stokes, 1997).

In sum, regardless of the particular linkage investigated, theoretical arguments exist for expecting a negative relationship between education and fertility. The problem, however, is that these arguments are not as precise in their predictions or as broad in their scope as the evidence they are required to organize. While this limitation is perhaps innocuous in interpreting the findings of a single study, it constrains the ability to reconcile findings from different settings. The main challenge, therefore, is to develop quantitative and contextual theories that will enable quantitative predictions regarding the mutual effects of education and fertility while recognizing the influence of socioeconomic context.

METHODOLOGICAL ADVANCES

Classic definitions of methodology emphasize its technical dimension, that is, the tools, rules, and procedures used to gather and analyze evidence. The dominant methodologies in education-fertility research include survey and ethnographic methods, each of which comprises distinct procedures for selecting and interrogating informants, as well as compiling and presenting the resulting information. However, methodology may also be viewed in a broader sense that includes the social organization of research. The present review adopts the latter perspective, and covers both technical and sociological changes in research practice.

Technical Changes

During the last three decades, the technical aspects of demographic research have markedly improved. Major advances concern both research tools and techniques, that is, both the hardware and software of demographic research. A major hardware change concerns the advent of computers and their extensive use in the analysis of demographic data. That computers have greatly facilitated data storage, retrieval, merging, computing, multivariate analysis, and reanalysis needs no elaboration. Demographers have also noted steady improvements in the statistical arsenal available for demographic analysis. Looking just at survey data, the commonly used tools have evolved progressively from simple correlations, to multiple regression, to path analysis, to contextual and dynamic modeling (Teachman et al., 1993). These statistical advances have facilitated the empirical distinction between correlation and causation in education-fertility research. Multivariate analysis enables extensive statistical controls, reducing the confounding effects of education correlates. Controls are further extended to unmeasured variables through the specification of fixed community or family effects, while other methods are used to address endogeneity (Bollen et al., 1995). Finally, longitudinal analyses consider the timing of fertility and schooling events, making it less likely that a spurious association will receive a causal interpretation.

While pervading all social sciences, these changes, especially the development of event-history methods, have profound implications for the study of education-fertility relationships, which involve two intrinsically dynamic, cumulative, and endogenous processes. In particular, the practice of using simple associations to draw causal inferences has become less acceptable. The change, it must be stressed, has been technical rather than epistemological: like current researchers, social scientists in the 1970s knew the distinction between correlation and causation. Lacking then, however, were the technical tools for choosing between competing interpretations of an observed correlation. Without these tools, researchers could more easily drift from (legitimately) considering causality as a possible interpretation to (abusively) retaining it as the final explanation. This drift may have been reinforced by an ideological belief in the efficacy of education (Carter, this volume) and by processes of "interactive myth-making"[5] through which researchers validate the thesis of a causal influence on the basis not of critical reviews of evidence, but the pronouncements of colleagues, themselves influenced by other colleagues' opinions.

At the same time, it is important to note that despite the availability of improved statistical tools, actual practices still lag behind cutting-edge methodology. For instance, the lack of schooling histories in most major data sets still limits the application of event-history techniques in studies of educational attainment. Likewise, little research on the effects of education on fertility in developing countries has adequately addressed endogeneity issues. Existing research contains "serious methodological problems that could invalidate the results" (Ainsworth et al., 1996). Overall, as noted earlier, the unfortunate consequence of the higher methodological standards has been to breed dissatisfaction with much of the previous evidence that was derived through less refined methods.

The Social Organization of Demographic Research

Since the 1970s, the makeup of the demographic research community has evolved substantially, notably with increasing numbers of women and researchers from developing countries. In themselves, such changes may have little influence on methodological practices and findings (Watkins, 1993). Perhaps more influential is the increasing bureaucratization of demographic research. Manifestations of this bureaucratization include the concentration of research production within a few institutions and a division of labor that has increasingly separated data collection from analysis. The first of these patterns is noted in the production of major research articles (Teachman et al., 1993),[6] as well as in the production of major data sets: DHS and World Bank data sets have thus far supported most large-scale studies on education and fertility in developing countries. And while 1970s researchers frequently collected and analyzed their own data, today's researchers are often spared the effort of designing questionnaires, constructing samples, training interviewers, and interacting with respondents.

---

[5]The term is used by Caldwell et al. (1987) in a paper addressing the mutual reinforcement of speculation and research in generating "knowledge." They suggest, for instance, that the disciplines of anthropology and demography often feed on each other, each accepting ideas from other disciplines more readily and less critically than it would accept ideas emerging from its own members. Something similar could be said about researchers' inclination to accept conclusions from colleagues even when aware of the limitations of the data. Often, the assumption may be that others must know something that one does not.

[6]As of 1992, for instance, more than 50 percent of all papers published in *Demography* were contributed by fewer than 10 percent of all organizations (Teachman et al., 1993).

Instead, they can concentrate on the ultimate phase of data analysis. Although this division of scientific labor presumably improves the efficiency of each activity in the research chain, it presents new challenges to researchers attempting to interpret data they did not collect or data originating from unfamiliar settings.

MOUNTING EVIDENCE

Because of the methodological improvements noted earlier, raw empirical evidence has accumulated, mostly in the form of correlations, regression coefficients, and odds ratios depicting micro-level associations between education and fertility. Beyond the sheer number of case studies, geographical coverage has improved markedly thanks to the implementation of WFS and DHS surveys throughout the developing world.[7] However, although empirical evidence is necessary to advance scientific knowledge, neither clarity nor consensus necessarily results from the mere accumulation of findings. This is especially the case when findings from individual studies do not warrant unambiguous interpretations or when findings appear to be inconsistent from study to study. To give meaning to raw findings, researchers must deal with problems of interpretation and generalization. As noted earlier, the term interpretation as used here refers to the meaning ascribed to the findings of a single study, while generalization denotes the overall picture framed by compiling all available evidence. The challenge of the workshop was precisely to reconcile the variety and richness of existing findings into a coherent, concise, and accurate summary.

As was argued earlier, methodological advances have improved researchers' capacity to arbitrate between alternative interpretations of observed associations. On the other hand, the reconciliation of findings from different settings has become increasingly difficult because of the geographic expansion of education-fertility research, the multiplication of substantive links of interest, and the lack of contextual theories. The expansion of geographic coverage has restricted broad generalizations by providing hard evidence of atypical patterns. On the other hand, the increasing policy attention to intergenerational links, to reverse effects, and to paths of influence has made it more difficult to summarize the complexity of the education-fertility relationship with a concise statement. Increasingly, qualifications are needed as to which path/link is being examined. Finally, the lack of contextual theories limits understanding of observed contextual variations. In the absence of such theories, researchers have resorted to meta-analysis to derive empirical generalizations (see Diamond et al., this volume; Jejeebhoy, 1995; Lloyd, 1994). However, such analyses are problematic

[7]As of 1997, about 42 WFS and 50 DHS surveys had been implemented in developing countries (Presser, 1997).

when they mix studies of varying methodological soundness (see Diamond et al. and Glewwe, this volume). Overall, as a result of these trends, summary statements on education-fertility relationships have tended to become more qualified and less definitive even as the volume of empirical evidence has expanded.

In contrast with these difficulties in generalization, methodological advances have progressively reduced the difficulties involved in interpreting the results of a single study. Yet even in this area, problems remain with concept clarification and data. First, greater attention needs to be paid to the local meaning and content of education. As the chapters by Carter, Diamond et al., and Glewwe in this volume suggest, little is known about the skills, knowledge, and attitudes pupils acquire in school and how they vary across different school institutions. Also, while dynamic modeling is widely advocated in education-fertility research, the major data sets that support these analyses do not contain schooling histories and thus do not allow the application of cutting-edge methodology (Lloyd and Blanc, 1996; Knodel and Jones, 1996). Overall, however, these difficulties of definition and data represent minor impediments, if only because their remedies are known and manageable. Certainly more daunting problems reside in explaining contextual variations.

SUMMARY, CONCLUSIONS, AND RESEARCH RECOMMENDATIONS

With a few exceptions, empirical studies around the world report negative statistical associations between education and fertility, both within and across generations. However, the meaning of these associations remains elusive and may in fact have become more so over the years. At issue are the twin difficulties of interpretation and generalization. Interpretation difficulties concern individual studies and the basis on which researchers determine whether an association between education and fertility reflects a causal influence, heterogeneity, reverse causation, or the endogeneity of schooling and fertility choices. Generalization difficulties concern how to reconcile findings from different studies. To date, both difficulties continue to plague education-fertility research despite policy interest in reliable interpretations, and despite the progress made since the publication of Cochrane's (1979) seminal work.

The purpose of this chapter has been twofold. First, it has reviewed some of the difficulties involved in ascribing meaning to education-fertility associations. More important, it has attempted to explain why these difficulties have persisted in spite of considerable research effort over the last three decades. The chapter's main argument has been that the enduring uncertainty about the meaning of education-fertility associations does not indicate a lack of scientific progress. Indeed, much progress has been achieved on all four pillars that sustain the education-fertility discourse: policy agenda, methodology, empirical evidence, and theories.

In particular, the policy issues underlying education-fertility research have expanded from an almost exclusive focus on high fertility to concern for women's educational attainment, children's welfare, labor force quality, and economic inequality. This expanding agenda has drawn attention to the multiple facets of the education-fertility relationship, including reverse and cross-generational effects, the paths through which education affects fertility, as well as to the particular features of the schooling experience that are most relevant to these effects. Over the same period, substantial methodological improvements have occurred, whether they concern the technical tools of research—the greater use of computers in demographic research, the development of statistical techniques to address problems of statistical control, unobserved heterogeneity, endogeneity, and the study of dynamic processes—or the social organization of demographic research, with a growing concentration of data and research production within a few institutions and an increasing separation of data collection and analysis activities. Finally, the implementation of large-scale surveys across the developing world has generated a voluminous database that permits extensive analyses and cross-country comparisons.

Yet, for all these methodological improvements, the scientific discourse on education-fertility relationships has remained surprisingly tentative. My interpretation is that this does not reflect an overall stagnation, but the fact that progress has been uneven. While advances have been achieved on the four pillars that sustain the education-fertility discourse, this progress has followed an odd sequence in which theory trails rather than leads empirical investigations, and in which methodological standards have surpassed the actual practices permitted by most existing data sets: while methods have drastically improved, the associated rise in methodological standards has bred dissatisfaction with previous findings that were based on less refined methods. While the specialization of data collection and analysis activities presumably improved the output efficiency of the demographic research industry, researchers now face the challenge of interpreting data that they did not collect or data that originated from unfamiliar settings. While the number, the geographical coverage, and the precision of empirical studies improved, researchers' ability to reconcile findings from different studies is restricted by the lack of quantitative, contextual theories that generate precise predictions about the expected contextual variations in education-fertility relationships. The ultimate outcome of this asynchronous evolution is that even though data have become more available and research tools have sharpened, the conclusions derived from existing evidence have become increasingly qualified and tentative.

A number of recommendations for future research flow from this diagnostic. One concerns data collection. Longitudinal data on the fertility and education experiences of both parents and children are needed. While fertility surveys contain fertility histories, similar historical data are not available for schooling, and cross-country differences in patterns of grade progression make it impossible to reconstruct schooling histories from available information. Where longitudinal surveys cannot be carried out, a retrospective reconstruction of schooling histories can provide a reasonable substitute. Such reconstruction can be facilitated by the design and use of life-history calendars and the combined use of ethnographic methods and survey techniques.

A second recommendation concerns the distribution of research effort across different facets of the education-fertility relationship. While the effort has become somewhat diversified, most of the emphasis remains on the effects of one's education on one's fertility. Even within this agenda, more studies should examine the specific schooling benefits that matter most to fertility outcomes. There is also a need for studies on the reverse linkage—the consequences of fertility for the educational attainment and other socioeconomic outcomes of young women. This research could build on the methodological experience of similar research in developed countries. Likewise, research must reexamine the effects of high fertility on schooling at the family level within a dynamic framework that acknowledges time variations in sibship size and family context, as well as unobserved heterogeneity in family background. Finally, very little research has examined the consequences of child schooling for parents' fertility.[8] This focus is particularly warranted by the current changes in schooling costs and returns in developing countries under structural adjustment.

A third broad class of recommendations concerns theory. Given the current state of methodological development, and assuming that longitudinal data become more available, theory is likely to become the key limiting factor. Without the guidance provided by good theory, empirical investigations are likely to proceed haphazardly, and generalizations will remain unduly constrained by the observation of contextual differences. The greatest theoretical challenge is to anticipate contextual variations in education-fertility relationships. This includes, for instance, variations across fertility transition stages and across educational development stages. Meta-analyses such as those attempted by Jejeebhoy (1995) and Diamond et al. (this volume) for contextual variations in education effects and by Lloyd (1994) for fertility effects on child schooling are steps in the appropriate direction. Ideally, however, such steps would be complemented by truly quantitative and contextual theories (see, e.g., Burch, 1996). Without significant theoretical developments, current methodological advances may not be put to their best use, making it likely that a decade from now, Cochrane's nagging question will resurface.

---

[8]See Axinn (1993) for an exception.

ACKNOWLEDGMENTS

I wish to thank the editors of this volume, workshop participants, and the anonymous reviewers, as well as Julie DaVanzo and Shannon Stokes, for their insights or comments. Remaining errors are my own.

REFERENCES

Ainsworth, M., K. Beegle, and A. Nyamete
1996 The impact of women's human capital on fertility and contraceptive use: A study of fourteen sub-Saharan countries. *World Bank Research Observer* 10(1):85-122.

Axinn, W.G.
1993 The effects of children's schooling on fertility limitation. *Population Studies* 47(3):481-493.

Babbie, E.
1989 *The Practice of Social Research.* Belmont, Calif.: Wadsworth Publishing Company.

Becker, G., and H. Lewis
1973 On the interaction between the quantity and quality of children. *Journal of Political Economy* 81(2):s279-s288.

Becker, G.S
1981 *A Treatise on the Family.* Cambridge, Mass.: Harvard University Press.

Bogue, Donald J.
1993 How demography was born. *Demography* 30(4):519-532.

Bollen, K.A., D.K. Guilkey, and T.A. Mroz
1995 Binary outcomes and endogenous explanatory variables: tests and solutions with an application to the demand for contraceptive use in Tunisia. *Demography* 2(1):111-131.

Burch, T.K.
1996 Icons, strawmen and precision: Reflection on demographic theories of fertility decline. *The Sociological Quarterly* 37(1):59-81.

Caldwell, J., P. Caldwell, and B. Caldwell
1987 Anthropology and demography: The mutual reinforcement of speculation and research. *Current Anthropology* 28(1):25-43.

Cochrane, S.H.
1979 *Fertility and Education. What Do We Really Know?* Baltimore, Md.: The Johns Hopkins University Press.

Crimmins, E.M.
1993 Demography: The past 30 years, the present and the future. *Demography* 30(4):579-591.

Eloundou-Enyegue, P., and C.S. Stokes
1997 Davis & Blake and Becker in Discrete-Time: From Verbal To Quantitative Theories Of Fertility. Paper presented at the 1997 Annual Meeting of the Population Association of America. Washington D.C., March 27-29.

Hanushek, E.
1992 The trade-off between child quantity and quality. *Journal of Political Economy* 100(1):84-117.

Jejeebhoy, S.J.
1995 *Women's Education, Autonomy and Reproductive Behavior: Experience from Developing Countries.* Oxford: Clarendon Press.

Kaplan, H.
1994 Evolutionary and wealth flows theories of fertility. *Population and Development Review* 20(4)753-791.

Knodel, J., and G.W. Jones
1996 Does promoting girls' schooling miss the mark? *Population and Development Review* 22(4):683-702.

Kuhn, T.S.
1970 *The Structure of Scientific Revolutions.* Chicago, Ill.: University of Chicago Press.

Lloyd, C.B.
1994 *Investing in the Next Generation: The Implications of High Fertility at the Level of the Family.* Working Paper No. 63. New York: The Population Council.

Lloyd, C.B., and A.K. Blanc
1996 Children's schooling in sub-Saharan Africa. *Population and Development Review* 22(2):265-298.

McNicoll, G.
1992 The agenda of population studies: A commentary and complaint. *Population and Development Review* 18(3):399-420.

Oliver, R.
1997 Fertility and women's schooling in Ghana. In P. Glewwe, ed., *The Economics of School Quality Investments in Developing Countries: An Empirical Study of Ghana.* London: MacMillan.

Presser, H.B.
1997 Demography, feminism and the science-policy nexus. *Population and Development Review* 23(2):295-331.

Preston, S.H.
1993 The contours of demography: Estimates and projections. *Demography* 30(4)593-606.

Samuel, J.
1990 The state of education in South Africa. In B. Nasson and J. Samuel, eds., *Education: From Poverty to Liberty.* Cape Town: David Philip.

Singh, S., and J. Casterline
1985 The socio-economic determinants of fertility. Pp. 199-222 in J. Cleland and J. Hobcraft, eds., *Reproductive Change in Developing Countries: Insights from the World Fertility Survey.* London: Oxford University Press.

Teachman, J.D., K. Paasch, and K.P. Carver
1993 Thirty years of demography. *Demography* 30(4):523-532.

Watkins, S.C.
1993 If all we knew about women was what we read in *Demography*, what would we know? *Demography* 30(4):551-578.

Index

A

D

H

I

N

P

Q

R

S

T

U

W

Z